Millets for Human Health and Disease

This book provides a comprehensive overview of the nutritional, therapeutic, and functional potential of millets, highlighting their role in promoting human health and preventing disease. The chapters cover the historical significance, classification, and compositional attributes of millets, including their macro- and micronutrient content, phytochemicals, and processing techniques. It further explores millet-based nutrition across life stages from infancy to pregnancy and lactation as well as their application in managing metabolic disorders such as diabetes, cardiovascular diseases, and obesity. Additionally, the book addresses millets as gluten-free alternatives for celiac disease and the current market trends in millet-based food products and presents a range of therapeutic and everyday recipes. With a focus on public health, sustainability, and value chain integration, this volume underscores the multifaceted benefits of millets in the modern diet and food system.

Key Features:

- Provides a holistic understanding of millets, covering their history, classification, nutritional composition, and global policy initiatives
- Discusses millet-based dietary strategies for infants, pregnant and lactating women, and individuals with metabolic disorders
- Explores therapeutic applications of millets in weight management, diabetes, cardiovascular diseases, cancer, and gluten-related disorders
- Examines processing technologies, value chain challenges, and the commercial potential of millet-based food products
- Includes traditional and modern recipes to promote millet consumption and practical dietary integration

This book is intended for researchers in food science, nutrition, public health, agriculture, and sustainable development.

Millets for Human Health and Disease

Edited by

Sarita Srivastava
Anju Bisht

CRC Press
Taylor & Francis Group
Boca Raton London New York

CRC Press is an imprint of the
Taylor & Francis Group, an **informa** business

Designed cover image: **Sarita Srivastava, Anju Bisht**

First edition published 2027
by CRC Press
2385 NW Executive Center Drive, Suite 320, Boca Raton FL 33431

and by CRC Press
4 Park Square, Milton Park, Abingdon, Oxon, OX14 4RN

CRC Press is an imprint of Taylor & Francis Group, LLC

ISBN: 9781041168485 (hbk)
ISBN: 9781041168492 (pbk)
ISBN: 9781003686668 (ebk)

DOI: 10.1201/9781003686668

Typeset in Times
by KnowledgeWorks Global Ltd.

Contents

Foreword vii
Message ix
Preface xi
About the Editors xiii
Contributors xv

Chapter 1 Millets: The Sri Anna 1
Neha Tiwari

Chapter 2 Millets Composition: Nutrients, Non-Nutrients, and Anti-Nutrients 14
Swati Shukla

Chapter 3 Millet-Processing Techniques: Feasibility and Gaps 33
Punjasthala Ravindrasingh Negi, Palak Tiwari, and Neelam Chaturvedi

Chapter 4 Policy Perspectives in Millets: Strengthening Production and Consumption in Millet Value Chains 45
Shefali Srivastava and Jayanti Kajale

Chapter 5 Millet-Based Nutrition for Infants: A Healthy Start 63
Surabhi Singh Yadav

Chapter 6 Millets During Pregnancy and Lactation: A Maternal Health Promoter 82
Neelam Chaturvedi

Chapter 7 Millets: An Immunity-Boosting Treasure 94
Bhavna, Shivangi Singh Chauhan, and Sangeeta C. Sindhu

Chapter 8 Millets' Role in Weight Management 110
Swati Shukla

Chapter 9 Anti-Diabetic Potential of Millets 139
Ayushi Joshi, Krati Goel, and Archana Kushwaha

Chapter 10 Cardioprotective and Anti-Cancer Effects of Millets 159
Alpana Joshi and Ayushi Joshi

Chapter 11 Millets for Celiac Disease 185
T. Tamilselvan and M. Badhani

Chapter 12 Millet-Based Food Options: A Review of Commercially Available Products 210
Shivli Srivastava and Shefali Srivastava

Chapter 13 Millet Magic: Healthy Recipes for Every Day 228
Tarvinder Jeet Kaur

Index 257

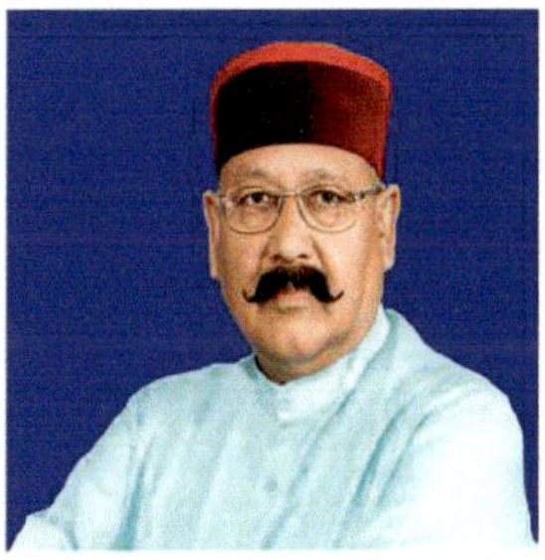

उत्तराखण्ड सरकार

लोक निर्माण विभाग, पर्यटन, सिंचाई, लघु सिंचाई
ग्रामीण निर्माण, पंचायती राज, जलागम प्रबंधन, संस्कृति, धर्मस्व
भारत-नेपाल उत्तराखण्ड नदी परियोजनायें
उत्तराखण्ड सरकार

Public Works, Tourism, Irrigation, Minor Irrigation
Rural Works Department, Panchayat RAj, Watershed Management, Culture
Flood Control, India-Nepal-Uttarakhand River Projects
Government of Uttarakhand

सतपाल महाराज
मंत्री
SATPAL MAHARAJ
Minister

Foreword

I commend this book titled *Millets for Human Health and Disease* by Dr. Sarita Srivastava and other co-authors for their dedication and their subject-matter expertise in compiling this compendium. Dr. Srivastava, who has been known to me for several years, is currently serving as Director of the Suvernada Foundation (NGO) at Udham Singh Nagar in Uttarakhand and had served until retirement as Professor and Head of the Department of Food & Nutrition at the renowned G. B. Pant University of Agriculture and Technology in Uttarakhand. This book would immensely increase awareness of this 'superfood' that is endowed with 'magical' properties to address most of the diseases related to gut health.

In India, millets have been the main staple since ancient times, and therefore, most of us grew up learning about millets as one of the healthiest staples, both from the point of view of gut health and sustainability! Millet cultivation and consumption until recently was largely restricted to the Indian subcontinent besides Africa. The three major millet crops grown in our country are *jowar* (sorghum), *bajra* (pearl millet), and *ragi* (finger millet); besides these, other varieties like *kodo*, *kutki*, *chenna*, and *samwa* are also consumed in small quantities.

It is only in the last two decades that its popularity has grown in the global markets. In a very short span of time, it has gained recognition as a 'superfood' because of its exceptional nutritional value and immense health benefits owing to its fiber content, proteins, and essential minerals. This book details the medical aspects of millets, derived from their rich dietary properties that aid digestion and keep the blood sugar and cholesterol levels in check. It is one of the cheapest sources of vitamin B complex and antioxidant properties, besides containing minerals like iron, calcium, zinc, magnesium, and phosphorus. It, in fact, is regarded as one of the best staples for protection against most metabolic disorders and cell damage in the body.

न त्वहं कामये राज्यं न स्वर्गं नापुनर्भवम्।
कामये दुःखतप्तानां प्राणिनामार्तिनाशनम्।।

कार्यालय - विधान सभा भवन, देहरादून दूरभाष : (0135) 2666377 फैक्स : (0135) 2666380 आवास - 17, सुभाष रोड़, देहरादून., दूरभाष : 9810990009, 8743880008
ई-मेल : writeto@satpalmaharaj.in वेबसाइट : www.satpalmaharaj.in

सतपाल महाराज
मंत्री
SATPAL MAHARAJ
Minister

त्तराखण्ड सरकार

लोक निर्माण विभाग, पर्यटन, सिंचाई, लघु सिंचाई
ग्रामीण निर्माण, पंचायती राज, जलागम प्रबंधन, संस्कृति, धर्मस्व
भारत-नेपाल उत्तराखण्ड नदी परियोजनायें
उत्तराखण्ड सरकार

Public Works, Tourism, Irrigation, Minor Irrigation
Rural Works Department, Panchayat RAj, Watershed Management, Culture
Flood Control, India-Nepal-Uttarakhand River Projects
Government of Uttarakhand

This 'wonder crop' requires significantly less water for cultivation as compared to any other major cereal. It is a boon in today's world as a drought-tolerant crop that can grow even in dry, low-fertility soil and mountainous areas. Its cultivation cost is frugal, demanding minimal input costs, be it fertilizers or pesticides. It addresses the need for providing food security, sustainability, and so forth, making its cultivation more pragmatic from the point of subsistence and affordability. Millets are resilient to harsh climates and offer more nutrition than rice or wheat. Agriculture experts say that millets are well-suited to the dryland regions of the world, which occupy 41 percent of the land surface, produce 44 percent of the crops, and provide livelihood to over 2 billion people. This is a win-win for all—the environment, the farmers, and the consumers!

It is only in the last couple of years that millets have gained popularity, and to promote it, the UN declared 2023 as the **International Year for Millets!** In fact, millets were the culinary masterpiece too during the **G20 Presidency Summit held in New Delhi in 2023!**

By synthesizing diverse perspectives and offering novel insights, all the co-authors of this marvelous work of research deserve tumultuous applause—providing one solution to mitigate several problems. This book, I am sure, will serve as a repository of real-world information and facts based on research data on millets to tackle the challenges of both the overdose of agricultural inputs and revolutionizing eating habits, thus making our world more sustainable and healthier too!

(Satpal Maharaj)

न त्वहं कामये राज्यं न स्वर्गं नापुनर्भवम्।
कामये दुःखतप्तानां प्राणिनामार्तिनाशनम्।।

कार्यालय - विधान सभा भवन, देहरादून दूरभाष : (0135) 2666377 फैक्स : (0135) 2666380 आवास - 17, सुभाष रोड़, देहरादून, दूरभाष : 9810990009, 8743880008
ई-मेल : writeto@satpalmaharaj.in वेबसाइट : www.satpalmaharaj.in

ICRISAT | INTERNATIONAL CROPS RESEARCH INSTITUTE FOR THE SEMI-ARID TROPICS
Transforming Dryland Agriculture

Message

In an era where hunger, malnutrition, and lifestyle-related diseases continue to challenge global health and productivity, the search for sustainable and nutritious food alternatives has become more critical than ever. Amidst the backdrop, millets (श्री अन्न) – the 'supergrains' – have emerged as a promising solution. Millets are nutrient-dense, climate-resilient, and economically viable, and have the potential to contribute meaningfully to global food and nutrition security.

This book serves as a complete guide to understanding the vast benefits of millets. It presents an in-depth insight into their nutritional composition, processing methods, and patterns of production–consumption. Readers are introduced to the vital role of millets in promoting health across the human lifespan and in managing conditions such as obesity, diabetes, cardiovascular diseases, and celiac disease.

Additionally, the distinctiveness of this book lies in its exploration of the expanding market for millet-based food products, while also emphasizing innovative recipe designs, further encouraging their adoption by consumers.

This work is a timely contribution to the ongoing dialogue on sustainable food systems and healthy eating. It not only serves as a rich resource for nutritionists, researchers, and health professionals but also motivates the readers to embrace millets as a staple in everyday diets.

I extend my heartfelt congratulations to the editors for curating a relevant and timely compilation that addresses a pressing need of the hour.

Dr Himanshu Pathak
Director General

Headquarters:
Patancheru 502 324, Telangana, India
Tel +91 8455683071, **Fax** +91 8455683074, +91 8455683075
E-mail icrisat-ind@icrisat.org
www.icrisat.org

Preface

In recent years, nutrition and health have received significant global attention, and the rising consumer awareness has led to a growing demand for healthy food options with therapeutic potential. The food industry's interest in developing novel, health-oriented products is expanding rapidly, while simultaneously facing challenges in meeting the nutritional needs of a growing population. To cater to the nutritional needs and overall well-being of mounting population throughout the globe, millets can be prudently explored.

Millets are among the earliest cultivated food grains known to humankind, sustaining civilizations across Asia and Africa for thousands of years. Despite their historical significance and exceptional nutritional value, millets gradually lost prominence with the advent of high-yielding cereal crops and changing dietary preferences. In recent decades, however, growing concerns regarding food security, climate resilience, lifestyle disorders, and sustainable agriculture have led to a renewed global interest in these ancient grains.

This book aims to present a comprehensive and scientifically grounded overview of millets, emphasizing their nutritional properties, therapeutic potential, and diverse culinary applications. Millets are rich sources of macronutrients, dietary fiber, essential minerals, vitamins, and bioactive compounds. Their low glycemic index, gluten-free nature, and antioxidant properties make them particularly valuable in the prevention and management of non-communicable diseases such as diabetes mellitus, cardiovascular disorders, obesity, cancer, and certain gastrointestinal conditions.

Beyond their nutritional advantages, millets play a crucial role in promoting sustainable food systems. They require minimal water inputs, thrive in marginal soils, and demonstrate remarkable resilience to climatic stress, making them ideal crops for ensuring food and nutritional security in the face of climate change. The inclusion of millets in regular diets not only supports human health but also contributes to environmental sustainability and rural livelihoods.

This book, *Millets for Human Health and Disease*, is divided into two sections. The first section introduces the readers to the millets and their significance in the human diet, highlighting health benefits of nutrient and non-nutrient components of millets. It also discusses viable processing techniques to harness the maximum potential of these underutilized healthy grains along with production–consumption of the millets and demand-supply gaps, and future projections. Further chapters in the first section deal with the significance of millet-based nutrition for infants and pregnant and lactating mothers and as an immunity booster for improving overall health throughout the lifespan.

The second section of the book includes chapters which deal with the role of millets in the management of diseased states, particularly weight management, diabetes, cardiovascular health, cancer, and celiac disease. The concluding chapters highlight the commercial availability of millet-based food products and provide practical guidance for incorporating millet-based healthy recipes into everyday diets.

It is hoped that this book will contribute to increased awareness, acceptance, and utilization of millets, fostering healthier dietary patterns and sustainable agricultural practices. By revisiting these resilient grains through the lens of modern science, this work aspires to support global efforts toward nutrition security, wellness, and ecological balance.

Designed for students, academicians, healthcare professionals, nutritionists, food technologists, and researchers, this book aims to serve as a valuable resource for understanding the multifaceted role of millets in health and disease. It is hoped that this work will encourage greater incorporation of millets into daily diets and public health strategies, thereby contributing to improved nutritional status, disease prevention, and sustainable food systems. The editors gratefully acknowledge the contributors for their sincere efforts and cooperation in the preparation of this book.

About the Editors

Sarita Srivastava is Director and Founder of an NGO, Suvernada Foundation, Rudrapur, Uttarakhand, India. She is retired Professor and Head of the Department of Foods and Nutrition at G. B. Pant University of Agriculture & Technology, Pantnagar, Uttarakhand, India. Dr. Sarita did her M.Sc. in Foods and Nutrition and her Ph.D. in Biochemistry from G. B. Pant University of Agriculture & Technology, Pantnagar, Uttarakhand, India and her Post-Doctorate from Technical University, Braunschweig, Germany (1988–89). She was a recipient of an FAO fellowship and worked under a UNDP project at Michigan State University, USA in 1993. She had been subject editor of *Pantnagar Journal of Research*. She has nearly 40 years of teaching experience. She has worked extensively on the nutritional quality of millets and product development for diversified uses, including food products for diabetics and celiac disease patients. In this area, she has guided 30 M.Sc. and 16 Ph.D. students. She is the editor of a book, *Small Millet Grains: The Superfoods in Human Diet*, published by Springer Nature. She authored a book, *Global Health Challenges: Nutrition and Management*, published by Taylor & Francis. Recently she authored a book, *Food Science and Nutrition: Comprehensive Guide*. Ninety-seven research papers and 42 popular articles are to her credit. Two patents on millet food products have been awarded to her by the Indian Government. Professor Sarita received several awards for excellence and appreciation of professional work. She received the Best Teacher Award from G. B. Pant University of Agriculture & Technology, Pantnagar, in 2002. She has also served as an expert in various national forums and international conferences.

Anju Bisht is Professor and Head of the Department of Home Science at M.B. Government P.G. College, Haldwani, Uttarakhand, India, under the Department of Higher Education, Government of Uttarakhand. She holds a Ph.D. in Human Nutrition and a postgraduate degree in Foods and Nutrition from G. B. Pant University of Agriculture and Technology, Pantnagar, Uttarakhand. With over two decades of teaching and research experience, her areas of research interest include community nutrition, development of millet-based functional and weaning foods, and nutrition management of lifestyle-related disorders. She has guided Ph.D. and postgraduate students and has published several research papers and book chapters with national and international publishers. Dr. Bisht has also contributed to authoring two books in the field of nutrition and health. She has served as a subject expert and resource person at various academic and professional forums and is a reviewer for reputed academic journals. She is a member of professional bodies, including the Nutrition Society of India and the Home Science Association of India.

Contributors

Bhavna
Department of Foods & Nutrition, CCS Haryana Agricultural University
Hisar, India

Mansi Badhani
Department of Food and Nutrition, College of Community Science, GBPUAT
Pantnagar, India

Neelam Chaturvedi
Department of Food Science and Nutrition, Faculty of Home Science, Banasthali Vidyapith
Rajasthan, India

Shivangi Singh Chauhan
Department of Foods & Nutrition, CCS Haryana Agricultural University
Hisar, India

Krati Goel
Department of Food and Nutrition, College of Community Sciences, G. B. Pant University of Agriculture and Technology
Pantnagar, India

Alpana Joshi
Department of Hospitality Management, Amrapali University
Uttarakhand, India

Ayushi Joshi
Department of Food and Nutrition, College of Community Sciences, G. B. Pant University of Agriculture and Technology
Pantnagar, India

Jayanti Kajale
Gokhale Institute of Politics and Economics
Pune, India

Tarvinder Jeet Kaur
Department of Home Science, Kurukshetra University
Kurukshetra, India

Archana Kushwaha
Department of Food and Nutrition, College of Community Sciences, G. B. Pant University of Agriculture and Technology
Pantnagar, India

Punjasthala Ravindrasingh Negi
Department of Food Science and Nutrition, Banasthali Vidyapith
Rajasthan, India

Swati Shukla
Department of Food and Nutrition, College of Community Sciences, G. B. Pant University of Agriculture and Technology
Pantnagar, India

Sangeeta C. Sindhu
Department of Foods & Nutrition, CCS Haryana Agricultural University
Hisar, India

Shefali Srivastava
Symbiosis Institute of International Business (SIIB), Symbiosis International (Deemed University)
Pune, India

Shivli Srivastava
Nestle Development Center
Gurugram, India

T. Tamilselvan
Flour Milling Baking and Confectionery Technology Department, CSIR-Central Food Technological Research Institute
Mysore, India

Neha Tiwari
Department of Home Science, R.C.U. Govt. P.G. College
Uttarakhand, India

Palak Tiwari
Department of Food Science and Nutrition, Banasthali Vidyapith
Rajasthan, India

Surabhi Singh Yadav
Nutrition and Dietetics Program, Symbiosis School of Culinary Arts and Nutritional Sciences (SSCANS), Symbiosis International (Deemed University) (SIU)
Pune, India

1 Millets
The Sri Anna

Neha Tiwari
Department of Home Science, R.C.U. Govt. P.G. College, Uttarkashi, Uttarakhand, India

1.1 INTRODUCTION

Millets are widely known as golden crops of India. They are highly nutritious and known as nutri-cereals. The interesting fact about millets is that they can survive in harsh climate with low water and input requirements. In the present times, the introduction of millets in our daily diet can be one of the best alternatives, as these miracle grains not only prove to be nutritious but also have a health-benefitting effect on our bodies. Due to the high content of nutrients and phytochemicals, they can fight against many diseases which are more prevalent nowadays. As there is a lack of awareness regarding numerous health advantages of millets among general population, the Government of India is now working to make millet-based foods more widely available in our everyday diets. Now millets are called "Sri Anna" which means superior to all grains. In Karnataka, millets are named "Siri Dhaanya." This name indicates that millets are not only known for their taste and good nutritional value but also possess medicinal value.

1.2 HISTORY OF MILLETS IN INDIA

Millets have been known for their existence since ancient time. Archaeological evidence suggests millet consumption during Indus Valley Civilization (3300–1300 BC). During this time, millets were the staple food of the civilization. In the Vedic period (1500–500 BC), especially in Rigveda, the cultivation of millets is mentioned. Millets were considered nutritious and versatile grains that could be used for various culinary purposes. Also, in ancient Tamil literature like the Sangam literature (300 BC to 300 CE), millets were found to be a part of South Indian cuisine. Among all the millets, ragi was the famous grain used to make various traditional dishes (Pokharia et al 2024). Cereals were divided into three categories by Sushruta (*Sushruta Samhita*, 600–500 BC): dhanyavarga, khudhanyavarga and samidhanyavarga. Among the millets that are part of Khudhaynavarga are *Coix* (gavedhuka), barnyard millet (syamaka) and kodo millet (kodrusaha).

Millets are also described in "Abhijnana Shakuntalam," the legendary masterpiece of Kalidasa (4–5th AD) where foxtail millets were given by sage Kanva while bidding farewell to Shakuntala in Dushyanta's court. This stipulates the propitious nature accredited to millets. The existence of millets is indicated in Varaha purana, where it is alluded that God Srinivasa is favourable to those who proffer foxtail millet (Bhadkariyaa and Khana 2023).

As stated by Dakar Bachan in early medieval Bengal (8–13th century AD), proso millet cultivation was recommended provided that rain occurred during the month of Falgun (February to March).

Pearl millet and sorghum, both originating in Africa, were also initiated concurrently apart from finger millet. Pearl millet was known in the later 3rd millennium BC in Saurashtra and moved to South India where it was known around 1800 BC. Pearl millets' existence was also found in both Neolithic South India (2000–1200 BC) and Narhan Culture (1300–800 BC).

Millets are mentioned in Ayurvedic texts from the 14th century AD, with the Sanskrit term "Nali" first appearing in Madanapala Nighantu (1374 AD). Regardless, archaeological evidence

DOI: 10.1201/9781003686668-1

exhibits finger millet was present in India much earlier, around 2300 BC in Hallur, Karnataka (Harappan levels). It was also found in late Harappan sites in Northern and Western India and was an essential food in Neolithic Karnataka.

The 15th-century Kannada poem composition "Ragi thandheera," written by Purandara Dasa from Karnataka, highlights the fame of finger millet (ragi) during those times. Srinatha, the Telugu poet from the 15th century, described the people's food habits of Palnadu area in Andhra, a part of the then Vijayanagara Empire, as entire survival on sorghum and pearl millet for porridge, fermented products, cooking etc. and that other than millets they have nothing to eat. Fernao Nuniz, a 16th-century Portuguese traveller, who visited Vijayanagar Kingdom, described that sorghum was the major food grain devoured in South India.

The 16th-century Kannada poet Kanakada's Ramadhanya Charithre has eternalized finger millets and symbolized the conflict between the upper and weak castes and classes, as an argument between two food grains, rice and finger millet (ragi), a most imaginative artistic piece with a strong social message. Sarvajna, a 17th-century Kannada poet, praised sorghum which was and is the staple food of the common people in North Karnataka districts (Bhadkariyaa and Khana 2023).

In Mughal India, during 16–17th century AD, millets like pearl millet, sorghum and finger millet were cultivated in dried areas of the northwest and western zones, in addition to wheat-dominant areas and other drier districts. In Ain-i-Akbari (16th century AD), Abul Fazl states that millets, which included sorghum, pearl millet, kodo millet, barnyard millet and finger millet, were part of kharif season and were grown in Malwa, Gujarat, Ajmer, Khandesh, Lahore, Agra, Allahabad, Awadh and Multan. Francisco Pelsaert of Dutch East Indian Company at Agra (1621–1627 AD) records that sorghum, pearl millet and foxtail millet were the food grains eaten by the poor in the 17th century.

Hyder Ali Khan (1720–1782), the Sultan of Mysore, would often eat dry roti of finger millet or sorghum with just water. James Scurry (1766–1822 AD), a British soldier who was held detained by Hyder Ali and Tipu Sultan for ten years (1780–1790) at Seringapatam, noted that during his footslog from Bengaluru prison to another place, he was given food made from finger millet flour.

1.3 CLASSIFICATION OF MILLETS

Millets are categorized into two major categories, i.e., major millets and minor millets (Figure 1.1).

1. Major millets
   a. Sorghum (jowar)
   b. Pearl millet (bajra)
   c. Finger millet (ragi)
2. Minor millets
   a. Foxtail millet (*kakum*)
   b. Kodo millet (kodon)
   c. Barnyard millet (sanwa)
   d. Little millet (*kutki*)
   e. Proso millet (chenna)

1.3.1 Sorghum

Sorghum is commonly known as jowar in India. The country's rice production is ranked first in the world, and sorghum is ranked fifth after rice, wheat, maize and barley. Sorghum is used as food for human consumption as well as nutritive forage to animals. The grains are also used for feed in poultry. Sorghum is mainly cultivated in Maharashtra, Karnataka and Tamil Nadu. It is rich in protein. The major portion of sorghum protein is prolamin (kafirin). Other than protein, sorghum is also rich in fibre, vitamins like thiamine and riboflavin, folic acid and β-carotene. The grain is also

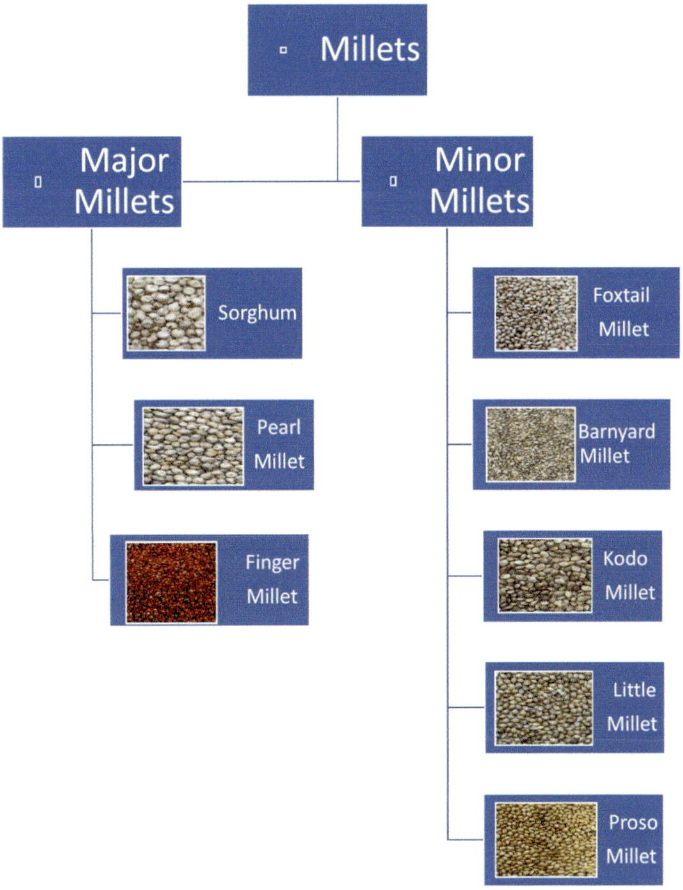

FIGURE 1.1 Classification of millets.

abundant in minerals like calcium, potassium, phosphorus, iron, zinc and sodium (www.fao.org/4/t0818e/T0818E0e.htm).

1.3.2 Pearl Millet

Pearl millet is called bajra. The niacin content of pearl millet is highest among all other cereals. It is also rich in other nutrients like protein (12–16%), lipids (4–6%) and dietary fibre (11.5%) (Hassan et al 2021). The energy content of pearl millet is also the highest as compared to other millets. It also contains folic acid, iron, calcium, zinc, magnesium, vitamin E and B-complexes. Pearl millet has a unique feature of having a high content of unsaturated fats which are beneficial for health.

1.3.3 Finger Millet

Finger millet is also known as ragi. It has the highest content of calcium (300–350 mg/100 g) as compared to other cereal grains which makes it a perfect source of calcium suitable for everyone, especially kids, teenagers, pregnant and lactating mothers (Devi et al 2011). Finger millet contains less amount of protein and fat than other common cereals. The uniqueness of finger millet protein is that it contains sulphur-rich amino acids. Finger millet also has high antioxidant activity. It has excellent malting properties which makes it suitable to make malted products, especially for kids.

1.3.4 Foxtail Millet

Foxtail millet, called kangni or kakum, is the most digestible and non-allergenic grain. It is cooked like rice or can be used to make other food items. They are also fermented to make vinegar or wines in some countries like China. Foxtail millet grain has a low glycaemic index (GI) which makes it suitable as an alternative for diabetics. It also has high fibre and protein content (Sharma and Niranjan 2017).

1.3.5 Kodo Millet

Kodo millet is known as kodon. It has high protein and high fibre content as well as contains high amount of lecithin which helps in strengthening the nervous system. It is rich in B vitamins like niacin, pyridoxine and folic acid (Bunkar et al 2021).

1.3.6 Barnyard Millet

India is the biggest producer of barnyard millet, the richest source of digestible protein, crude fibre and iron. It is generally known as sanwa and jhangora. It is widely grown across India, China and Korea. Basically, it is used for food and fodder. Barnyard millet is a rich source of both soluble and insoluble dietary fibre. Gamma-aminobutyric acid (GABA) and beta-glucan are found in barnyard millet which makes it an ideal source for controlling blood glucose levels and lipid levels. In India, it is mainly cultivated in Uttarakhand, Tamil Nadu, Andhra Pradesh and Karnataka (Mhaske et al 2025).

1.3.7 Little Millet

Little millet is commonly called *kutki*. Little millet and proso millet share some common characteristics except that the plant is generally shorter in stature, has smaller panicles and seeds and is grown on a limited scale voluntarily or with minimum care on poor lands. It is cooked just like rice. It is rich in many nutrients, particularly iron and antioxidants, and, in India, is mainly cultivated in Madhya Pradesh, Odisha, Jharkhand and Uttar Pradesh (Anbukkani et al 2017).

1.3.8 Proso Millet

It is also known as chenna and *barri* and can be grown in low-rain areas. It is a drought-resistant crop and can tolerate harsh climatic conditions. It is rich in calcium, so it can be used as the best alternative for bone growth and maintenance. It is also good for heart patients as it is low in cholesterol. It is also a rich source of manganese and is generally grown in northern states of India (Calinova 2007).

1.4 NUTRITIONAL IMPORTANCE OF MILLETS

Millets are popularized due to their high nutritional value and health benefits. They can grow in areas with low rainfall which makes them popular for attaining food and nutritional security. In developing countries, millets are primarily consumed by humans, whereas in developed countries, they're mainly used as animal feed. Millets are rich in protein, micronutrients and phytochemicals, making them a nutritional powerhouse. They typically contain 7–12% protein, 2–5% fat, 65–75% carbohydrates and 15–20% dietary fibre. The protein in millets is also highly digestible due to lower levels of cross-linked prolamins, making them a great option compared to other cereal grains.

The nutritional composition of various millets is summarized in Table 1.1, while their vitamin and mineral content is outlined in Table 1.2.

TABLE 1.1
Proximate Composition of Millets (per 100 g)

Millets	Moisture (g)	Protein (g)	Ash (g)	Fat (g)	Dietary Fibres (g)			Carbohydrates (g)	Energy (kcal)
					Total	Insoluble	Soluble		
Bajra (*Pennisetum typhoideum*)	08.97 ± 0.60	10.96 ± 0.26	1.37 ± 0.17	5.43 ± 0.64	11.49 ± 0.62	9.14 ± 0.58	2.34 ± 0.42	61.78 ± 0.85	347.99 ± 18
Sorghum (*Sorghum vulgare*)	09.01 ± 0.77	09.97 ± 0.43	1.39 ± 0.34	1.73 ± 0.31	10.22 ± 0.49	8.49 ± 0.40	1.73 ± 0.40	67.68 ± 1.03	334.13 ± 13
Ragi (*Eleusine coracana*)	10.89 ± 0.61	07.16 ± 0.63	2.04 ± 0.34	1.92 ± 0.14	11.18 ± 1.14	9.51 ± 0.65	1.67 ± 0.55	66.82 ± 0.73	320 ± 10
Little millet (*Panicum miliare*)	14.23 ± 0.45	08.92 ± 1.09	1.72 ± 0.27	2.55 ± 0.13	06.39 ± 0.60	5.45 ± 0.48	2.27 ± 0.52	65.55 ± 1.29	346.31 ± 19
Kodo millet (*Paspalum scrobiculatum*)	14.23 ± 0.45	08.92 ± 1.09	1.72 ± 0.27	2.55 ± 0.13	06.39 ± 0.60	4.29 ± 0.82	2.11 ± 0.34	66.19 ± 1.19	331.70 ± 10
Foxtail millet (*Setaria italica*)	10.45 ± 0.14[a]	11.50 ± 1.08	0.47 ± 0.03[a]	2.38 ± 0.03[a]	14.06 ± 0.04[b]	13.25 ± 0.05[b]	0.81 ± 0.03[b]	73.33 ± 0.03[a]	331 ± 5
Barnyard millet (*Echinochloa esculenta*)	9.4 ± 0.2[b]	5.1 ± 0.1[b]	2.2 ± 0.1[b]	2.9 ± 0.1[b]	12.34 ± 0.05	8.19 ± 0.05	4.15 ± 0.03	65.55 ± 0.5	307 ± 10
Proso millet (*Panicum miliaceum*)	–	12.50 ± 0.05	–	1.10 ± 0.01	11.53 ± 0.03	9.48 ± 0.45	2.05 ± 0.55	70.04 ± 0.75	341 ± 10

Source: Gopalan et al (2007).
[a] Mohamed et al (2009).
[b] Chouhan et al (2016).

TABLE 1.2
Vitamin and Mineral Contents of Millets (mg/100 g)

Millets	Calcium (mg)	Chromium (mg)	Cobalt (mg)	Copper (mg)	Iron (mg)	Zinc (mg)	Thiamine (mg)	Riboflavin (mg)	Niacin (mg)
Bajra (*Pennisetum typhoideum*)	27.35 ± 2.16	0.025 ± 0.006	0.030 ± 0.015	0.54 ± 0.11	6.42 ± 1.04	1.7–2.4	0.24 ± 0.02	0.18 ± 0.02	0.9 ± 0.11
Sorghum (*Sorghum vulgare*)	27.60 ± 3.71	0.010 ± 0.003	0.012 ± 0.007	0.45 ± 0.11	3.95 ± 0.94	2.0–3.0	0.38 ± 0.01	0.15 ± 0.01	2.15 ± 0.34
Ragi (Eleusine coracana)	364 ± 58	0.032 ± 0.019	0.022 ± 0.009	0.67 ± 0.22	4.62 ± 0.36	2.5–2.8	0.37 ± 0.02	0.19 ± 0.02	2.12 ± 0.24
Little millet (*Panicum miliare*)	16.06 ± 154	0.016 ± 0.006	0.001 ± 0.00	0.34 ± 0.08	1.26 ± 0.44	2.2–8.0	0.24 ± 0.04	0.04 ± 0.002	1.56 ± 0.41
Kodo millet (*Paspalum scrobiculatum*)	15.27 ± 1.28	0.021 ± 0.027	0.005 ± 0.003	0.26 ± 0.05	2.34 ± 0.46	0.5–0.75	0.26 ± 0.04	0.18 ± 0.02	1.52 ± 0.31
Foxtail millet (*Setaria italica*)	54.85±0.04[a]	0.030	–	1.40	4.53±0.07[a]	2.3–4.1[a]	0.45 ± 0.05	0.13 ± 0.03	3.45 ± 0.26
Barnyard millet (*Echinochloa esculenta*)	18.8 ± 0.1[b]	0.090	–	0.60	11.1 ± 0.2[b]	4.20–6.0	0.3 ± 0.01[c]	0.15 ± 0.04[c]	4.86 ± 0.43[c]
Proso millet (*Panicum miliaceum*)	14.20 ± 0.02	0.020	–	1.60	3.8 ± 0.30	1.5–3.2	0.41–0.63[d]	0.22–0.28[d]	1.32–4.50[d]

Source: Gopalan et al (2007).
[a] Arora et al (2023).
[b] Chouhan et al (2016).
[c] Kalaiarasi et al (2024).
[d] Das et al (2019).

The above table showed that protein is highest in proso millet (12.50 g/100 g), followed by foxtail millet (11.50 g/100 g) (Gopalan et al 2007). The protein content is lowest in barnyard millet (5.1 g) and ragi (7.16 g) as compared to other millets (Mohamed et al 2009). The total dietary fibre (per 100 g) is highest in foxtail millet (14.06 g), followed by barnyard millet (12.34 g), proso millet (11.53 g) and bajra (11.49 g), in which the maximum content is of soluble dietary fibre (Chouhan et al 2016). The per cent energy content of barnyard millet (307 kcal) and ragi (320 kcal) is lower as compared to other millets, which makes them a good alternative to incorporate in the diet for those who wants to reduce weight.

Table 1.2 showed that among all the minerals, the iron content is highest in barnyard millet (11.1 mg/100 g), followed by bajra (6.42 mg/100 g), ragi (4.62 mg/100 g) and foxtail millet (4.53 mg/100 g). Ragi is called the powerhouse of calcium (364 mg/100 g). The high calcium content in ragi is beneficial for various age groups, especially among children and pregnant women. Millets are also a source of cobalt, an essential mineral that forms a core component of vitamin B12, which helps in the formation of healthy red blood cells. Among all millets bajra contains 0.030 mg/100 g of cobalt, followed by ragi (0.020 mg/100 g). Other millets like foxtail millet, barnyard millet and proso millet are not considered a good source of cobalt (Kalaiarasi et al 2024). Copper is an essential mineral that plays a vital role in human body, viz., energy production, iron metabolism and red blood cell formation. Table 1.2 shows that among all millets, proso millet and foxtail millet are rich sources of copper as compared to other millets. Millets are also a good source of vitamins like thiamine, riboflavin and niacin. The thiamine content is highest in foxtail millet (0.45 mg), proso millet (0.41) and sorghum (0.38). Proso millet and barnyard millet have higher riboflavin content compared to other types of millets. Among all millets, barnyard and foxtail millets are a good source of niacin as compared to others (Gopalan et al 2007; Kalaiarasi et al 2024).

1.5 THERAPEUTIC IMPORTANCE OF MILLETS

Millets are called the powerhouse of nutrients. They contain many nutrients which prove to be beneficial in many health conditions. They contain insoluble dietary fibre which has high antioxidant properties (Himanshu et al 2018). Due to high antioxidant properties, they are proving to be beneficial in many degenerative diseases like cancer, neurological concerns and gastrointestinal diseases. Figure 1.2 enlists the different health benefits of millets (Dayakar et al 2017; Chaurasia and Anichari 2023; Sharma et al 2021).

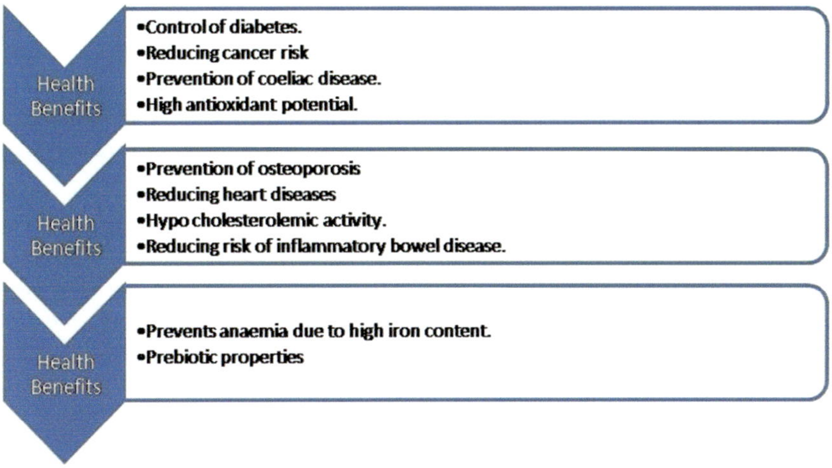

FIGURE 1.2 Health benefits of millets.

1.5.1 Cardiovascular Diseases

Millets have been proved to be very beneficial for heart as they contain significant amounts of minerals like magnesium and potassium. Magnesium plays a role in lowering blood pressure and reducing the risk of heart stroke. Along with magnesium, potassium acts as a vasodilator and helps in reducing blood pressure. The fibre content of millets is significantly higher than other cereal grains, which helps in reducing LDL cholesterol and increasing the HDL cholesterol (Saini et al 2021).

1.5.2 Diabetes mellitus

Diabetes mellitus is a metabolic condition denoted by high blood sugar levels (hyperglycaemia) and affects not only the metabolism of carbohydrates but also protein and fat metabolism. Millets are rich in fibre, which helps lower blood glucose levels and thus helps those with diabetes. Daily consumption of millet-based foods has been proved to be beneficial for people suffering from diabetes (Sharma et al 2021). Sorghum is a good source of slow-digestible fibre, which slows down carb digestion and absorption in the intestine. It also has low GI which helps the diabetics and hyperlipidaemic persons (Shinde et al 2023). Other millets like pearl millet, barnyard millet, proso millet, finger millet and foxtail millet also have low GI and high fibre content. They also contain phytonutrients which act as antioxidants.

1.5.3 Gastrointestinal Disorders

The fibre in millets can help relieve issues like constipation, bloating, gas and cramping. In addition, millets are naturally gluten-free, unlike some other grains. Gluten is a protein found in wheat, barley and rye that triggers an abnormal immune system reaction in people with coeliac disease. This reaction damages the small intestine, preventing the body from absorbing nutrients from food. Being gluten-free, millets are boon for those suffering from coeliac diseases (Saini et al 2021).

1.5.4 Cancer

Phenolic acids, tannins and phytate found in millets help prevent cancers like colon and breast cancer (Gupta et al 2023).

1.5.5 Antioxidant Properties (Detoxification)

Millets are also rich in many antioxidants which have a positive effect as they neutralize the free radicals. These free radicals can lead to cancer by eliminating other toxins. Compounds like quercetin, curcumin, ellagic acid and catechins help remove toxins and foreign agents from the body by supporting excretion and regulating enzyme activity. This is the reason that tremendous attention has been given to polyphenols due to their roles in human health (Chandrasekara and Shahidi 2012).

1.6 GLOBAL INITIATIVES AND POLICIES IN PROMOTING MILLETS

The Government of India, in its endeavour to fortify the magical millets into the Indian diets, is driving initiatives for promoting the consumption and manufacturing of millets. India's Aadi Mahotsav, a celebration of tribal spirit, is proud to promote millets, benefitting farmers, food security and nutrition. We're advancing millet value chains, supporting farmers and nourishing communities. By establishing Van Dhan Vikas Kendras in tribal areas, we aim to boost economic development and ensure national security for tribal populations. These examples bear witness to the active efforts of the Government of India in the promotion of millets in diet, notably through the tribal route. In Uttarakhand, the Government of India is focusing on improving, enhancing and promoting millet consumption among general people. For this a special event named "garh bhoj" is organized by all the higher institutes focusing on promoting local food items specially made of millets and locally grown crops (Azmi 2023).

In 2018, millets were classified as nutri-cereals by the Government of India to recognize their nutritional value and climate resilience. In the same year the Government of India celebrated the National Year of Millets to create domestic and global demand for millets. The Indian Institute of Millet Research (IIMR) in Hyderabad empowers farmers, women and entrepreneurs with skills to create value-added millet products, fostering sustainable businesses and livelihoods. The Government of India nominated the United Nations to declare 2023 the International Year of Millets. The UN General Assembly passed the resolution, and the year was celebrated with events to encourage millets and advance their recipes and supplementary products. The Regional Research Centre for Bajra was inaugurated in Gudamalani, Rajasthan in September 2023. Different policies taken by the government are described below.

1.6.1 Nutri-Cereals under National Food Security Mission (NFSM)

Millets were classified as nutri-cereals by the government in 2018 because of their nutritional benefits. During the years 2018–2019, the Department of Agriculture and Farmers Welfare (DA&FW) executed the Sub-Mission on Nutri-Cereals (Millets) as part of the National Food Security Mission (NFSM). The main objective of this institute was to intensify the millet cultivation area; production and manufacturing are on the rise. The millets included in this category were sorghum (jowar), pearl millet (bajra), finger millet (ragi), foxtail millet (kangani), proso millet (cheena), kodo millet (kodo), barnyard millet (sawa), little millet (kutki), in addition to two pseudo millets, buckwheat (kuttu) and *Amaranthus* (chaulai), which are nurtured across 212 districts which stress over 14 states. The goal of the mission was to develop a market-driven strategy dealing with production, demand and research challenges, aimed to elevate the production of nutri-cereal in specific districts of the country by implementing sustainable methods to swell the cultivation area and enhancing productivity. Furthermore, the mission aimed to strengthen the nutri-cereals system by enhancing the supply of seeds and adding value to the post-harvest process, eventually leading to better price understanding for farmers through efficient market connections (MoA&FW (Ministry of Agriculture & Farmers Welfare), 2021).

1.6.2 PLI Scheme on Millet

On March 31, 2021, the government granted approval for a central sector programme entitled the "Production Linked Incentive (PLI) scheme for Food Processing Industry," with the allocated budget of INR 10,900 crores. The mission will be carried out over a span of seven years, starting from the academic years 2021–2022, and will wrap up in 2026–2027. With the motive of boosting India's food manufacturing sector and promoting Indian food brands globally, with a focus on millet-based products. Essential support is provided for the development of recipes and other various products that promote the utilization of millets to various start-ups and entrepreneurs. The Ministry of Food Processing Industries took an initiative that aims to provide incentives to the large-scale food industry referred to as the Production Linked Incentive Scheme for Millet-Based Goods (PLISMBP); it promotes the use of millet-based products (MoA&FW (Ministry of Agriculture & Farmers Welfare), 2022).

1.6.3 Promoting Millets in Public Distribution System (PDS)

The Government of India embedded millets into the public distribution system with the aim of enhancing their availability and affordability. In addition to this, for the transportation of millets, the government has eased inter-state transportation rules. In order to fulfil the pre-procurement need of the consuming state, the Food Corporation of India (FCI) has included the transportation of surplus millets across state borders (www.mofpi.gov.in).

1.6.4 Promotion of Millet by MWCD in Supplementary Nutrition Program (SNP)

The Ministry of Women and Child Development has put forward that states and UTs include millets in meals under the Anganwadi Services' Supplementary Nutrition Program to boost nutrition. As part of Mission Saksham Anganwadi & Poshan 2.0, a millet-based dish is now a must in the weekly take-home ration for beneficiaries as per the suggestion of the Ministry of Women and Child.

1.6.5 Support for Millet Research

The government has set up the IIMR in Hyderabad to promote millets. It aims to transform millets from subsistence farming to a globally competitive industry through cost-effective and ecofriendly practices. IIMR's Nutrihub incubator supports it by funding and providing trainings to entrepreneurs in the nutri-cereal sector. The Indian Council of Agricultural Research (ICAR) has joined with 45 centres to develop new millet varieties and improve processing technologies, focusing on small millets, sorghum and pearl millet. These hybrid millet varieties and equipment used to process them into high-value products are developed by national research institutions focused on targeting urban markets and export opportunities and the advancement of new millet varieties as part of the All India Coordinated Research Project (AICRP) focused on small millets, sorghum and pearl millet (www.aicpmip.res.in/index.html).

1.6.6 Support to States

The Department of Agriculture (MoA&FW) supports the states through the centrally sponsored scheme known as "Support to State Extension Programme for Extension Reforms." This scheme encloses a range of add-on activities, such as farmers' training, site visits, practical knowledge, kisan mela, kisan goshthi, farmers–scientists interaction, organizing farmers' interest groups and setting up of farm schools, primarily focusing on engaging awardee/progressive farmers in the field.

1.7 MILLETS IN COMBATING FOOD AND NUTRITIONAL INSECURITY

Nowadays millets are being considered superfoods that meet the requirements of both environment and human health. They are known as miracle grains because of their low resource necessity as well as nutritional benefits, making them the best option for food insecurity and achieving sustainable development goals (SDGs). Popularizing millet-incorporated value-added food products can reduce the overdependence on a few plant species and help in attaining food and nutrition security (Arya and Bisht 2022). Millets play a crucial role in attaining food security, especially in those regions which are more prone to food shortages (Saxena et al 2018).

There are numerous reasons for calling millets the best option for achieving nutritional security. One of them is that they provide heterogeneity to our daily diet. They can be used to cook different food products, likely porridge, bread and roti and can even be fermented and baked, leading to less dependency on other refined grains and staple cereals. People today are moving more towards baked food items in their daily diet like bread, buns, cakes and biscuits. Replacement of refined flour with millet flour may be the best option for attaining nutritional security. Since these foods are made from millet, they are not only tasty but also more nutrient-dense than their refined counterparts.

Millets are highly nutritious, having essential vitamins, minerals, dietary fibre and antioxidants. Millets contribute to a balanced and nutrient-rich diet, helping fight malnutrition and making sure that people receive the required nutrients for good health. In modern civilization people are facing many health problems. One of them is coeliac disease, in which people are gluten-sensitive and are not able to eat wheat-based food products. For these people, millets are boon as they are gluten-free. This expands food options for those with dietary restrictions, contributing to their food security (Hassan et al 2021).

Along with their nutritional and medicinal benefits, they are rainfed crops that can be cultivated in hostile climates with unpredictable rainfall and high temperatures. Many specific circumstances are not needed for their cultivation. Millets are not affected by dry landscapes as they require less water compared to traditional staples like rice and wheat. This property is mostly important in regions with water scarcity, as it assures a steady source of food. The risk of crop failure due to pests, diseases or changing environmental conditions can be reduced by the cultivation of a variety of millet species, increasing food security. Crop diversity not only supports biodiversity but also helps to build a safety net for communities dependent on agriculture. These practices promote soil health and reduce the need for chemical inputs, contributing to long-term food security by ensuring the adaptability of agricultural systems. An Export Promotion Forum has been formed to promote Indian millets globally, focusing on marketing, development and export growth.

FSSAI's Eat Right campaign fosters millets as a healthy diet option. A Millets Experience Centre at Dilli Haat, New Delhi, raises awareness and motivates millet adoption. Government offices are advised to serve Shree Anna snacks and meals in canteens. The Department of Agriculture and Farmers Welfare is boosting millet production through the Sub-Mission on Nutri-Cereals, covering 28 states and two UTs under National Food Security Mission. The nutri-cereals (millets) such as sorghum (jowar), pearl millet (bajra), finger millet (ragi/mandua) and minor millets, i.e., foxtail millet (kangani/kakun), proso millet (cheena), kodo millet (kodo), barnyard millet (sawa/sanwa/jhangora), little millet (kutki) and two pseudo millets, buckwheat (kuttu) and *Amaranthus* (chaulai) are covered under NFSM programme. Under NFSM-Nutri Cereals, farmers get incentives for acquiring best practices, like certified seeds, combined nutrient management and improved farm tools. They also receive training and support for crop presentations, water-saving tech etc.

The Government of India has given the states the flexibility under Rashtriya Krishi Vikas Yojana (RKVY) to promote millets, with approval from the state-level committee. Several states like Assam, Bihar, Karnataka, Chhattisgarh, Madhya Pradesh, Maharashtra, Odisha, Rajasthan, Tamil Nadu, Uttarakhand and Uttar Pradesh have launched millet missions. Production of nutri-cereals and bajra rose by 8 and 17% in 2022–2023, reaching 173.20 lakh tonnes and 114.31 lakh tonnes, respectively, as compared to 160 lakh tonnes and 97.81 lakh tonnes during 2021–2022. Bajra production saw a notable uptick during 2022–2023 compared to previous years except during 2021–2022. This upward trend was shown in Bajra in comparison to other millets.

1.8 CONCLUSION

In conclusion, because of their ability to grow in adverse situations and good nutritional content, millets are a top pick for food and nutrition security, and being gluten-free and having a low GI, they offer numerous health benefits. They are perhaps a beneficial supplement to a well-balanced diet, promoting better health and general wellbeing. Millets are rich in protein, dietary fibre, vitamins and minerals like iron, magnesium and phosphorus. Additionally, they include a variety of phytochemicals that have antioxidant property and thus have the ability to improve health and fight against diseases. Millets are quite compatible and can be added to a variety of foods, including breads, snacks and porridges. Millets provide wholesome, climate-resilient and commercially viable food sources, making them a feasible solution to the problem of food insecurity. They are an important resource for ensuring food security and enhancing livelihoods, particularly in areas experiencing food shortages and nutritional inadequacies, due to their high nutritional content and capacity to flourish in harsh settings. Although they are very healthy and nutrient-dense grains, they are sometimes underutilized by consumers because of the indifferent attitude towards millets. Millets are promoted in government programmes because of their high nutritional content, ability to withstand drought and potential to increase food security. In order to increase their awareness and make them popular, the Government of India has taken many initiatives and policies so that they can be consumed by the majority of population. Millets can be the best option for attaining nutritional and food security by utilizing them to maximum. They are a sustainable and adaptable food source that can help create a more sustainable future and a healthier diet.

REFERENCES

www.aicpmip.res.in/index.html
www.fao.org/4/t0818e/T0818E0e.htm
www.mofpi.gov.in
www.wcd.gov.in

Anbukkani, P., Balaji, S. J., and Nithyashree, M. L. 2017. Production and consumption of minor millets in India: A structural break analysis. *Ann. Agric. Res. New Series.* 38(4): 1–8.

Arora, L., Aggarwal, R., Dhaliwal, I., Gupta, O. P., and Kaushik, P. 2023. Assessment of sensory and nutritional attributes of foxtail millet-based food products. *Front. Nutr.* 10:1146545. doi: 10.3389/fnut.2023.1146545.

Arya, C., and Bisht, A. 2022. Small millets: Path to food and nutrition security. In *Small millet grains: The superfood in human diet*, edited by S. Srivastava. Springer, Singapore, 161–182 pp. doi: 10.1007/978-981-16-9306-9_8

Azmi, H. (2023, February 19). 'Garh Bhoj': A social activist's mission to popularise traditional Uttarakhand foods. *The Hindu.* pp. 6–7. www.thehindu.com/news/national/other-states/garh-bhoj-a-social-activists-mission-to-popularise-traditional-uttarakhand-foods/article66528114.ece

Bhadkariyaa, S., and Khana, A. 2023. History and domestication of millet crops. *Millets: The ancient grain for the future.* Kripa Drishti Publication, Pune, pp. 62–71. ISBN: 978 81 19149 19 3

Bunkar, S. D., Goyal, S., Kumar, K., and Kamalvanshi, V. 2021. Nutritional, functional role of kodo millet and its processing: A review. *Int. J. Curr. Microbiol. App. Sci.* 10(01): 1972–1985.

Calinova, J. 2007. Nutritionally important components of Proso millet (*Panicum miliaceum* L.). *Food.* 1(1): 91–100.

Chandrasekara, A., and Shahidi, F. 2012. Bio accessibility and antioxidant potential of millet grain phenolics as affected by simulated in vitro digestion and microbial fermentation. *J. Funct. Foods.* 4: 226–237.

Chaurasia, R. K., and Anichari, N. 2023. Nutritional and health benefits of millets: A review. *Pharma Innov. J.* 12(6): 3360–3363.

Chouhan, E., Yadav, S., and Negi, N. 2016. Proximate, phytochemical and antinutrient analysis of unprocessed and processed barnyard millet flours. *Int. Ayurvedic Med. J.* 4(8): 2482–2487.

Das, S., Khound, R., Santra, M., and Santra, D. K. 2019. Beyond bird feed: Proso millet for human health and environment. *Agriculture.* 9(3): 64.

Dayakar, B., Bhaskarachary, K., Arlene, G. D., Devi, G., and Vilas, A. 2017. *Nutritional and health benefits of millets.* ICAR_Indian Institute of Millets Research (IIMR) Rajendranagar, Hyderabad, PP 112. ISBN: 81-89335-68-5

Devi, P. B., Vijayabharathi, R., Sathyabama, S., Malleshi, N. G., and Priyadarisini, V. B. 2011. Health benefits of finger millet (*Eleusine coracana* L.) polyphenols and dietary fiber: A review. *J. Food Sci. Technol..* 51(6): 1021–1040.

Gopalan, C., Ramasastri, B. V., and Balasubramanian, S. C., 2007. *Nutritive value of Indian foods.* National Institute of Nutrition, Indian Council of Medical Research, Hyderabad.

Gupta, M., Asfaha, D., and Ponnaiah, G. 2023. Millets: A nutritional powerhouse with anti-cancer potential. *Cureus.* 15(10): e47769. doi: 10.7759/cureus.47769.

Hassan, Z. M., Sebola, N. A., and Mabelebele, M. 2021. The nutritional use of millet grain for food and feed: A review. *Agric. Food Secur.* 10: 1–14.

Himanshu, M., Chauhan, S., Sachin, K., and Arya, S. S. 2018. Nutritional and nutraceutical properties of millets: A review. *Clin. J. Nutr. Diet.* 1(1): 1–10.

Kalaiarasi, G., Jayabalan, K., Muthu, K., and Pandiyan, A. 2024. Comparative study on nutrition properties of different types of millet powder. *Food Nutr. Sci.* 15(12): 12–20.

Mhaske, P. S., Nathan, B., Nallusamy, S., Raman, R., Sampathkumar, V., Kathirvel, P., Ravikumar, C. N., Sathyaseelan, C., and Selvakumar, D. 2025. Exploring the anti-diabetic potential of barnyard millet: Insights from virtual screening, MD simulation and MM-PBSA. *J. Biomol. Struct. Dyn.* 14: 1–15. doi: 10.1080/07391102.2025.2478466.

MoA&FW (Ministry of Agriculture & Farmers Welfare). 2021. Creating awareness among farmers for nutri cereals (Millets). Available from: https://pib.gov.in/PressReleaseIframePa

MoA&FW (Ministry of Agriculture & Farmers Welfare). 2022. Government to roll out several programmes in the country and abroad for popularizing millets and other nutri cereals. Available from: https://pib.gov.in/PressReleaseIframePa

Mohamed, T., Zhu, K., Amadou, I., and Fatmata, T. 2009. Functionality, in vitro digestibility and physicochemical properties of two varieties of defatted foxtail millet protein concentrates. *Int. J. Mol. Sci. (IJMS).* 10: 5224–5238. 10.3390/ijms10125224.

Pokharia, K., Anil, K., Singh, J., and Srivastava, A. 2024. Archaeobotanical evidence of millets in the Indian subcontinent with some observations on their role in the Indus civilization. *J. Archaeol. Sci.* 42(1): 442–455.

Saini, S., Saxena, S., and Samtiya, M. 2021. Potential of underutilized millets as nutri-cereal: An overview. *J. Food Sci. Technol.* 58: 4465–4477. doi: 10.1007/s13197-021-04985-x.

Saxena, R., Vanga, S. K., Wang, J., Orsat, V., and Raghavan, V. 2018. Millets for food security in the context of climate change: A review. *Sustainability.* 10(7): 2228. doi: 10.3390/su10072228

Sharma, N., and Niranjan, K. 2017. Foxtail millet: Properties, processing, health benefits, and uses. *Food Rev. Int.* 34(4): 329–363. doi: 10.1080/87559129.2017.1290103

Sharma, R., Sharma, S., Dar, B. N., and Singh, B. 2021. Millets as potential nutri cereals: A review of nutrient composition, phytochemical profile and techno functionality. *Int. J. Food Sci. Technol.* 56(8): 3703–3718.

Shinde, R. M., Shende, R. T., Wasule, D. L., Gaharwar, M., and Parlawar, N. D. 2023. Millets in India: A nutritional powerhouse for sustainable agriculture and food security. *Agri Articles.* 03(04): 379–382.

2 Millets Composition
Nutrients, Non-Nutrients, and Anti-Nutrients

Swati Shukla
Department of Food and Nutrition, College of Community Sciences, G.B. Pant University of Agriculture & Technology, Pantnagar, Uttarakhand, India

2.1 INTRODUCTION TO MILLETS

2.1.1 History and Importance of Millets

2.1.1.1 Ancient Cultivation and Cultural Relevance of Millets

Millets have been cultivated in India since the Neolithic era, about 10,000 years ago, marking one of the earliest transitions to settled agriculture. Archaeobotanical evidence confirms millet cultivation in China around 8000 years ago, with its spread to India through ancient trade. Indian Neolithic sites like Burzahom and Chirand, and Harappan sites such as Mohenjo-Daro and Lothal, have unearthed millet grains, underscoring their early agricultural and dietary significance.

Species like little millet and browntop millet were cultivated in Harappan times (2500–2000 BC), while sorghum, finger millet, and pearl millet became widespread between 1700 BC and the Mughal period. Millets also found royal and scholarly mention—from being part of Mysore Sultan Hyder Ali's diet to Canadian scientist Leslie Coleman's studies.

Ancient scriptures like the Vedas and Arthashastra focus on and mention the traditional and nutritional value of the millets. Ayurveda categorized millets as "Kshudradhanya" (small grains), describing their light and digestive properties (Veerabadhran et al 2023).

Millets hold deep cultural significance across India. They feature in temple rituals, drought food reserves, and seasonal festivals. Communities in Tamil Nadu, Odisha, Nagaland, Andhra Pradesh, and Karnataka have traditions involving millet-based rituals and recipes. Folklores, songs, and dances—like "Bajre Da Sitta" in Punjab or mulaipari songs in Tamil Nadu—further reflect their place in rural life and storytelling (Elasi et al 2023; Tripathi and Vyas 2023).

Globally, millets are recognized for their resilience and nutritional richness. With declining cultivation and awareness, India declared 2018 the "National Year of Millets" and led the UN to declare 2023 the "International Year of Millets," supported by 70 countries. Millets, often called "nutricereals," offer sustainable solutions to food security and climate-resilient agriculture (Elasi et al 2023).

2.1.1.2 Role in Sustainable Agriculture and Food Security

As depicted in Figure 2.1, millets have long been valued by early agricultural communities for their remarkable adaptability to diverse environmental conditions, particularly in arid and semi-arid regions. These resilient grains thrive in marginal soils and require significantly less water, fertilizers, and chemical inputs compared to conventional staple crops. Their hardy nature makes them especially suitable for regions vulnerable to climate change and environmental degradation (Tripathi and Vyas 2023; Veerabadhran et al 2023).

As we approach a future where the global population is projected to reach nearly 10 billion by 2050, the challenge of producing enough food sustainably—while protecting ecosystems and

 DOI: 10.1201/9781003686668-2

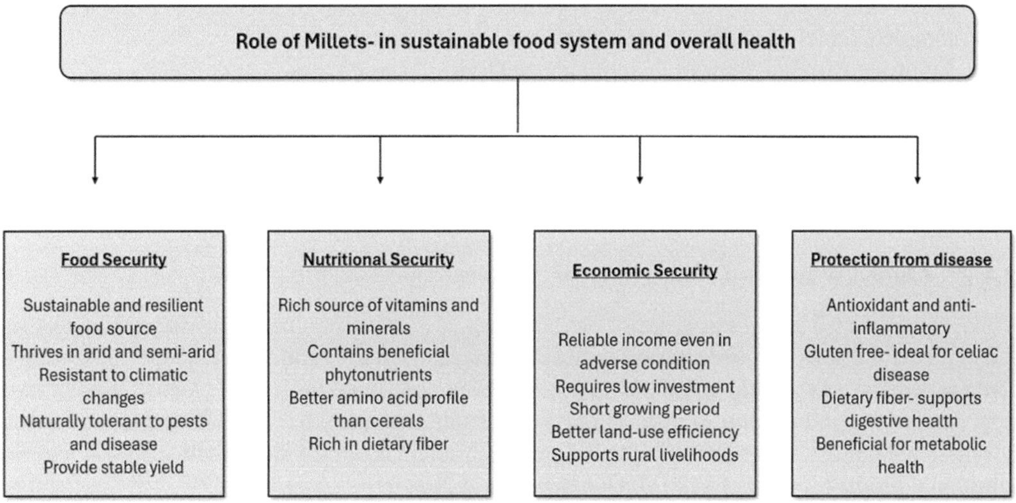

FIGURE 2.1 Role of millets in sustainable food system and health. (Source: Kumar et al 2018.)

preparing for climate-related disruptions—has never been more pressing. Agricultural systems are already under strain due to increasing temperatures, erratic rainfall, rising sea levels, and more frequent extreme weather events. These climate changes are expected to severely impact crop yields, particularly in dryland areas.

Historically, a heavy focus on a few high-yielding, input-intensive crops like rice, wheat, and maize has contributed to increased food production. However, this has also led to a narrow concentration of food sources—these three crops alone provide around 60% of the world's dietary energy intake. Such dependence makes global food systems more vulnerable to shocks, especially under worsening climate conditions.

Millets, on the other hand, offer a convincing substitute. As climate-resilient and nutrient-dense crops native to several G20 countries, they have the potential to diversify food systems, strengthen resilience, and support both environmental and human health. Millets can tolerate high temperatures, low rainfall, and poor soil quality, making them a sustainable option for farmers in climate-stressed areas.

For small-scale and marginalized farmers, millet cultivation offers numerous advantages. The low input requirements—minimal need for irrigation, fertilizers, or pesticides—make it economically viable for those with limited resources. In addition to improving livelihoods and farmer income, millets play a crucial role in enhancing food and nutritional security at the community level (Tripathi and Vyas 2023).

From a food security perspective, millets are particularly valuable (Arya and Bisht 2022). They grow well where conventional crops like rice and wheat may struggle, especially in regions facing water scarcity or soil degradation. Their resistance to pests and diseases also reduces the reliance on chemical pesticides, further contributing to environmentally sustainable practices.

Beyond their agronomic benefits, millets are packed with health-promoting nutrients.

- They are naturally gluten-free, making them suitable for people with celiac disease.
- They have high fiber content, low glycemic index, and rich mineral profile—including iron, zinc, and calcium.
- Support the prevention and management of non-communicable diseases such as diabetes, obesity, cardiovascular conditions, and high blood pressure.

- When consumed with legumes, as commonly done in India, millets also provide a more complete protein profile, enhancing their nutritional value.
- All millet varieties show high antioxidant activity.

Furthermore, millet cultivation has a lower carbon footprint compared to water- and energy-intensive crops, supporting broader climate goals and contributing to environmentally conscious food systems (Food Safety and Standards Authority of India (FSSAI) 2023).

2.1.2 Overview of Millet Varieties

Millets, categorized as "minor cereals" or "Nutri cereals," are listed as the world's sixth most significant cereal grains and are clubbed with oats, sorghum, maize, and barley under the section of "coarse cereals" (Satyavathi et al 2021). Although they contribute just 2% to global cereal production, nearly 95% of the world's millet output comes from Asia and Africa. Belonging to the Poaceae (Gramineae) family, millets are ancient, indigenous grains known for their small seed size and rich nutritional profile (Saleem et al 2023; Gahalawat et al 2024).

The term "millet" is derived from the Latin word *Millium*, meaning tiny seeds, and is also linked to the French word *Mille*, referring to the thousands of seeds found in a handful.

Food Safety and Standards Authority of India (FSSAI) (2023) and Nautiyal et al (2023) elaborate on the categorization of these nutrient-dense grains based on size (Figure 2.2; Table 2.1).

Major millets—consisting of millets like sorghum, pearl millet or Bajra, and finger millet or Ragi—are one of the most extensively cultivated and consumed as staple and are relatively big in size.

Sorghum is a highly nutritious, traditional staple crop predominantly grown in the dryland regions of the world. As a warm-season cereal, it thrives in hot climates, showing resilience to pests and diseases, but is sensitive to low temperatures. Worldwide, sorghum stands fifth in production among cereal crops and occupies fourth position in India. Remarkably, it accounts for over 60% of total millet production worldwide.

In India, sorghum is primarily cultivated in states like Maharashtra, Karnataka, Telangana, Andhra Pradesh, Tamil Nadu, and Madhya Pradesh. It serves as a dietary mainstay for around 300 million people across the globe. Known for its health benefits, sorghum supports blood circulation,

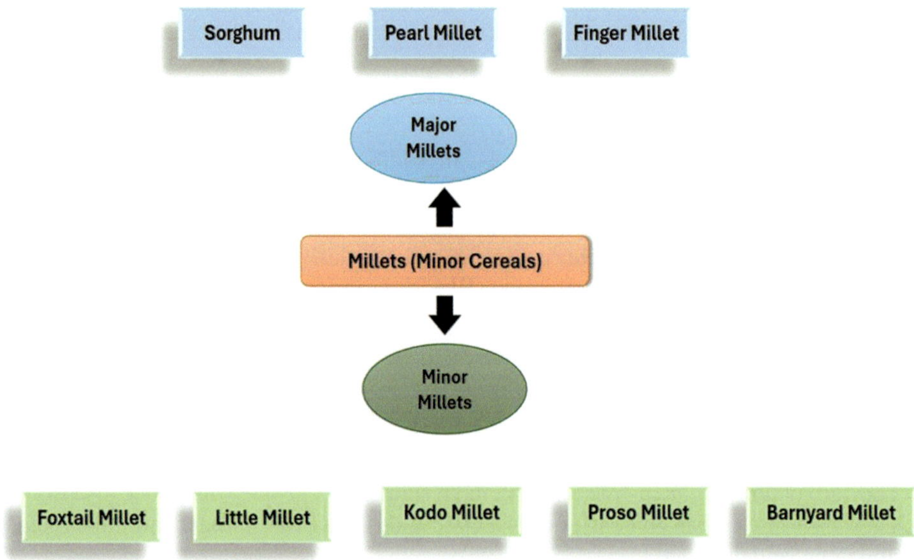

FIGURE 2.2 Classification of millets.

TABLE 2.1
Classification of Millets

Type	Millets	Scientific Name	Common Name
Major	Sorghum	*Sorghum bicolor*	Jowar, Cholam, Milo, Milo-maize, Kaoliang
	Pearl millet	*Pennisetum glaucum*	Bajra, babala, bulrush, cumbu, dukhn, gero, sajje
	Finger millet	*Eleusine coracana*	Ragi, Aariyam, Panjapule, maduva, nachani
Minor	Foxtail millet	*Setaria italica*	Italian/German millet, Kangni, Navane, thinai, kang
	Little millet	*Panicum sumatrense*	kutki, sama, gindi, mutaki
	Kodo millet	*Paspalum scrobiculatum*	Koden, Kodra, Harka, Koovaragu, Varagu, Arikelu, Kodua
	Proso millet	*Panicum miliaceum*	Cheena, common millet, hog millet, broom corn, yellow hog, Hershey, and white millet
	Barnyard millet	*Echinochloa esculenta*	Sanwa, oodalu, Kavadapullu, Kuthiravali, Udalu, Kira, Jhangora

aids in weight management, and promotes cell regeneration. Sorghum is also versatile in culinary use, being prepared in forms such as dosa, upma, roti, rice, cookies, and salads.

Nutrient value per 100 g: Energy—334 kcal, Protein—9.9 g, Fat—1.73 g, Carbohydrate—67.7 g, Calcium—27.6 mg, Iron—3.9 mg, Folic acid—39.4 µg (Food Safety and Standards Authority of India (FSSAI) 2023)

Pearl Millet is the sixth most important cereal globally in terms of area and production, known for its exceptional drought tolerance—the highest among all millets. In India, it ranks just after rice and wheat in terms of cultivation and is one of the most commonly consumed millets. This greenish grain is predominantly grown in Rajasthan, Haryana, Gujarat, Maharashtra, Uttar Pradesh, and Punjab.

Rich in protein, pearl millet also provides essential minerals like zinc, copper, and magnesium, along with beneficial phytochemicals and heart-healthy unsaturated fats. It supports several health functions, including lowering cholesterol, strengthening bones, improving heart health, and aiding in weight management. Pearl millet is a multipurpose grain and is generally included in a variety of dishes like flatbreads, upma, khichdi, beverages, idlis, and snacks like khakhra.

Nutrient value per 100 g: Energy—347 kcal, Protein—10.9 g, Fat—5.43 g, Carbohydrate—61.8 g, Calcium—27.4 mg, Iron—6.4 mg, Folic acid—36.1 µg (Food Safety and Standards Authority of India (FSSAI) 2023)

Finger Millet, commonly known as *ragi*, is a hardy crop that grows well across a wide range of altitudes—from sea level up to the Himalayan hills—but performs best in well-drained, loamy soils. Karnataka leads its cultivation in India, producing about 50% of the country's output, which accounts for nearly 34% of global production. The plant is a dwarf, highly tillering species, ranging in height from 30 to 150 cm. Its tiny seeds resemble mustard in size and vary in color from light or dark brown to white.

This reddish grain is a nutritious, protein-rich alternative to wheat and rice. It is abundant in dietary fiber and a good source of micronutrients like vitamins A and B. It also contains the essential amino acids, making it a relatively good quality protein source, which can help with satiety and metabolic health.

Nutrient value per 100 g: Energy—320 kcal, Protein—7.2 g, Fat—1.92 g, Carbohydrate—66.8 g, Calcium—364 mg, Iron—4.6 mg, Folic acid—34.7 µg (Food Safety and Standards Authority of India (FSSAI) 2023)

Minor millets: They are a group of small-grained cereal crops that are less commonly cultivated and consumed compared to major millets. Despite their limited global production, they play a vital role in many regional diets due to their resilience to harsh environmental conditions and notable nutritional value. This category includes foxtail, little, kodo, proso, and barnyard millet.

Foxtail millet: One of the ancient, harvested millets, it stands as the third-largest grown millet crop across the globe, typically in the semi-arid tropics of Asia. In India, it is cultivated in Tamil Nadu, Andhra Pradesh, Karnataka, Odisha, Maharashtra, and Madhya Pradesh. The grains resemble paddy rice in structure and require the removal of the outer husk before consumption. If eaten regularly, this millet provides about twofold the protein content (12%) as compared to rice.

Nutrient value per 100 g: Energy—331 kcal, Protein—12.3 g, Fat—4.3 g, Carbohydrate—60.1 g, Calcium—31 mg, Iron—2.8 mg, Folic acid—15 µg (Food Safety and Standards Authority of India (FSSAI) 2023)

Foxtail millet, rich in calcium, iron, and copper, is ideal for pregnant women and malnourished children, supporting strength and immunity. It benefits the nervous system, muscle health, heart health, and immunity. It can be used in dosas, cheelas, chapatis, kheer pudding, and pancakes.

Little Millet, grown in Karnataka, Tamil Nadu, Maharashtra, Madhya Pradesh, Uttar Pradesh, and Uttarakhand, is rich in dietary fiber, antioxidants, and iron.

It is smaller than proso millet, with shorter panicles and seeds. Often grown alongside other millets, pulses, and oilseeds, it is commonly used as a rice substitute in various dishes due to its small size and quick cooking time.

Nutrient value per 100 g: Energy—346 kcal, Protein—10.1 g, Fat—5.89 g, Carbohydrate—65.5 g, Calcium—16.1 mg, Iron—1.2 mg, Folic acid—36.2 µg (Food Safety and Standards Authority of India (FSSAI) 2023)

Kodo Millet was domesticated in India nearly 3000 years ago and is grown in regions like Maharashtra, Odisha, Uttar Pradesh, Tamil Nadu, Andhra Pradesh, and Telangana. Known for its hardiness, drought resistance, and ability to thrive on stony or gravelly soils unsuitable for other crops, Kodo millet is an annual grass that can grow up to 90 cm tall. The grains range in color from light red to dark grey.

Naturally gluten-free, Kodo millet is an excellent choice for those with celiac disease or gluten sensitivity and can serve as a wheat substitute. With a low glycemic index, it releases glucose into the bloodstream slowly. Additionally, Kodo millet is rich in magnesium, selenium, and a good source of thiamine, riboflavin, copper, and zinc.

Nutrient value per 100 g: Energy—331 kcal, Protein—8.9 g, Fat—2.55 g, Carbohydrate—66.2 g, Calcium—15.3 mg, Iron—2.3 mg, Folic acid—39.5 µg (Food Safety and Standards Authority of India (FSSAI) 2023)

Proso Millet is cultivated in regions like Uttarakhand, Uttar Pradesh, Haryana, Gujarat, Rajasthan, Maharashtra, and Karnataka. It is a short-season crop suited for low rainfall areas and can be cultivated alongside red gram, maize, and sorghum. Proso millet is high in protein and calcium, promoting heart health and lowering cholesterol.

It is also rich in iron, potassium, phosphorus, zinc, magnesium, and B vitamins. Commonly used in dishes like idli, khaja, and burfi.

Nutrient value per 100 g: Energy—341 kcal, Protein—12.5 g, Fat—2.55 g, Carbohydrate—70.4 g, Calcium—14 mg, Iron—0.2 mg, Folic acid—39.5 µg (Food Safety and Standards Authority of India (FSSAI) 2023)

Barnyard Millet is grown in Uttar Pradesh, Rajasthan, Madhya Pradesh, Gujarat, Karnataka, and Tamil Nadu, thriving at higher elevations and maturing in three to four months. It is cultivated on marginal land unsuitable for other crops and is the fourth most produced minor millet, with India being the largest producer.

Rich in soluble and insoluble fiber, protein, iron, zinc, calcium, magnesium, fat, vitamins, and essential amino acids, it provides valuable nutrition and supports food security for many people globally.

Nutrient value per 100 g: Energy—307 kcal, Protein—11.2 g, Fat—2.2 g, Carbohydrate—65.5 g, Calcium—11 mg, Iron—15.2 mg, Folic acid—15.2 µg (Food Safety and Standards Authority of India (FSSAI) 2023)

2.1.3 Global Production and Distribution of Millets

Millets are primarily grown in developing countries in Asia and Africa, as shown in Figure 2.3, accounting for approximately 94% of global production, which totals around 28 million tons. The highest production is contributed by pearl millet, followed by foxtail, proso, and finger millet. Globally, millets are grown on about 34.1 million ha, with 97% of production taking place in developing nations, largely by marginal farmers. Among the 93 countries cultivating millets, 7 exceed 1 million ha each, and around 25 nations report areas larger than 0.1 million ha (FAOSTAT 2018).

As per the report by the Food and Agriculture Organization (FAO), global millet production was 26.7 million metric tonnes in 2009, led by Africa as the largest producer and followed by Asia and India. Production of pearl millet declined from 32.8 million tonnes in 2010 to 28.4 million tonnes in 2014, with Asia and Africa contributing over 98% of global output. The share of African countries decreased, while Asia's contribution grew. Similarly, sorghum production, while significant, remains fifth in global cereal production (Dayakar Rao et al 2017).

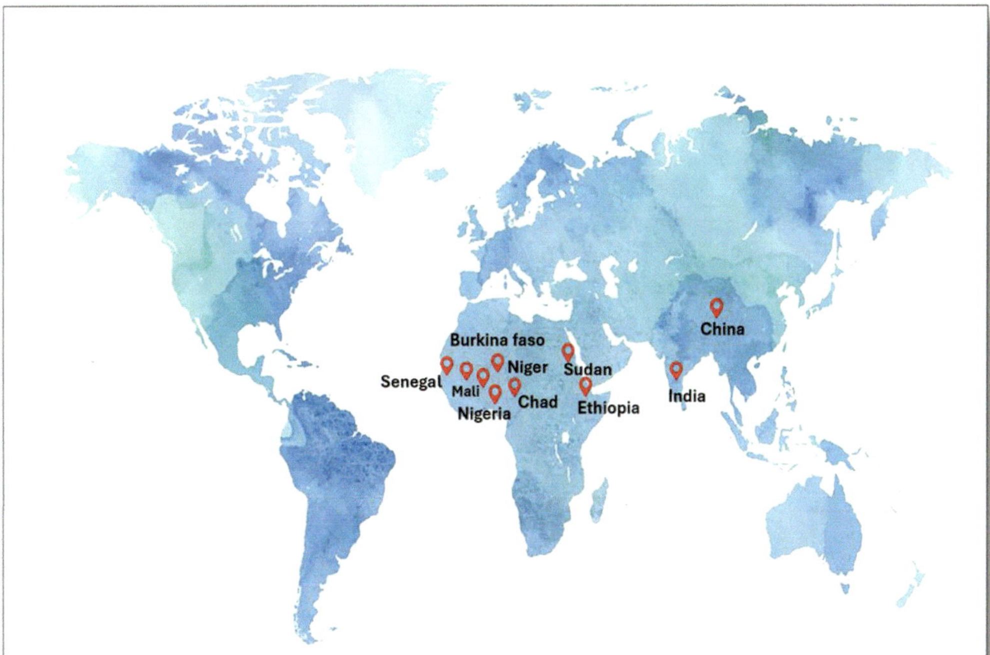

FIGURE 2.3 Top seven millet-producing countries in the world. (Source: Kheya et al 2023.)

India is a major player in millet production, accounting for 40.51% of the world's pearl millet in 2020. Key producing states include Rajasthan, Maharashtra, Uttar Pradesh, Karnataka, and Madhya Pradesh, which together contribute almost 98% of India's millet output. India is also the largest global grower of millets, covering 26.6% of global and 83% of Asia's millet-growing areas (Kane-Potaka et al 2021).

In recent years, millet production and consumption have surged in India, driven by health benefits and environmental awareness. Surveys show that many consumers are adopting millets due to health concerns, weight management, and taste preferences. There is also growing recognition of millet cultivation's environmental benefits, though marketing challenges remain, with some consumers feeling that millets are overly marketed as health-specific foods (Shah et al 2024).

2.2 NUTRIENT COMPOSITION OF MILLETS

Minor millets are termed "nutri-cereals" for their rich content of proteins, fiber, essential nutrients, and antioxidants. They are distinguished by their high dietary fiber, protein, and beneficial phytochemicals, making them more nutritious than many other cereals (Saleem et al 2023; Jacob et al 2024).

Millets play a vital role in promoting food and nutritional security and are widely used in nutrient-rich, multigrain, and gluten-free foods. The high content of polyphenols and bioactive compounds in these grains helps lower the glycemic index, benefiting those with diabetes and heart conditions.

Millets consist of three main parts:

1. *Endosperm*: It is the major proportion of millet with starch as the principal content, and very little proteins and B vitamins
2. *Germ*: It is a nutrient-dense core rich in B and E vitamins, minerals, fats, and phytochemicals; and
3. *Bran*: It is the outermost coating of the seed meant for its safety. It primarily contains the highest fiber along with B-vitamins, minerals, and phytonutrients (Food Safety and Standards Authority of India (FSSAI) 2023) (Figure 2.4).

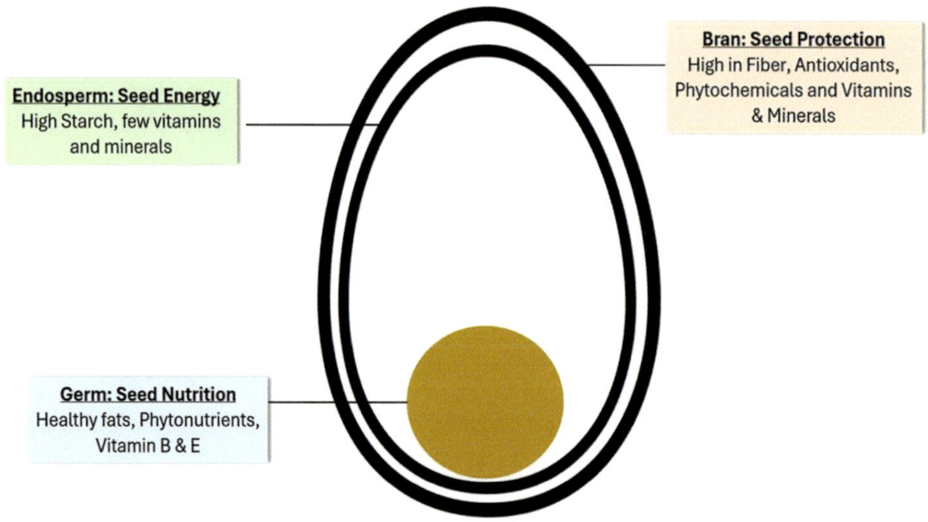

FIGURE 2.4 Composition of millet seed.

While widely consumed in developing countries, millets have been underutilized in developed nations, where they are mostly used as animal feed. Nutritionally, millets rival major cereals, offering 7–12% protein, 2–5% fat, 65–75% carbohydrates, and 15–20% fiber. Pearl millet is protein- and lipid-rich, while finger millet stands out for its high calcium content. Millets also offer a better essential amino acid profile than maize and pair well with legumes to create complete, high-quality protein sources (Dayakar Rao et al 2017).

2.2.1 Macronutrients in Millets

Carbohydrates: They form the largest component of millet grains, comprising about 65% of the total weight, though this varies among different millet varieties. A significant portion of these carbohydrates is in the form of non-starchy polysaccharides and dietary fiber, contributing to millets' health benefits. The carbohydrates in millets are categorized into structural—which are principally part of structural components like cellulose and pectin; and non-structural—which are more focused around nutritional aspects such as starch and sugars, and serve as the main source of energy reserve. It is made up of amylose and the more abundant amylopectin, arranged in structured granules (Jacob et al 2024).

Pigments in the grain's pericarp can sometimes influence starch color, yielding pink, yellow, or green hues.

Soluble sugars in millets—mainly sucrose, glucose, and fructose—fluctuate during grain development, with mature grains containing about 1.3% on average. High-lysine and sugary cultivars of millets tend to have higher levels of these sugars. The digestibility of millet starch is relatively low (15–25%) compared to rice or wheat, partly due to the influence of millet proteins, which may inhibit starch gelatinization or form complexes that limit digestibility.

Starch in millets can be categorized into rapidly digestible starch (RDS), slowly digestible starch (SDS), and resistant starch (RS). SDS is particularly beneficial for stabilizing blood sugar and insulin levels, making millets a good dietary option for managing diabetes and cardiovascular conditions. Additionally, the fiber and complex carbohydrates in millets support digestive health, reduce cholesterol levels, and help prevent conditions like constipation, ulcers, and metabolic disorders (Dayakar Rao et al 2017).

Protein: Its content in millets can vary significantly depending on environmental and agronomic factors such as water availability, soil fertility, temperature, and conditions during grain development, as well as the crop's genetic makeup. Most of the protein in millets is found in the endosperm (around 80%), followed by the germ (16%) and the pericarp (3%). The major protein fractions in millets include prolamins (particularly kafirins) and glutelins, while albumins and globulins are mainly concentrated in the germ (Sahu and Tripathi 2023).

Although millets are not particularly rich in lysine—a limiting essential amino acid—they can be nutritionally balanced when paired with lysine-rich foods like legumes or animal proteins. Millet protein fractions differ in amino acid content. While the endosperm is typically lower in lysine, cystine, methionine, and threonine, the bran and germ are richer in lysine, arginine, and glycine (Dayakar Rao et al 2017) and lower in amino acids like phenylalanine, leucine, and isoleucine.

The albumin and globulin fractions, which range from about 11.6 to 29.6% in different millet types, contain higher levels of essential amino acids. Despite variations in amino acid distribution across different parts of the grain, the overall protein quality of millets is enhanced when they are consumed as part of a diverse diet.

Fats: Millets contain a moderate amount of fats, generally ranging from 2 to 8% of the grain's weight, with pearl millet having the highest content. These fats are primarily composed of unsaturated fatty acids like linoleic and oleic acids, which are beneficial for health (Jacob et al 2024).

The scutellar region of the germ is where the lipids are mostly concentrated, which implies that this fat content is significantly reduced during the milling process, especially where the germ portion is removed, as in the case of decortication.

TABLE 2.2
Micronutrient Content in Millets (Per 100 g)

Micronutrients	Pearl Millet	Finger Millet	Sorghum	Little Millet	Kodo Millet
Iron (mg)	6.42	4.62	3.95	1.26	2.34
Calcium (mg)	27.35	364	27.6	16.06	15.27
Magnesium (mg)	124	146	133	91.4	122
Zinc (mg)	2.76	2.53	1.96	1.82	1.65
Thiamin (mg)	0.25	0.37	0.35	0.26	0.29
Riboflavin (mg)	0.20	0.17	0.14	0.05	0.20
Niacin (mg)	0.86	1.34	2.1	1.29	1.49

Source: Longvah et al (2017).

Millet lipids are categorized into nonpolar, polar, and non-saponifiable types. Nonpolar lipids, which dominate at 70–80%, mainly consist of triglycerides (85%), followed by sterols and diglycerides. These act as energy stores, especially during germination. Polar lipids, including phospholipids (17–25%) and glycolipids (2.5–6.2%), play essential biochemical roles. The non-saponifiable fraction (3–5%) includes health-promoting compounds such as carotenoids, tocopherols, and phytosterols. The fatty acid profile of millets is mostly unsaturated (78–82%), with saturated fats making up about 17.9–21.6%, contributing to both nutritional quality and functional health benefits (Dayakar Rao et al 2017; Sahu and Tripathi 2023).

2.2.2 Micronutrients in Millets

Millets are packed with essential micronutrients (Table 2.2), including key B vitamins like niacin, riboflavin, and thiamin that support metabolism and overall well-being. They are also rich in important minerals such as iron, calcium, and magnesium, which are crucial for maintaining healthy bones, producing red blood cells, and supporting muscle function (Chandrakar and Shahi 2023).

Millets have a significantly higher mineral content compared to common staple cereals. Their mineral concentration ranges from 1.7 to 4.3 g/100 g, which is notably greater than that of wheat (1.5%) and rice (0.6%) (Kumar et al 2018).

2.3 NON-NUTRIENT COMPONENTS IN MILLETS

2.3.1 Dietary Fiber and Its Health Benefits

Millets are a valuable source of dietary fiber, contributing around 15–20%—nearly twice the amount found in rice and comparable to that of whole wheat. This fiber is present in both soluble forms (such as β-glucans, arabinoxylans, and pectins) and insoluble forms (including cellulose and hemicellulose), primarily concentrated in the seed coat and bran (Jacob et al 2024).

Dietary fibre components exert their beneficial effects mostly by way of their swelling properties, and by increasing transit time in the small intestine (Table 2.3).

Dayakar Rao et al (2017) have explained how fiber in millets plays a crucial role in maintaining digestive health, regulating blood sugar levels, lowering cholesterol, and supporting healthy body weight. Soluble fibers undergo complete fermentation in the colon, producing short-chain fatty acids like butyrate that help regenerate gut lining and reduce the risk of colon cancer. Insoluble fibers improve bowel regularity and undergo partial fermentation.

Additionally, fiber helps slow down glucose absorption, making it beneficial for managing diabetes, and binds to bile salts to support cholesterol reduction. However, it may interfere with the

TABLE 2.3
Properties of Dietary Fibre and Its Health Consequences

Properties	Health Consequences
Water solubility and bulk formation	Supports regularity, better digestive health, prevents constipation
Improved transit time of food in gut	Reduce risk of IBD (Inflammatory Bowel Disease)
Slowed carbohydrate digestion and release into bloodstream	Stable blood sugar levels, better diabetes management, improved metabolic health feeling of satiety, helps control appetite and calorie intake
Acts as prebiotic; used by gut bacteria	Release SCFA; support gut health, regulates inflammation and improves immunity

absorption of minerals such as calcium, iron, and zinc. Among various millet types, barnyard millet stands out for its particularly high crude fiber content (Mishra et al 2022).

2.3.2 Phytochemicals in Millets

Millets are a significant supplier of numerous phytochemicals, including flavonoids, tannins like proanthocyanidins, phenolic compounds, phytosterols, and lignin. These phytochemicals have a potential positive impact on human health. All millet grain and especially sorghum fractions possess high antioxidant activity in vitro relative to other cereals and fruits. The principal phytochemicals in millets are Phenolic compounds with a variation based on bioavailability, size, and even levels of phenolic acids, flavonoids, and condensed tannins. These phytochemicals exhibit various health benefits due to their antioxidant and anti-inflammatory properties, which help them to combat oxidative stress and reduce the risk of chronic diseases (Chandrakar and Shahi 2023).

2.3.2.1 Phenolic Compounds

Phenolic compounds encompass the phenol functional group as a central component. These are secondary metabolites of plants responsible for color, nutritional, and antioxidant properties. These phenolic compounds can be as simple molecules or clustered, complex molecules, exhibiting health benefits (Figure 2.5). For instance, these are efficient antioxidant and anti-inflammatory agents that

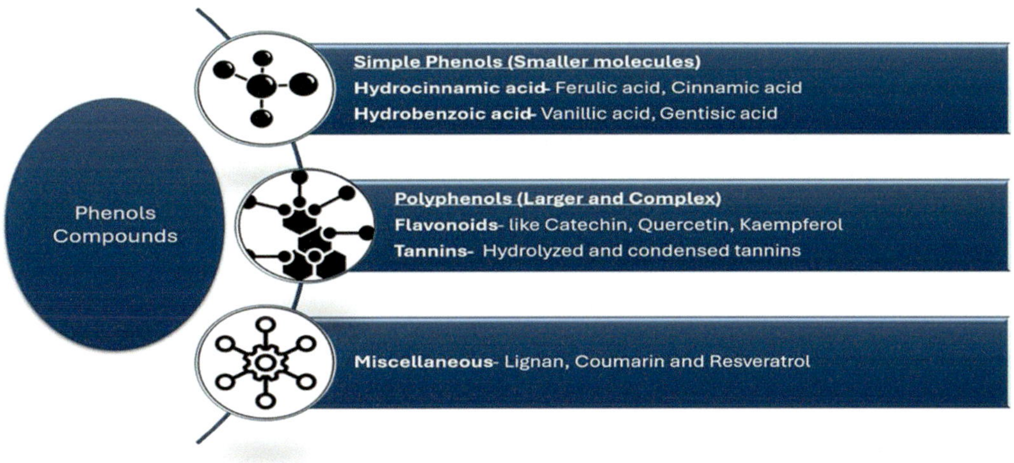

FIGURE 2.5 Different phenolic compounds in millets.

help with the prevention of oxidative stress-associated damage. These powerful compounds can interact with digestive enzymes, alpha-amylase, and glucosidase and thus help in better glucose management, supporting insulin signaling pathways and insulin response.

2.3.2.2 Flavonoids

These are natural elements found in a diverse form in plants and their parts and considered as more potent antioxidants than vitamin C and E. Apigenin, catechin, quercetin, and kaempferol are the commonly found flavonoids in millets. Along with polyphenols and flavonoids, the presence of carotenoids and vitamin E enhances the antioxidant capacity of millets (Mishra et al 2022).

2.3.2.3 Condensed Tannins

Tannins constitute important secondary metabolites in plants and are classified under polyphenols with high molecular weight, such as proanthocyanidins (Smeriglio et al 2017). Besides their antimicrobial potential, these molecules are also established antioxidants as they prevent the oxidative stress-associated damage, scavenge free radicals, and even ameliorate the inflammation. These are also well-known anti diabetic agents because of their potential to inhibit the activity of enzymes like α-amylase and α-glucosidase and thus, regulate glucose metabolism (Zhu 2018).

2.3.2.4 Phytosterols

These are plant-derived sterols that naturally occur and are chemically similar to mammalian sterols such as cholesterol. These are present in all the plant tissues as part of the membrane, maintaining the phospholipid layer, and in cellular organelles, acting as signaling molecules. Besides their nutritional value, these compounds also provide health benefits as functional foods. For instance, these sterols are known to lower serum cholesterol levels. These are also anti-inflammatory in nature, known to support gut health by reducing inflammation, enhancing cell regeneration, and improving gut motility. Thereby, it helps support conditions like gastric ulcers and IBD (Inflammatory Bowel Disease) (Miszczuk et al 2024).

2.3.2.5 Lignan

These are constituents of dietary fiber which are water-insoluble and cannot be digested by endogenous enzymes in the digestive tract, but still play a crucial role in human health. These compounds trap the toxic substances and act as detoxifying agents. Lignin also plays a crucial role in cardiovascular health by reducing the coronary blockage, lowering the LDL (Low-Density Lipoprotein) cholesterol levels, acting as a vasodilator, and lowering the elevated blood pressure. Therefore, with these mechanisms, lignan helps maintain overall metabolic health (Kuchipudi 2023).

2.3.3 Bioactive Peptides

Protein is one of the key macronutrients essential for the human body, playing a crucial role in growth, development, regulation of bodily functions, and maintenance of overall health. Millets are a valuable source of plant-based proteins. The typical protein profile in millet seeds includes various fractions such as albumin, globulin, cross-linked prolamin, β-prolamin, and glutelin. The composition and concentration of these proteins can vary significantly based on the millet variety.

In recent years, scientific interest has grown around a specific class of protein derivatives known as bioactive peptides (BAPs). These are short chains of amino acids, typically fewer than 20 residues and smaller than 10 kDa, and are released from their parent proteins during digestion or enzymatic hydrolysis.

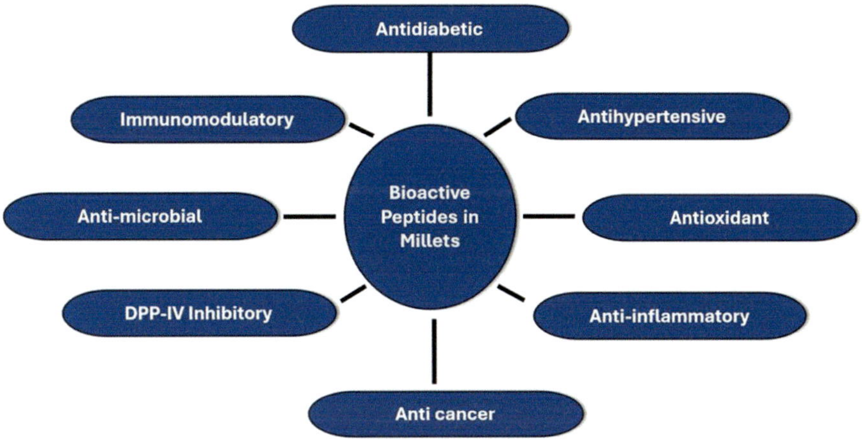

FIGURE 2.6 Health benefits of millet-based bioactive peptides.

BAPs derived from millet proteins have gained attention for their positive physiological effects. They may support bodily functions and help manage or prevent certain health conditions, making millets a promising functional food in nutrition and health science (Xu et al 2019; Majid and Priyadarshini 2020; Aderinola and Duodu 2022).

These BAPs act as an anti-microbial agent as they inhibit the viral replication as well as prevent the growth of various fungi and bacteria. Rich in peptidic amino acids, these BAPs are capable of transferring electrons to free radicals. Hence, they act as strong antioxidants and anti-inflammatory agents, preventing the spread of oxidative stress and related inflammation and inflammatory markers (Figure 2.6).

In the context of elevated blood pressure, the BAPs exhibit efficient anti-hypertensive activity by inhibiting the Angiotensin Converting Enzyme (ACE). ACE is the crucial enzyme that converts angiotensin I (ANG I) to produce angiotensin II (ANG II), which in turn, is a powerful active compound that raises blood pressure by narrowing blood vessels. BAPs also have antidiabetic properties, attributed to mechanisms like inhibiting the activity of DPP-IV (dipeptidyl peptidase 4), which consequently stimulates secretion of GLP-1. This GLP-1 molecule helps in insulin release, improves insulin sensitivity, and ultimately, better glucose utilization. Owing to its antioxidant property, these BAPs can contain the damage associated with oxidative stress, and cancer can be one of the aspects. It is seen that these peptides can inhibit the growth and proliferation of uncontrolled multiplying cells, which is a hallmark of cancer development and progression.

2.3.4 Anti-Nutrients in Millets

Antinutrients are naturally occurring phytochemical compounds that plants synthesize as part of their defense strategy against herbivores, insects, and pathogens. These secondary metabolites help the plant survive in harsh environments, but when consumed by humans—especially in raw or unprocessed forms—they can interfere with the absorption and bioavailability of essential nutrients. This reduced nutrient uptake can contribute to conditions such as bloating, nutritional deficiencies, and even micronutrient malnutrition.

Plant-based foods often contain a range of antinutritional factors, including phytates, oxalates, tannins, saponins, and various enzyme inhibitors like protease and amylase inhibitors. While these compounds can provide some health benefits or protective roles for plants, they may also pose challenges for human digestion and nutrient utilization (Paschapur et al 2021; Gowda et al 2022).

2.3.4.1 Phytates (Phytic Acid)

Phytic acid, also known as inositol hexaphosphate (IP6), is a major antinutrient found in millets, legumes, cereals, oilseeds, and nuts, where it serves as the primary storage form of phosphorus (1–5% by weight). It is a highly negatively charged molecule that chelates essential bivalent minerals such as zinc (Zn^{2+}), iron ($Fe^{2+/3+}$), and calcium, making them less bioavailable for human absorption. Since humans lack the enzyme phytase, we cannot hydrolyze phytate efficiently, which limits our ability to extract these minerals.

Several food processing techniques, such as soaking, germination, malting, and autoclaving, can significantly reduce phytate levels. For instance, raw finger millet has around 676.7 mg phytic acid, which reduces to 587 mg/100 g after 12 hours of soaking and further reduces to 238.4 mg/100 g after 36 hours of germination (Bheemaiah et al 2024).

2.3.4.2 Enzyme Inhibitors

Enzyme inhibitors are another class of antinutrients that interfere with digestive processes:

- *Protease inhibitors*: These are typically found in seeds and tubers and account for up to 10% of their total protein content. Protease inhibitors block enzymes like trypsin and chymotrypsin, impeding protein digestion. Trypsin inhibitors specifically bind to peptides after lysine or arginine, reducing the effectiveness of protein metabolism.
- *Amylase inhibitors*: Millets are known to contain alpha-amylase inhibitors, which disrupt carbohydrate digestion by inhibiting starch breakdown. Processing methods such as coarse grinding, soaking, germination, and autoclaving are effective in reducing amylase inhibitor activity (Paschapur et al 2021).

2.3.4.3 Tannins

Tannins are polyphenolic compounds found in plant leaves, fruits, and bark. Their ability to form complexes with proteins reduces protein digestibility and the availability of essential amino acids. Tannins may form reversible or irreversible bonds with proteins, thereby impairing their nutritional value. While they do have antioxidant properties, their role in reducing nutrient absorption makes them a concern in unprocessed diets (Samtiya et al 2020).

2.3.4.4 Oxalates

Oxalates are the antinutrients present in millets, but relatively in smaller amounts. These compounds, such as oxalic acid, bind with minerals like calcium, magnesium, sodium, and phosphorus and form oxalate salts. Subsequently, this results in their hindered absorption and bioavailability (Akbar 2022).

2.3.4.5 Saponins

Saponins are surface-active glycosides found in over 100 plant families, particularly in legumes, oilseeds, and some cereals. These compounds are known to cause hemolysis by interacting with cholesterol in red blood cell membranes. Saponins also inhibit digestive enzymes, including amylase, lipase, and proteases, potentially contributing to indigestion and nutrient malabsorption. They may form complexes with fat-soluble vitamins and sterols, further interfering with their absorption (Samtiya et al 2020).

2.3.4.5.1 Mitigation Strategies

To reduce the antinutrient content in plant-based foods, several processing techniques are recommended:

- Soaking
- Germination
- Malting

- Autoclaving
- Decortication (removal of seed coat)

These methods enhance nutrient availability and improve digestibility without compromising the overall health benefits of these foods.

2.4 PROCESSING AND ITS EFFECT ON MILLET COMPOSITION

Millets are typically processed before consumption to remove undesirable components, enhance shelf life, and improve their nutritional and sensory properties. These grains are rich in phenolic compounds, particularly tannins and phenolics, with smaller amounts of flavonoids. While these compounds have antioxidant properties, they also act as antinutrients by binding with essential minerals like iron and zinc, thus reducing their bioavailability. Another key antinutrient in millets is phytic acid, which binds to proteins and minerals, further hindering nutrient absorption.

Shelf life is another critical factor in millet processing. Whole millets can be stored for four to five years using traditional techniques like mud rhombuses, underground pits, and aerial bundles, as these prevent insect infestation and moisture buildup. However, once millets are milled into flour, their structural integrity is lost, making them more vulnerable to spoilage. The breakdown of lipids by lipase enzymes and microbial contamination are primary reasons for the shorter shelf life of millet flour. For instance, pearl millet flour, due to its higher fat content, begins to deteriorate within 10–15 days under normal storage conditions.

To address these challenges, various processing methods are employed (Bisht 2022). Traditional methods like decortication, roasting, boiling, puffing, and milling can help reduce the antinutrient levels. Processes like Soaking/germination or fermentation not only reduce the anti-nutrient levels but also enhance the flavor, nutritional value, and shelf life. This process improves millet's digestibility by partially predigesting proteins and carbohydrates while increasing the bioavailability of vitamins and minerals.

To extend shelf life, processing strategies such as heat treatments, mechanical processing, and the use of preservatives are applied to inhibit enzyme activity and microbial growth. Thermal processes like microwave processing and non-thermal processes like cold plasma, ultrasound processing, or pulse light processing techniques not only enhance storage stability by inactivating *microbes* and preventing microbial contamination but also improve the bioavailability of nutrients.

However, it's important to note that processing can also lead to nutrient loss. Techniques such as dehulling, milling, and high-temperature treatments like roasting and puffing can strip away the bran and germ, reducing fiber, micronutrients, and fats. Oxidation and lipolysis during thermal processing may also lead to rancidity. On the contrary, methods like germination, soaking, and malting sustain nutritional integrity while improving the digestibility of proteins, carbohydrates, and better bioavailability of minerals (Ravi and Rana 2024).

2.4.1 Impact on Nutritional Profile and Reduction of Anti-Nutrients

Impact on nutrients:

- *Protein*: Millets are rich in protein, offering a plant-based alternative with less saturated fat and more dietary fiber. Processing methods like soaking, germination, and malting enhance protein digestibility and increase protein content. Germination and fermentation degrade antinutritional factors, improving protein availability.
- *Carbohydrates*: Millets consist of 60–75% carbohydrates. Germination and fermentation increase soluble sugars by breaking down complex starches, improving carbohydrate digestibility, and making millets more energy-dense.

- *Dietary fiber*: The bran fraction of millets is a major source of dietary fiber, but dehulling reduces fiber content. Germination increases fiber due to changes in cell wall structure and biosynthesis. Fiber lowers the risk of type 2 diabetes with better blood glucose regulation and also ensures better gut health, lowering the risk of conditions like constipation.
- *Minerals*: Millets are rich in minerals like potassium, magnesium, iron, calcium, and zinc. Processing methods like soaking, germination, and decortication improve mineral bioavailability by reducing antinutrients like phytates that inhibit mineral absorption. Germination activates phytase enzymes, enhancing mineral release.
- *Vitamins*: Milling reduces vitamin content by removing the bran and germ. The process of germination has been shown to elevate the levels of vitamins, such as vitamin C, in finger millet. However, refined millets (polished/debranned) lose significant vitamin content, particularly in the bran layer.
- *Fats*: Fat content decreases during germination, malting, and high-pressure soaking due to lipid hydrolysis. High-temperature processing like cooking and popping also reduces fat content. This makes millets a potential source of low-fat food products (Dayakar Rao et al 2017; Gowda et al 2022).

Effect on anti-nutrients:

- *Reduction of anti-nutrients*: Processing methods like soaking, germination, malting, roasting, and popping reduce antinutrients (e.g., phytates, tannins, trypsin inhibitors) in millets, improving nutrient bioavailability.
- *Germination and fermentation*: These processes specifically degrade antinutrients, enhancing the availability of proteins and minerals such as iron and manganese. For instance, malting boosts the iron bio-availability by 300% and manganese by 17% (Paschapur et al 2021).

2.5 HEALTH IMPLICATIONS OF MILLETS' COMPOSITION

Urbanization has greatly influenced consumption patterns in India, leading to a decline in the consumption of cereals like millets and an increase in the intake of animal-based products, oils, refined sugars, fats, and alcohol. This shift in diet plays a significant role in promoting oxidative stress, which occurs when there is an imbalance between the production and accumulation of reactive oxygen species (ROS) in the body. These ROS, in turn, can contribute to cellular aging, DNA damage, disturbed metabolic health, and associated disorders and even carcinogenesis.

To combat oxidative stress, the body utilizes antioxidants—either produced naturally or supplied through food—which act as free radical scavengers, preventing and repairing damage caused by ROS. This, in turn, strengthens the immune system and reduces the risk of degenerative diseases. Millets, being a rich source of antioxidants, help reduce ROS levels and play a key role in preventing and treating radical-mediated diseases, thus reducing the risk of various degenerative conditions.

Millets offer more than just basic nutrition. They are rich in phytochemicals, including antioxidants, that can help prevent diseases such as cancer and cardiovascular conditions. Research shows that regular millet consumption can lower the risk of heart disease, diabetes, and metabolic syndrome, improve digestion, detoxify the body, enhance immunity, and protect against degenerative diseases like Parkinson's disease. Additionally, millets can help control blood pressure, reduce heart disease risks, prevent cancer, and promote digestive health by slowing gastric emptying. These benefits make millets an essential part of a health-conscious diet, aiding in the prevention and management of diseases such as cardiovascular disease, diabetes, obesity, and celiac disease (Mishra et al 2022) (Table 2.4).

TABLE 2.4
Components in Millets and Their Health Benefits

Components in Millets	Health Benefits
Dietary fiber (Soluble and Insoluble)	• Improves gut health and promotes the growth of good bacteria • Slows down carbohydrate digestion; better blood sugar regulation • Provides satiety and helps in weight management
Dietary fiber and resistant starch	• Contributes to the low glycemic index of millets • Provides sustained energy release • Beneficial against diabetes mellitus • Helpful in cardiovascular health • Support healthy gut and microbiome, better immunity
Protein	• Provides satiety and better energy expenditure • Supports immune function • Healthy addition to a vegetarian and vegan diet
Micronutrients (Vitamins and Minerals)	• Help bridge the micronutrient gap • Supports metabolic reactions, nervous health • Improved immunity
Phytonutrients	• Act as antioxidants; combat oxidative stress and inflammation • May help reduce the risk of chronic diseases • Help with overall health and wellbeing
Low fat with beneficial unsaturated fats	• May help with lipid-lowering properties • May contribute to overall cardiovascular health

Source: Tripathi et al (2023) and Jacob et al (2024).

2.6 FUTURE PERSPECTIVES AND RESEARCH DIRECTIONS

2.6.1 Advancements in Millet Breeding and Biofortification

Nutritional insecurity remains a significant global challenge, particularly in regions where populations rely heavily on cereal-based diets that are often deficient in essential micronutrients. Millets, next to cereals, are a primary source of energy in semi-arid and drought-prone regions of Asia and Africa. These grains are nutritionally superior, offering high levels of protein, essential amino acids, minerals, and vitamins. Biofortification of staple crops has been confirmed to be a cost-effective strategy to address micronutrient malnutrition.

Ensuring nutritional security is crucial for improving global health, as plant-based diets serve as the primary source of essential nutrients for normal growth and development. Yet, nearly half of the global population, particularly in Asia and Africa, suffers from nutritional deficiencies due to their reliance on cereal crops.

Biofortification provides a sustainable, food-based solution to combat nutrient deficiencies by delivering nutrient-rich crops directly to underprivileged populations.

Biofortified crops have largely been developed through conventional breeding techniques that leverage natural genetic variation, with Golden Rice being a notable exception. Millets reflect noteworthy genetic variation in crucial minerals like iron, zinc, and calcium compared to other cereals. Their drought resistance and resilience to pests and diseases make them ideal for regions vulnerable to crop failure. Despite these advantages, only pearl millet has been prioritized for iron biofortification in India, leaving untapped potential in other millets for biofortification. Two primary strategies for biofortification in millets include: (1) enhancing nutrient accumulation in milled grains and (2) reducing antinutrients to increase mineral bioavailability (Vinoth and Ravindhran 2017).

2.6.2 Expanding Millet Consumption in Modern Diets

2.6.2.1 Incorporating Millets in Gluten-Free and Plant-Based Diets

Over the past few years, the demand for millets has increased as gluten-free and plant-based alternative, driven by increased awareness around health, gluten sensitivity, and sustainability benefits of plant-derived food options.

Millets fit exceptionally well based on these criteria as-

- *Gluten-free by nature*: Wheat is a staple for the vast majority of the population, but owing to its gliadin and glutenin protein content, many people with gluten sensitivity are restricted from consuming this conventional crop. Millet, owing to its gluten-free nature, not only protects against such sensitivity but also provides equal or superior nutrient supply (Asrani et al 2022). A study published in the *Journal of Drug Research in Ayurvedic Sciences* highlighted that gluten-free nature of millets helps maintain gut health intact by reducing gluten-induced inflammation and also prevents triggering of adverse immune responses (Singh et al 2023)
- *Nutrient-dense alternative*: Millets have equal or superior nutritional quality based on different nutritive aspects. These grains are abundant in dietary fiber, antioxidants as phytonutrients, and RS, which helps in better metabolic health, providing better satiety and improved glycemic control. These also offer a wide array of vitamins and minerals like calcium, iron, and zinc, which makes them a potential agent of bridging the nutrition gap and helps support preventing the scenario of malnutrition. These also have comparable and superior, in some cases, better amino acid profiles, supplying essential amino acids—making them a healthier alternative for vegans and vegetarians.
- *Culinary versatility*: Millets are a versatile grain that can go well with a variety of dishes, including soups, porridges, stir-fried, flatbreads, baked goods, fermented and steamed options, and snacks. This can enable value addition to your regular meals, providing variety and enhancing the nutritional value, overcoming the monotony of regular meal options and narrow nutrient availability.

2.6.2.2 Potential for Millets as Functional Foods

Millets are often recognized as "Shree Anna" owing to their rich nutritional profile and potential health benefits. Because of its unique composition with nutrients and phytonutrients, millets can serve as functional foods

- *Rich in phytonutrients*: Millets contain bioactives like phenols, anthocyanidins, flavonoids, which act as strong antioxidants and anti-inflammatories. This helps reduce oxidative stress and supports metabolic health.
- *Dietary fiber and resistant starch*: This acts as a prebiotic, promotes the growth of healthy gut microbiome, and enhances gut health, immunity, and inflammation. These also provide a feeling of satiety with better blood sugar management because of their low glycemic index property.
- *Vitamins and minerals*: Millets are a good source of vitamins and minerals supporting various metabolic pathways and system health.

Given these attributes, millets can be positioned as functional foods that not just nourish but also prevent or manage metabolic disorders while promoting overall health.

2.7 CONCLUSION

Millets are nutrient-rich, sustainable, and climate-resistant grains with a rich historical and cultural legacy. These offer long-lasting alternatives to staple cereals, promoting food security and environmental sustainability with stable yield. They supply high-quality protein, dietary fiber, essential minerals and vitamins, phytonutrients, and BAPs and thus support metabolic health and systemic functioning. Processing techniques like germination and fermentation can contribute to improving the nutrient bioavailability while reducing antinutrients. Regular inclusion in the diet can help prevent the risk of lifestyle-related diseases and support long-term well-being.

REFERENCES

Aderinola, T.A., and K.G. Duodu. 2022. Production, health-promoting properties and characterization of bioactive peptides from cereal and legume grains. *BioFactors 48*(5): 972–992. https://doi.org/10.1002/biof.1889

Akbar, N. 2022. Nutrients anti-nutrients interaction in millets and its effect on malnutrition. *Acta Scientific Nutritional Health 6*(12).

Arya, C., and A. Bisht. 2022. Small millets: Path to food and nutrition security. In *Small Millet Grains: The Superfoods in Human Diet*. Springer Nature Singapore, Singapore, pp. 161–182.

Asrani, P., A. Ali, and K. Tiwari. 2022. Millets as an alternative diet for gluten-sensitive individuals: A critical review on nutritional components, sensitivities and popularity of wheat and millets among consumers. *Food Reviews International 39*(6): 3370–3399. http://dx.doi.org/10.1080/87559129.2021.2012790

Bheemaiah, B.S., N.A.N. Gowda, J. Subbiah, S. Chakraborty, P.V.V. Prasad, and K. Siliveru. 2024. Physiochemical, bio, thermal, and non-thermal processing of major and minor millets: A comprehensive review on antinutritional and antioxidant properties. *Foods 13*(22): 3684. https://doi.org/10.3390/foods13223684

Bisht, A. 2022. Processing of small millets. In *Small Millet Grains: The Superfoods in Human Diet*. Springer Nature Singapore, Singapore, pp. 49–73.

Chandrakar, L., and S. Shahi. 2023. Millets and their nutritional value: A review. *Journal of Advanced Zoology* 44: 1690–1697. https://doi.org/10.17762/jaz.v44iS3.2387

Dayakar Rao, B., K. Bhaskarachary, G.D. Arlene Christina, G. Sudha Devi, and V.A. Tonapi. 2017. *Nutritional and Health Benefits of Millets*. ICAR–Indian Institute of Millets Research (IIMR), Hyderabad, pp. 1–112

Elasi, S., T. Ramamoorthy, and V. Kowsalya. 2023. Cultural heritage of millets. *Farm Chronicle – An Agriculture Newsletter 2*(Special Issue): 77–81.

FAOSTAT. 2018. *Production-Yield Quantities of Millets in World + (Total) 1962–2018*. http://www.fao.org/faostat/en/data/QC/visualize

FSSAI (Food Safety and Standards Authority of India). 2023. *Millets – Nutritious Cereal of India*. Eat Right India. https://eatrightindia.gov.in/millets2023/assets/documents/Millets%20-%20Nutritious%20Cereal%20of%20India.pdf

Gahalawat, P., N. Lamba, and P. Chaudhary. 2024. Nutritional and health benefits of millets: A review article. *Journal of Indian System of Medicine 12*: 4–11.

Gowda, N.A.N., K. Siliveru, P.V.V. Prasad, Y. Bhatt, B.P. Netravati, and C. Gurikar. 2022. Modern processing of Indian millets: A perspective on changes in nutritional properties. *Foods 11*(4): 499. https://doi.org/10.3390/foods11040499

Jacob, J., V. Krishnan, C. Antony, M. Bhavyasri, C. Aruna, K. Mishra, T. Nepolean, C.T. Satyavathi, and K.B.R.S. Visarada. 2024. The nutrition and therapeutic potential of millets: An updated narrative review. *Frontiers in Nutrition 11*: 1346869. https://doi.org/10.3389/fnut.2024.1346869

Kane-Potaka, J., S. Anitha, T.W. Tsusaka, R. Botha, M. Budumuru, S. Upadhyay, P. Kumar, K. Mallesh, R. Hunasgi, A.K. Jalagam, and S. Nedumaran. 2021. Assessing millets and sorghum consumption behavior in urban India: A large-scale survey. *Frontiers in Sustainable Food Systems 5*: 680777. https://doi.org/10.3389/fsufs.2021.680777

Kheya, S.A., S.K. Talukder, P. Datta, S. Yeasmin, M.H. Rashid, A. Hasan, M. Anwar, A.K.M.A. Islam, and A.K.M.M. Islam. 2023. Millets: The future crops for the tropics—Status, challenges and future prospects. *Heliyon 9*: e22123. https://doi.org/10.1016/j.heliyon.2023.e22123

Kuchipudi, J.D. 2023. Nutritional aspects & health benefits of millets. *Just Agriculture 3*(5): 306–311.

Kumar, A., V. Tomer, A. Kaur, V. Kumar, and K. Gupta. 2018. Millets: A solution to agrarian and nutritional challenges. *Agriculture & Food Security 7*(31). https://doi.org/10.1186/s40066-018-0183-3

Longvah, T., R. Ananthan, K. Bhaskarachary, and K. Venkaiah. 2017. *Indian Food Composition Tables*. National Institute of Nutrition, Indian Council of Medical Research, Hyderabad.

Majid, A., and C.G.P. Priyadarshini. 2020. Millet derived bioactive peptides: A review on their functional properties and health benefits. *Critical Reviews in Food Science and Nutrition 60*(19): 3342–3351. https://doi.org/10.1080/10408398.2019.1686342

Mishra, A., B. Pattnaik, T. Dutta, and I. Baitharu. 2022. Nutritional values and potential health benefits of millets: A review. *Journal of Nutrients 8*(1): 9–26. https://doi.org/10.18488/87.v8i1.3176

Miszczuk, E., A. Bajguz, L. Kiraga, K. Crowley, and M. Chłopecka. 2024. Phytosterols and the digestive system: A review study from insights into their potential health benefits and safety. *Pharmaceuticals 17*(5): 557. https://doi.org/10.3390/ph17050557

Nautiyal, J.P., A.M. Lone, T. Ghosh, M. Sharma, V.R. Tiwari, C. Ramesh, and K. Ramesh. 2023. *The Millets of India*. EIACP Centre (MoEFCC), Wildlife Institute of India, Dehradun, Uttarakhand.

Paschapur, A., D. Joshi, K. Mishra, L. Kant, V. Kumar, and A. Kumar. 2021. Millets for life: A brief introduction. *Millets for Life* 1–20. https://doi.org/10.1007/978-981-16-0676-2_1

Ravi, J.L., and S.S. Rana. 2024. Maximizing the nutritional benefits and prolonging the shelf life of millets through effective processing techniques: A review. *ACS Omega 9*(37): 38327–38347. https://doi.org/10.1021/acsomega.4c03466

Sahu, K., and R. Tripathi. 2023. Millets: Nutritional composition—A review. *International Journal of Creative Research Thoughts (IJCRT) 11*(11).

Saleem, S., N.U. Mushtaq, W.H. Shah, A. Rasool, K.R. Hakeem, C.S. Seth, I. Tahir, and R.U. Rehman. 2023. Millets as smart future food with essential phytonutrients for promoting health. *Journal of Food Composition and Analysis 124*: 105669. https://doi.org/10.1016/j.jfca.2023.105669

Samtiya, M., R.E. Aluko, and T. Dhewa. 2020. Plant food anti-nutritional factors and their reduction strategies: An overview. *Food Production, Processing and Nutrition* 2(6). https://doi.org/10.1186/s43014-020-0020-5

Satyavathi, C.T., S. Ambawat, V. Khandelwal, and R.K. Srivastava. 2021. Pearl Millet: A climate-resilient nutricereal for mitigating hidden hunger and provide nutritional security. *Frontiers in Plant Science 12*. https://doi.org/10.3389/fpls.2021.659938

Shah, P., N. Mehta, and S. Shah. 2024. Exploring the factors that drive millet consumption: Insights from regular and occasional consumers. *Journal of Retailing and Consumer Services 76*: 103598. https://doi.org/10.1016/j.jretconser.2023.103598

Singh, S.B., A.K. Meena, B.S. Sisodia, S. Sharma, M.M. Sharma, and P. Mansoria. 2023. From farm to gut: Unraveling the role of millets in promoting metabolic well-being via gut microbiota. *Journal of Drug Research in Ayurvedic Sciences 8*(Suppl 1): S50–S54.

Smeriglio, A., D. Barreca, E. Bellocco, and D. Trombetta. 2017. Proanthocyanidins and hydrolysable tannins: Occurrence, dietary intake and pharmacological effects. *British Journal of Pharmacology 174*(11): 1244–1262. https://doi.org/10.1111/bph.13630

Tripathi, G., H.J. Patel, A. Borah, D. Nath, H. Das, S. Bansal, N. Singh, and B.V. Singh. 2023. A review on nutritional and health benefits of millets. *International Journal of Plant & Soil Science 35*(19): 1736–1743.

Tripathi, T., and S. Vyas. 2023. From ancient grains to modern solutions: A history of millets and their significance in agriculture and food security. *International Journal of Home Science* 9(2): 72–78.

Veerabadhran, V., H.R. Palakuru, G.P. Pratap, B. Rajeshwari, G.P. Prasad, N. Srikanth, and R. Acharya. 2023. A critical review of the history and practices of millets in India. *Journal of Drug Research in Ayurvedic Sciences 8*(Suppl 1): S18–S25. https://doi.org/10.4103/jdras.jdras_113_23

Vinoth, A., and R. Ravindhran. 2017. Biofortification in millets: A sustainable approach for nutritional security. *Frontiers in Plant Science 8*: 29. https://doi.org/10.3389/fpls.2017.00029

Xu, Q., H. Hong, J. Wu, and X. Yan. 2019. Bioavailability of bioactive peptides derived from food proteins across the intestinal epithelial membrane: A review. *Trends in Food Science & Technology 86*: 399–411.

Zhu, F. 2018. Proanthocyanidins in cereals and pseudocereals. *Critical Reviews in Food Science and Nutrition 59*(10): 1521–1533. https://doi.org/10.1080/10408398.2017.1418284

3 Millet-Processing Techniques
Feasibility and Gaps

Punjasthala Ravindrasingh Negi, Palak Tiwari, and Neelam Chaturvedi
Division of Food Science and Nutrition, Faculty of Home Science, Banasthali Vidyapith, Tonk, Rajasthan, India

3.1 MILLETS: A NUTRIENT-PACKED ANCIENT GRAIN

Millets have been grown since ancient times in the arid and semi-arid regions of Asia, Africa, and Europe. They are drought-resistant, nutrient-rich, and small-seeded grains which are generally regarded as "smart grains" (Kanojia et al 2024). Being adaptive to harsh climatic conditions, they are suitable for areas with low rainfall and less fertile soil (Srivastav and Chauhan 2024). These crops are members of family Poaceae, including pearl millet (*Pennisetum glaucum*), finger millet (*Eleusine coracana*), foxtail millet (*Setaria italica*), proso millet (*Panicum miliaceum*), little millet (*Panicum sumatrense*), kodo millet (*Paspalum scrobiculatum*), and barnyard millet (*Echinochloa frumentacea*) (Amadou et al 2013). Over time, other cereals like wheat, maize, and rice have been more extensively cultivated diminishing the importance of millet grains. A recent shift has been noticed in consumer preferences towards sustainable and healthier food options. They have also been termed as "nutricereals" due to their high nutrient values, bio-active compounds, and low glycaemic index (GI) (Sharma et al 2023). Since underutilized millets have health benefits, the Indian government has taken initiatives to promote their use, and as a result, they are gradually making their way into the mainstream of dietary choices (Ministry of Agriculture and Farmer's Welfare 2023). Millets have now been recognized as an integral part in addressing issues related to food security, reducing malnutrition, and promoting sustainable farming practices globally (Kanojia et al 2024). The types, names and importance of different types of millets have been described below in table 3.1.

3.2 CLASSIFICATION OF MILLETS

The two main categories of millets are major millets, which include pearl millet, finger millet, and sorghum, and minor millets, including foxtail millet, barnyard millet, proso millet, little millet, and kodo millet (depicted in the figure 3.1). They are essential staple crop in regions with less fertile soil and low rainfall as they require minimal farming input and accommodate extreme climatic conditions (Sun et al 2023).

3.3 NUTRITIONAL PROFILE AND HEALTH BENEFITS OF MILLETS

Packed with essential nutrients like vitamins, minerals, protein, and dietary fibre, millets are an ideal choice for daily consumption (Kanojia et al 2024). The flavonoids and phenolic compounds which are beneficial against oxidative stress, diabetes and certain cancers also constitute their nutritional profile. Millets are an optimal choice for diabetic patients and individuals with gluten sensitivity or celiac disease due to their low GI and gluten-free characteristics (Koduru et al 2018). They also have high fibre content which makes them suitable for weight management and good digestion.

DOI: 10.1201/9781003686668-3

TABLE 3.1
Types, Names, and Importance of Millets

Type of Millets	Common Name	Botanical Name	Importance
Major millets	Jowar (Sorghum)	*Sorghum bicolor*	Well known for its high fibre and antioxidant properties
	Bajra (pearl millet)	*Pennisetum glaucum*	Rich in iron and calcium and can withstand drought conditions
	Ragi (finger millet)	*Eleusine coracana*	Rich in calcium, protein, and essential amino acids
Minor millets	Kangni (foxtail millet)	*Setaria italica*	Rich in iron, magnesium, fibre and well suited for people with celiac disease as it is gluten-free
	Kutki (little millet)	*Panicum sumatrense*	Rich in fibre, folate, niacin, and minerals like magnesium, iron, zinc, and phosphorous
	Kodra (kodo millet)	*Paspalum scrobiculatum*	It is well suited for diabetic patients as it has low glycaemic index
	Sanwa (banyard millet)	*Echinochloa frumentacea*	It is the fastest-growing millet with good protein content and minerals like zinc, iron, magnesium, and phosphorous
	Barri (porso millet)	*Panicum miliaceum*	Rich in vitamin B complex, iron, and calcium

Source: Tripathi et al (2023).

Millets are gaining attention for their major contribution towards overall health as they offer a wholesome alternative to refined grains (Tripathi et al 2023).

3.4 ANTI-NUTRITIONAL PROFILE OF MILLETS

Despite having a rich nutritional profile, millets also contain certain anti-nutritional factors like phytic acid, tannins, and polyphenols that can impair digestion, absorption, and overall consumption of the other essential nutrients (Popova and Mihaylova 2019).They have been shown to lower the risk of coronary heart disease, breast cancer, and inflammation when consumed in moderation; however, those whose diets heavily rely on cereals and grains may be adversely affected by these antinutrients. These antinutrients found in millets can be reduced through techniques such as germination, fermentation, soaking, malting, and cooking (Patterson et al 2017).

3.5 PRIMARY PROCESSING TECHNIQUES

Millets are an excellent source of protein, minerals, vitamins, and dietary fibre, but for their consumption they need to undergo processing. Processing converts the raw millet grains into their

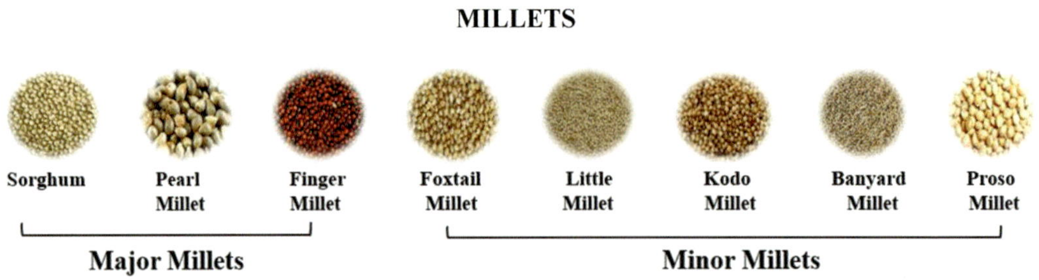

FIGURE 3.1 Classification of millets.

edible form, which results in improved nutritional profile, quality, and sensory appeal (Sarita and Singh 2016). In order to enhance digestion, micronutrient availability, and overall palatability of millet, dehulling, milling, malting, and fermentation are the most common techniques employed on the grains. While milling reduces the nutrient content by removing the germ and bran, they may also eliminate the indigestible elements and impurities from the grains, ensuring the production of value-added millet-based products suitable for varied culinary applications (Kang et al 2024). The stages of millet processing techniques have been explained in figure 3.2 below.

3.5.1 Decortication

De-cortication refers to the partial removal of the outer layer of the millets, typically the seed coat. While it was traditionally achieved through hand pounding, it is now performed using rice dehullers or abrasive dehullers (Jaybhaye et al 2014). This process enhances the bioavailability of nutrients, digestibility, and consumer acceptability by lowering anti-nutritional factors and cellulose content while improving the solubility and palatability of the grains. However, it can also result in the loss of fat, protein, and polyphenols, necessitating optimization to maintain a balance between nutrient retention and improved cooking qualities (Wilson et al 2022).

3.5.2 Dehulling

Dehulling is an important processing technique that removes the hull and pericarp of the grains, in order to make them edible (Taylor and Duodu 2015). At the domestic level, dehulling was traditionally accomplished by hand pounding; however, for more efficient processing, modern methods like centrifugal shellers, abrasive mills, and rice mills have been introduced. These methods can remove 12–30% of the outer layer of the grains, but excessive dehulling may also lead to a reduction in the nutritional content such as essential amino acids, dietary fibre, bio-active materials, and phenolic compounds (Rani et al 2018). Moreover, the combination of hydrothermal treatment with dehulling can also have a negative impact on the phenolic compounds and antioxidant potential of the grains making it essential to increase the efficiency of these techniques to reduce the nutrient losses (Jaybhaye et al 2014).

3.5.3 Milling

Milling is a process where germ and bran are separated from the millet and then the grains are converted into fine flour through grinding and sieving in a hammer mill. This technique helps in the

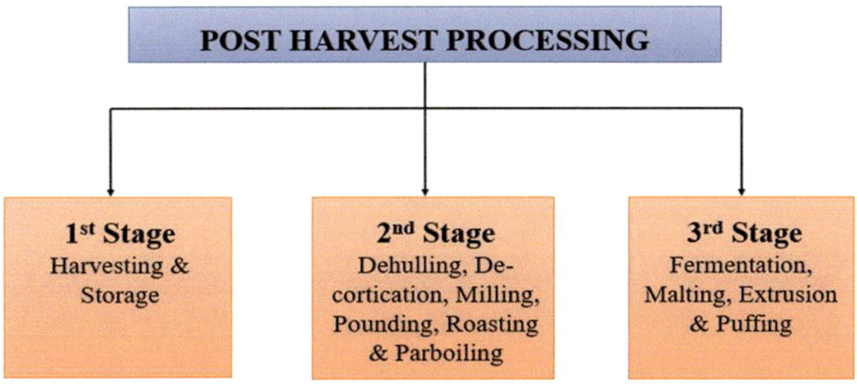

FIGURE 3.2 Stages of millet-processing techniques.

problems associated with coarse seed coat, coloured pigments, and astringent flavour of the millets. Milling not only enhances the bioavailability of the essential nutrients and consumer acceptability of the millet grains but also streamlines their production. Despite various advantages, there are certain limitations of this technique as it leads to a considerable loss in the nutrient content of the millet grains such as dietary fibre, protein, vitamins, and minerals. However, a more efficient milling technique needs to be established for the variety of millets with very small kernels like pearl millet in order to enhance the quality of their products, as their endosperms are tightly attached to the germ (Rani et al 2018).

3.5.4 Pounding

Pounding is an age-old processing technique where millets are pounded wet, dry, or moistened in a wooden mortar or a stone using a wooden pestle, and the starchy hard endosperm is separated from the fibrous bran with the addition of water. While reducing the stickiness of cooked porridge, parboiling improves the effectiveness of dehulling. The labour-intensive process of hand pounding, which is usually carried out by women, entails crushing grains with a hand-held stone against a lower stone (Chapke et al 2020).

3.5.5 Parboiling

Parboiling refers to partial cooking of millet grains while preserving their bran or husk intact, which is followed by drying, dehusking, and decortication (Chapke et al 2020). This technique retains the nutrient-rich components like bran, while improving the biochemical characteristics of millets and increasing milling efficiency. Parboiling increases the phenolic and antioxidant content of the grains, lowers the GI, and decreases the amount of easily digested starch, which makes them advantageous for people with metabolic disorders like diabetes and cholesterol (Gowda et al 2022). The detailed process of parboiling has been explained in the figure 3.3.

3.5.6 Roasting

Traditionally millet grains are roasted to enhance their aroma and flavour by browning the seed coat by exposing them to high heat (160–200°C) and thus making them more appealing and palatable. In this, millets are pre-soaked to maintain the moisture content, followed by drying in the shade, and thereafter, roasting is performed. Roasting makes dehusking or pearling more feasible, as it loosens the husk from the cotyledon (Kate and Singh 2021). The modern roasting equipment has helped in controlling the time and temperature, which ensures consistent roasting of various grains, including rice, millets, and chickpeas (Kang et al 2024).

3.6 SECONDARY PROCESSING TECHNIQUES

The secondary processing techniques convert primary raw materials into ready-to-eat (RTE) or ready-to-cook (RTC) products, thereby reducing the cooking time and improving the convenience. The efficient processing of millet grains can be done by using a combined method of contemporary

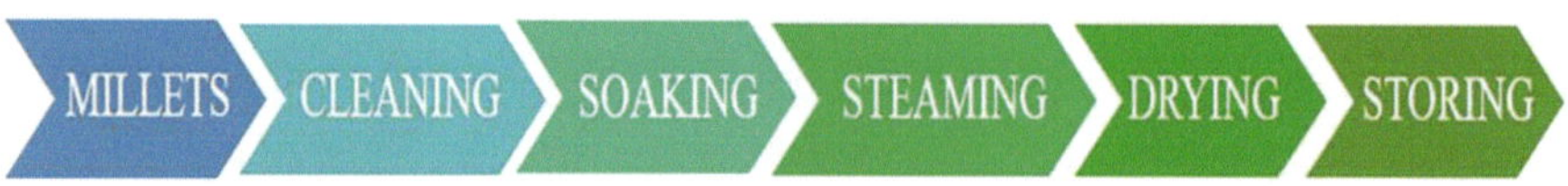

FIGURE 3.3 Process of parboiling.

techniques like extrusion cooking and roller drying with more conventional techniques like popping and flaking (Chapke et al 2020).

3.6.1 Fermentation

Fermentation is a very old technique of food preservation where the enzymes present in the grains break down the soluble sugars and starch found in them, thus improving the physicochemical properties of their end product. This process takes place in the presence of a fermenting medium like yeast or lactobacilli which are the living organisms, and these microbial strains help in preservation of the flavour (Rai et al 2008). Fermentation also reduces the anti-nutritional factors present in the grains, thereby improving digestibility and protein content, and enhances the overall nutritional quality of the millets (Kate and Singh 2021).

3.6.2 Malting

Malting is known as one of the oldest techniques in the processing of millets, where the grains undergo sprouting under controlled temperature and humidity. These sprouts are then dried carefully in order to prevent the enzymatic reactions. Malting reduces the anti-nutritional factors like phytates present in the millets, thus improving the nutritional quality, digestibility, and sensory attributes, thereby making them an ideal choice for consumption (Singh and Saini 2012). This technique constitutes three major steps: steeping, where the millet grains are soaked in water; germination, where the grains are allowed to germinate by activating the enzymes; and kilning in which enzyme activity and further sprouting are stopped, and the grains are dried to remove the excessive water present in them. Malting is an essential technique, as it leads to improved nutrient quality in the millet grains (Kumar et al 2016).

This traditional method of malting is more complex and time-consuming, whereas in the modern malting technique all these three steps (steeping, germination, and kilning) have been combined together, making it more efficient and simpler. In this single system, millet grains are evenly layered on the sieves, and water is been sprinkled over them for thorough soaking. In this process of steeping, there is continuous drainage of water to facilitate aeration establishing an ideal environment for germination. Once the germination process is done, hot air is passed through the sieves to make the grains dry for the further process of kilning. This modern technique is more efficient in yielding premium malts as it enhances the flavour, texture and also improves the nutritional quality of various food products (Kate and Singh 2021). The steps involved in the process of malting is depicted in the figure 3.4.

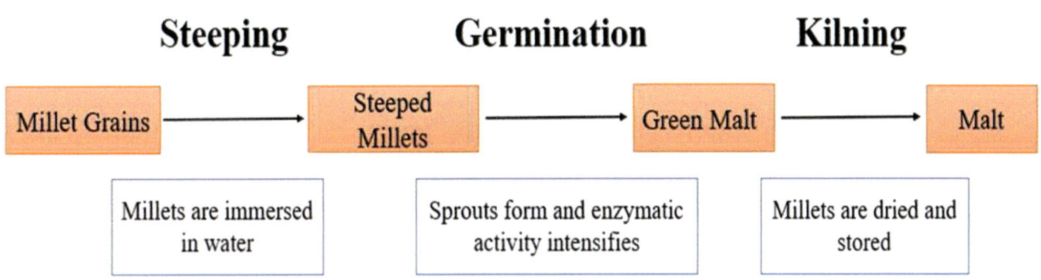

FIGURE 3.4 Sequential steps involved in the malting of millets.

3.6.3 Puffing

Puffing or popping is the most common practice to produce porous, crisp and RTE breakfast snacks and cereals (Lehmann and Robin 2007). In this process, millets are subjected to high temperature (230–250°C) for 20–30 seconds. The protein and starch present in it undergo multiple changes, which results in them expanding and creating that porous, crisp, and light texture. Puffing improves the digestibility of proteins and carbohydrates, enhances mineral bioavailability, and also reduces the anti-nutritional factors such as tannins and phytates. Maillard reaction also takes place due to the high heat, adding the appealing aroma to the product (Nirmala et al 2000). Moreover, fat and moisture content are reduced, whereas dietary fibre and mineral profile are enhanced. Mostly sorghum, pearl millet, and finger millets are used for puffing. The modern techniques of puffing use a hot air popping gun which provides small-scale and industrial options for yielding products with improved physical and nutritional attributes (Kate and Singh 2021). Figure 3.5 represents the process of making puffs from sorghum.

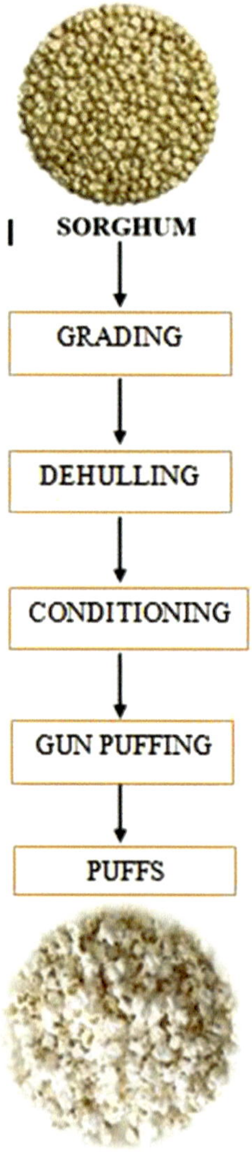

FIGURE 3.5 Schematic representation of puffing.

3.6.4 Extrusion

Extrusion is a method that uses high temperature for a short period of time (HTST) for quick cooking and shaping the millets into products like snacks, pasta, breakfast cereals, and baby foods. In this process, the ingredients are pushed through a machine at high temperature and pressure with great mechanical force for cooking. The required temperature is reached through steam, heated barrels, or the heat created inside the machine (Jaybhaye et al 2014). This method improves the nutritional quality of millets by making their starch easier to digest and increasing the fibre content, antioxidants, and water absorption. It also helps create a crisp texture by boosting the natural phenolic compounds (Patel et al 2018). Conditions such as temperature, pressure, feed rate, and how long the material stays in the machine affect changes in the protein, fats, and starch content of the millets. Overall, extrusion is a flexible and efficient technique that allows the production of many nutritious millet-based foods with different textures (Kate and Singh 2021).

3.7 EFFECTS OF PROCESSING ON NUTRITIONAL PROPERTIES OF MILLETS

3.7.1 Proteins

Millets are an excellent source of protein which makes them suitable for vegan people who rely wholly on plant-based products for meeting their protein requirement. Along with the good amount of protein, these grains also constitute minimal saturated fats with some anti-nutritional factors like trypsin inhibitors and phytates which may hinder the protein uptake and inhibit its absorption and utilization in the body. This can be prevented through simple processes such as soaking, germination, milling, dehulling, heating, and fermentation, as they improve protein digestibility, thereby reducing the amount of anti-nutritional factors present in them (Sharma et al 2015). Moreover, through the action of microbial proteolytic enzymes, fermentation reduces phytates and converts insoluble proteins into soluble forms (Rani et al 2019). The other techniques like soaking, malting, and popping have shown significant improvements in protein content and in vitro protein digestibility (IVPD). Controlled decortication results in the removal of antinutrients while preserving the essential amino acids, thereby improving protein digestibility. These low-cost techniques are effective for developing protein-rich foods and combating protein-energy malnutrition, particularly in underdeveloped nations (Gowda et al 2022).

3.7.2 Carbohydrate

The starch is the primary carbohydrate present in millets ranging from 60 to 75% and its availability is highly influenced by processing methods such as sprouting, cooking, and soaking (Dayakar Rao et al 2017). While decortication increases the total carbohydrate content of the millet grains by removing the seed coat, germination on the other hand enhances the concentration of soluble sugars due to the breakdown of starch and improves carbohydrate digestibility, making them suitable for energy-dense foods like infant formula. Parboiling reduces starch digestibility and GI by leaching out starch, suggesting its potential for formulating products suited for people with diabetes and other metabolic disorders (Bora et al 2019).

3.7.3 Dietary Fibre

Millets are a rich source of dietary fibre that provides roughage and is found majorly in the bran of the grains. They are not readily digestible in the body as our body lacks the enzymes which are responsible for the breakdown of these complex polysaccharides. Primary processing techniques like decortication/dehulling reduce the fibre content of the millets as the bran is separated from the endosperm, with the loss of fibre being more prominent when dehulling exceeds 30% (Yousaf et al 2021). According to several studies, while some processes such as milling, dehulling reduce the insoluble fibre content (cellulose, hemicellulose, and lignin) of the grains, the other techniques like fermentation and germination can improve soluble dietary fibre (Sharma et al 2015). However, thermal processing (e.g., extrusion, puffing, popping, and roasting) degrades dietary fibre, particularly in the outer layer of the bran, due to heat-induced polysaccharide breakdown. The fibre present in the bran helps in managing type 2 diabetes and constipation, making it essential to reduce polishing during milling and promote the consumption of whole millets and their by-products for a healthier diet (Gowda et al 2022).

3.7.4 Vitamins

The vitamin content present in the millet grains is significantly affected due to processes such as milling, de-branning, and polishing, as they eliminate the bran and germ components which are rich in vitamin E, riboflavin, niacin, and thiamine. Germination and fermentation result in an increase in the vitamin content of millet grains, whereas on the other hand certain processes like dehulling and milling cause considerable loss of vitamin content, as most vitamins are concentrated in the outer layers of the grain (Shahidi and Chandrasekara 2015). The incorporation of millet flour along with probiotic fermentation in food products like biscuits has also shown enhanced vitamin levels. Thus, fermentation and germination offer efficient strategies to improve the vitamin profile of millet-based foods, mitigating the losses caused by conventional processing techniques (Gowda et al 2022).

3.7.5 Minerals

Minerals are majorly accumulated in the pericarp, aleurone, and germ part of the millet grains (Dayakar Rao et al 2017). Even though soaking improves mineral bioavailability of the millets, certain minerals like zinc and iron may leach into the soaking water. Techniques like fermentation and germination significantly enhance mineral availability by reducing inhibitors like phytic acid and activating enzymes such as phytase. Germination increases minerals like iron, calcium, and magnesium, while fermentation enhances phosphorous, calcium, and iron bio-accessibility. However, decortication reduces total mineral content (e.g., calcium by 40%, iron by 50%) but improves mineral bio-accessibility by reducing antinutrient factors (Sharma et al., 2015). Acid treatments and organic acids like hydrochloric acid improve mineral extractability and bio-accessibility. Composite millet flour enriched with skimmed milk or vegetables has also shown an increase in calcium, copper, and zinc content. Therefore, germination, fermentation, and controlled processing can enhance the bioavailability of minerals, offering potential for value-added millet-based products (Gowda et al 2022).

3.7.6 Bio-Active Compounds

The millet grains possess a wide range of bio-active compounds which are crucial for sustaining human health. These bio-active compounds majorly include polyphenols (naturally occurring plant-based antioxidants) such as flavonoids, hydroxycinnamic acids, and hydroxybenzoic acid (Shahidi and Chandrasekara 2013). Apart from these polyphenols, millets also contain bio-active compounds such as inulin, lignan, resistant starch, β-glucan, phytates, and feraxans (Saleh et al 2013). The techniques and severity in millet processing have a significant effect on the functionality and bioavailability of bio-active compounds, where milling may result in enhancing the glycaemic response, while other processing techniques may reduce the stability and bioactivity of these beneficial bio-active compounds in the millet grains (Pradeep and Sreerama 2015). As phenolic compounds are majorly found in the seedcoat of the millets, processes like dehulling and decortication, where seed coats are separated from the grains have shown to reduce total phenols, tannins, and antioxidant activity of the millet grain (Chethan et al 2008). A study carried out on the malting of finger millet has reported a threefold decrease in protocatechuic acid after malting for 96 h, whereas other phenolic compounds such as gallic, ferulic, coumaric, and vanillic acids have increased (Subba Rao and Muralikrishna 2002). The effect of processes such as fermentation, hydrothermal treatment, and germination depends upon the factors like temperature, pH, and kind and count of zymophyte. Some studies have elucidated that soaking had a negative effect on the total phenol, total flavonoid, tannins, β-carotene, vitamin E, antioxidant activity, β-glucosidase, and amylase inhibitory activities of the millet grains. Steaming process (100°C for 50 mins) has been shown to reduce the total flavonoid and total phenol content, whereas roasting has been shown to increase the total phenols in the millet grains (Li et al 2022).

3.8 INDUSTRIAL FEASIBILITY AND ADVANCEMENTS OF MILLET PROCESSING

There have been several studies on the advancements in the millet-processing techniques in order to increase the efficiency, digestibility, nutrient quality, and overall consumer acceptability. Moreover, the limitations of the traditional processing methods have been mitigated through their new modernized versions resulting in enhanced sensory attributes of the millets while maintaining their nutritional integrity. Innovative processes such as extrusion, fortification, and puffing have been introduced to create diverse millet-based products, including snacks, baked goods, and beverages, offering a convenient and nutritious alternative to refined grain-based foods (Saini et al 2021). Additionally, extrusion technology has revolutionized the market with expanded, shelf-stable snacks and crispy, making millet-based foods increasingly popular.

The emerging technologies like fermentation, and vacuum and modified atmosphere packaging, have further resulted in the enhanced nutritional profile and extended the shelf-life of millet-based foods (Kanojia et al 2024). Furthermore, automation and digital technologies in processing facilities have improved efficiency, product consistency, and quality control. These innovations have diversified and commercialized millet-based products, making them more accessible and appealing globally, while contributing to food security and public health (Kumari et al 2020).

3.9 CHALLENGES AND GAPS IN MILLET PROCESSING

1. *Decline in cultivation and productivity*: In recent years, the area under millet cultivation has drastically reduced as they are time-consuming, gives low yields, labour-intensive and limited marketing of their products. Moreover, the productivity of certain varieties like sorghum and pearl millet has either stagnated or declined over years.
2. *Lack of awareness and demand*: There is less awareness among the consumers about the nutritional content and health benefits of the millet grains, resulting in negative impact about their taste and texture which affects their acceptance in daily diets and thus leads to low demands.
3. *High-cost and limited market presence*: Millets usually have a higher price as compared to the staples like rice and wheat, which makes them less affordable to the population with low income. Moreover, their accessibility in the markets, including e-commerce platforms, is limited, which further leads to a barrier for the consumers to purchase them.
4. *Inefficient processing techniques*: As the millet-processing techniques are inefficient and complex due to various factors such as variability in grain size, husk-grain bonding, and hardness, it becomes practically difficult to produce them on a large scale.
5. *Lack of government support and shelf-life challenges*: There has been lack of support from the government in India, leading to the hinderance in millet cultivation, processing their

consumption. Also, due to the enzyme activity, lipid oxidation, and susceptibility to rancidity, the shelf-life of processed millets becomes limited for which better pre-treatments and storage techniques need to be employed in order to extend the shelf-life and storage stability of the millets.

3.10 FUTURE OF MILLET PROCESSING IN THE SUSTAINABLE WORLD

As a sustainable solution, millets play a vital role in addressing global problems in food security and public health. These drought-resistant crops can withstand harsh climatic conditions, which include marginal areas and drought-prone regions, with very little water and minimal farming input requirements (Hu et al., 2022). Unlike staple crops such as rice and wheat, millets do not require extensive irrigation processes or large number of chemical fertilizers resulting in enhanced agricultural sustainability. Their rich nutritional profile and ability to withstand adverse environmental conditions make them an essential resource in low-income and resource-constrained regions, combating malnutrition and micronutrient deficiencies. Moreover, they serve as the best option suited for individuals with celiac disease or gluten intolerance due to their gluten-free nature, further broadening their appeal (Ramarathnam & Ochi 2018).

3.11 CONCLUSION

Millets are a valuable gift by nature as they offer numerous health benefits contributing towards the overall well-being of humans. Their excellent drought-resisting capacity and adaptability to extreme climatic conditions have made them the best staple crops to be grown in areas with very little rainfall and low fertile soil. Millets have various health benefits which make them suitable for diabetic patients and their gluten-free nature helps people with gluten intolerance and celiac disease. As these grains cannot be directly consumed in their raw, harvested form, they need to undergo extensive processing before they can be consumed. There are various traditional processing techniques such as pounding and dehulling employed with certain modern techniques such as extrusion in order to make millets desirable for human consumption by reducing the anti-nutritional factors present in them. This cannot be achieved through any one of the processing methods but with the combination of traditional methods with the modern ones. Despite exceptional qualities, there are many challenges which are seen in the processing of these grains namely lack of awareness, negative perceptions about the taste, limited processing equipment, high price, and limited market accessibility which hinders millet consumption and their incorporation in daily diet. There are many millet-based products available in the market such as puffs, malts, dosas, but due to low acceptance and less awareness, it has not been able to become a part of daily life. Also, advancements in the processing techniques such smart processing techniques with the integration of artificial intelligence (AI) in the cultivation of millets and more focus on the research and development in the field of millet processing would lead to high efficiency and productivity. The government initiatives in order to encourage millet cultivation, distribution, and consumption would further enhance techniques in millet processing with quality equipment and cost-effective solutions in the processing of millets. This would result in increased awareness and cultivation of millets resulting in their adoption into the mainstream of the daily diet, ensuring food security and sustainability.

REFERENCES

Amadou, I., Gounga, M. E., & Le, G. 2013. Millets: Nutritional composition, some health benefits and processing – A Review. *Emirates Journal of Food and Agriculture*, *25*(7), 501. https://doi.org/10.9755/ejfa.v25i7.12045

Bora, P., Ragaee, S., & Marcone, M. 2019. Characterisation of several types of millets as functional food ingredients. *International Journal of Food Sciences and Nutrition*, *70*(6), 714–724.

Chapke, R. R., Shyam Prasad, G., Das, I. K., Hariprasanna, K., Singode, A., Kanthi Sri, B. S., & Tonapi, V. A. 2020. *Latest millet production and processing technologies*. ICAR-Indian Institute of Millets Research.

Chethan, S., Dharmesh, S. M., & Malleshi, N. G. 2008. Inhibition of aldose reductase from cataracted eye lenses by finger millet (*Eleusine coracana*) polyphenols. *Bioorganic & Medicinal Chemistry*, *16*(23), 10085–10090.

Dayakar Rao, B., Bhaskarachary, K., Arlene Christina, G. D., Sudha Devi, G., Vilas, A. T., & Tonapi, A. 2017. Nutritional and health benefits of millets. *ICAR_Indian Institute of Millets Research (IIMR) Rajendranagar, Hyderabad*, *2*, 38–57.

Fox, G. 2017. Starch in brewing applications. In *Elsevier eBooks* (pp. 633–659). https://doi.org/10.1016/b978-0-08-100868-3.00016-0

Gowda, N. N., Siliveru, K., Prasad, P. V., Bhatt, Y., Netravati, B. P., & Gurikar, C. 2022. Modern processing of Indian millets: A perspective on changes in nutritional properties. *Foods*, *11*(4), 499.

Hu, Q., Zhao, Y., Hu, X., Qi, J., Suo, L., Pan, Y., …, & Chen, X. 2022. Effect of saline land reclamation by constructing the "Raised Field-Shallow Trench" pattern on agroecosystems in Yellow River Delta. *Agricultural Water Management*, *261*, 107345.

Jaybhaye, R. V., Pardeshi, I. L., Vengaiah, P. C., & Srivastav, P. P. 2014. Processing and technology for millet based food products: A review. *Journal of Ready to Eat Food*, *1*(2), 32–48.

Kang, P., Krishnanand, A. K., Kaur, S., Rasane, P., Singh, J., Nanda, V., Assouguem, A., Lahlali, R., Ullah, R., & Alqahtani, A. S. 2024. Minor millets: Processing techniques and their nutritional and health benefits. *Open Agriculture*, *9*(1). https://doi.org/10.1515/opag-2022-0324

Kanojia, S., Gomadhi, G., Kamalasundari, S., Malathi, G., Krishnaveni, S. A., Ramasamy, M., Dhanalakshmi, K., Chitra, K., & Debnath, A. 2024. Exploring millet grains: nutritional benefits, processing advancements, and future directions for food security and health improvement. *European Journal of Nutrition & Food Safety*, *16*(5), 101–108. https://doi.org/10.9734/ejnfs/2024/v16i51426

Kate, A., & Singh, A. 2021. Processing technology for value addition in Millets. In *Springer eBooks* (pp. 239–254). https://doi.org/10.1007/978-981-16-0676-2_11

Koduru, U., Jiménez, M., Chang, G., Thomas C., Kumar, T. K., & Singh J. 2018. Structural modification of zein for the development of functional materials. *Biopolymers*, *90*(6), 819–831.

Kumar, S., Singh, A., Kohli, D., & Mishra, R. 2016. Fabrication of integrated malting unit for production of malts. *International Journal of Engineering Research and Applications*, *6*(8), 33–36.

Kumari, S., Kumar, G., & Singh, U.K. 2020. Nutritional potential, biofunctionalities, limitations, and utilization of legumes as a source of human food. *Journal of Food Biochemistry*, *44*(9), 13332.

Lehmann, U., & Robin, F. 2007. Slowly digestible starch – Its structure and health implications: A review. *Trends in Food Science & Technology*, *18*(7), 346–355.

Li, Z., Zhao, X., Zhang, X., & Liu, H. 2022. The effects of processing on bioactive compounds and biological activities of sorghum grains. *Molecules*, *27*(10), 3246.

Press Information Bureau. (2023, March 18). *International year of millets: India leading the way*. Ministry of Information and Broadcasting, Government of India. https://static.pib.gov.in/WriteReadData/specificdocs/documents/2023/mar/doc2023318173501.pdf

Nirmala, M., Rao, M. S., & Muralikrishna, G. 2000. Carbohydrates and their degrading enzymes from native and malted finger millet (Ragi, *Eleusine coracana*, Indaf-15). *Food Chemistry*, *69*(2), 175–180.

Patel, A., Parihar, P., & Dhumketi, K. 2018. Nutritional evaluation of Kodo millet and puffed Kodo. *International Journal of Chemical Studies*, *6*(2), 1639–1642.

Patterson, C. A., Curran, J., & Der, T. 2017. Effect of processing on antinutrient compounds in pulses. *Cereal Chemistry*, *94*(1), 2–10.

Popova, A., & Mihaylova, D. 2019. Antinutrients in plant-based foods: A review. *The Open Biotechnology Journal*, *13*(1), 68–76. https://doi.org/10.2174/1874070701913010068

Pradeep, P. M., & Sreerama, Y. N. 2015. Impact of processing on the phenolic profiles of small millets: Evaluation of their antioxidant and enzyme inhibitory properties associated with hyperglycemia. *Food Chemistry*, *169*, 455–463.

Rai, K. N., Gowda, C. L. L., Reddy, B. V. S., & Sehgal, S. 2008. Adaptation and potential uses of sorghum and pearl millet in alternative and health foods. *Comprehensive Reviews in Food Science and Food Safety*, *7*(4), 320–396.

Ramarathnam, N., & Ochi, H. 2018. Nutritional and health-promoting attributes of millets. *Nutritional and Health Aspects of Food in Western India*, 41–61.

Rani, M., Amane, D., & Ananthanarayan, L. 2019. Impact of partial replacement of rice with other selected cereals on idli batter fermentation and idli characteristics. *Journal of Food Science and Technology*, *56*, 1192–1201.

Rani, S., Singh, R., Sehrawat, R., Kaur, B. P., & Upadhyay, A. 2018. Pearl millet processing: A review. *Nutrition & Food Science*, *48*(1), 30–44. https://doi.org/10.1108/nfs-04-2017-0070

Saini, P., Kumar, N., Kumar, S., Mwaurah, P. W., Panghal, A., Attkan, A. K., …, & Singh, V. 2021. Bioactive compounds, nutritional benefits and food applications of colored wheat: A comprehensive review. *Critical Reviews in Food Science and Nutrition*, *61*(19), 3197–3210.

Saleh, A. S., Zhang, Q., Chen, J., & Shen, Q. 2013. Millet grains: Nutritional quality, processing, and potential health benefits. *Comprehensive Reviews in Food Science and Food Safety*, *12*(3), 281–295.

Sarita, E. S., & Singh, E. 2016. Potential of millets: Nutrients composition and health benefits. *Journal of Scientific and Innovative Research*, *5*(2), 46–50.

Shahidi, F., & Chandrasekara, A. 2013. Millet grain phenolics and their role in disease risk reduction and health promotion: A review. *Journal of Functional Foods*, *5*(2), 570–581.

Shahidi, F., & Chandrasekara, A. 2015. Processing of millet grains and effects on non-nutrient antioxidant compounds. In *Processing and impact on active components in food* (pp. 345–352). Academic Press.

Sharma, A., Dongre, P., Harsha, H., Ausari, P. K., & Devendra, D. 2023. Horticulture horizons an exploring advanced technologies in plant cultivation. *Plant Science Archives*, *8*(2), 13–14. https://doi.org/10.51470/psa.2023.8.2.13

Sharma, N., Sahu, J. K., Bansal, V., Esua, O. J., Rana, S., Bhardwaj, A., Bangar, S. P., & Adedeji, A. A. 2022. Trends in millet and pseudomillet proteins – Characterization, processing and food applications. *Food Research International*, 164, 112310. https://doi.org/10.1016/j.foodres.2022.112310

Sharma, S., Saxena, D. C., & Riar, C. S. 2015. Antioxidant activity, total phenolics, flavonoids and antinutritional characteristics of germinated foxtail millet (*Setaria italica*). *Cogent Food & Agriculture*, *1*(1), 1081728.

Singh, N. B., & Saini, R. S. 2012. Products, diversification, marketing and price discovery of pearl millet in India.

Srivastav, S., & Chauhan, E. S. 2024. Browntop millet (*Brachiaria ramosa*): An overview of the underutilized miraculous multifunctional millet. *International Journal of Health Sciences and Research*, 14(5), 181–187.

Subba Rao, M. V. S. S. T., & Muralikrishna, G. 2002. Evaluation of the antioxidant properties of free and bound phenolic acids from native and malted finger millet (Ragi, *Eleusine coracana*, Indaf-15). *Journal of Agricultural and Food Chemistry*, *50*(4), 889–892.

Sun, M., Yan, H., Zhang, A., Jin, Y., Lin, C., Luo, L., Wu, B., Fan, Y., Tian, S., Cao, X., Wang, Z., Luo, J., Yang, Y., Jia, J., Zhou, P., Tang, Q., Jones, C. S., Varshney, R. K., Srivastava, R. K., …, Huang, L. 2023. Milletdb: A multi-omics database to accelerate the research of functional genomics and molecular breeding of millets. *Plant Biotechnology Journal*, *21*(11), 2348–2357. https://doi.org/10.1111/pbi.14136

Taylor, J. R., & Duodu, K. G. 2015. Effects of processing sorghum and millets on their phenolic phytochemicals and the implications of this to the health-enhancing properties of sorghum and millet food and beverage products. *Journal of the Science of Food and Agriculture*, *95*(2), 225–237.

Tripathi, G., Jitendrakumar, P. H., Borah, A., Nath, D., Das, H., Bansal, S., Singh, N., & Singh, B. V. 2023. A review on nutritional and health benefits of millets. *International Journal of Plant & Soil Science*, *35*(19), 1736–1743. https://doi.org/10.9734/ijpss/2023/v35i193722

Wilson, A., Elumalai, A., Moses, J. A., &Anandharamakrishnan, C. 2022. Effect of processing on functional characteristics, physiochemical properties, and nutritional accessibility of millets. In *Handbook of millets-processing, quality, and nutrition status* (pp. 205–229). Singapore: Springer Nature Singapore.

Yousaf, L., Hou, D., Liaqat, H., & Shen, Q. 2021. Millet: A review of its nutritional and functional changes during processing. *Food Research International*, *142*, 110197.

4 Policy Perspectives in Millets
Strengthening Production and Consumption in Millet Value Chains

Shefali Srivastava[1] and Jayanti Kajale[2]
[1] Symbiosis Institute of International Business (SIIB), Symbiosis International (Deemed University), Pune, Maharashtra, India
[2] Gokhale Institute of Politics and Economics, Pune, Maharashtra, India

4.1 INTRODUCTION

Millets are often referred to as "nutri-cereals" or "superfoods". They are also known as "Shree Anna" which means the best among all the food grains because of their valuable nutritional content and historical significance, making them essential to combat malnutrition and diseases related to lifestyle choices. Millets contain a wealth of vital nutrients, including proteins, dietary fibres, vitamins (particularly from the B-complex group), and minerals such as calcium, iron, zinc, potassium, and magnesium (Bisht et al 2022).

Millets possess a lower glycaemic index, which aids in regulating blood sugar levels, making them beneficial for individuals with diabetes. In addition to this, millets are inherently gluten-free and demonstrate potential to manage celiac disease, blood pressure, and cholesterol levels. Thus, millets offer greater nutritional benefits, especially as compared to wheat and rice (Arya and Bisht 2022). Therefore, given their multifarious benefits, they are regarded as "Shree Anna" (Singh et al 2025).

As millets are climate-resilient crops, they can flourish in a wide range of challenging environmental conditions, which positions them as a sustainable alternative in the context of climate change. Millets can thrive in environments with minimal water, demanding considerably less rainfall and irrigation than water-guzzling crops like rice. These crops typically require fewer synthetic fertilisers and pesticides, which not only reduces costs for farmers but also diminishes agriculture's environmental impact. As C4 crops, millets exhibit a greater rate of converting carbon dioxide to oxygen, assisting in the battle against climate change (Brown 1999). They also bolster soil health and fertility through carbon sequestration (Vidhya and Pragasan 2022).

Their non-substitutable role calls for strengthening their value chains as well as their demand and supply. This chapter explores the production and consumption aspects of millets in the post-independence period and discusses the inefficiencies that need to be eliminated to strengthen the millet value chain. The chapter analyses the post-independence trends in millet area, production, and yield while examining the role of policies, initiatives, and programmes that have shaped these patterns over time. The chapter mainly relies on secondary data sources such as datasets published by the Government of India and Food and Agriculture Organization (FAO) as well as various research papers.

4.2 GLOBAL SCENARIO OF MILLETS

India holds the first position worldwide in both the area under millet cultivation and its production. According to FAOSTAT, the other major millet-producing countries in 2023 were Niger, China, Mali, and Nigeria. Between 2015 and 2023, India has experienced growth in both millet area,

DOI: 10.1201/9781003686668-4

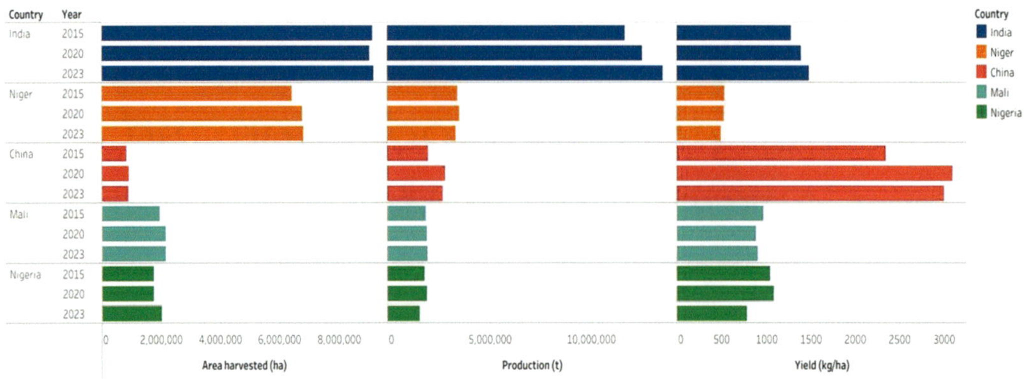

FIGURE 4.1 Area, production, and yield of millet for top five producing countries. (Data source: Authors' computation based on Food and Agriculture Organization (FAO) (2023).)

production, and yield. This can be observed from Figure 4.1. Nevertheless, while there has been an improvement in millet yield, it still falls short compared to China's yield. Figure 4.2 focuses on the ranks of various countries in millet production and their respective yield levels. It indicates that if India had yield equivalent to China, it would produce twice the quantity of millets than it is producing now from the same land area.

4.3 MILLET PRODUCTION IN INDIA: AN OVERVIEW

Millets have had an eventful history, transitioning from staple to obscurity and back to prominence. Prior to the Green Revolution, the cropping system in India featured a significantly greater proportion of millets, pulses, and oilseeds. Evidently, the acreage under nutri-cereals almost halved between the periods 1962–65 and 2012–14 in absolute terms (Shah and Vijayshankar 2022). These crops were well-suited to the varied agricultural conditions across India, particularly in semi-arid and rainfed areas. Staple foods for millions included millets like jowar (sorghum), bajra (pearl millet), and ragi (finger millet), along with various small millets. The millets were valued for their drought resistance, minimal input needs, and a rich nutritional profile, offering vital minerals and fibre to the diets of rural populations.

The launch of high-yielding rice and wheat varieties in the 1960s and 1970s, along with the expansion of irrigation, subsidized inputs, and government procurement policies favouring these grains, resulted in a declining trend in the area and production of millets (Figure 4.3). However, this was a necessary response at the time to address food insecurity. Farmers transitioned to cultivating rice and wheat because of guaranteed markets and price support. Over time, millets gradually became sidelined from public procurement, school meals, and family diets. This led to a decrease in dietary diversity, the diminishing of local food customs, and contributed to escalating nutritional issues (Shah and Vijayshankar 2022).

Annual per capita consumption of millet is shown in Figure 4.4. As it is evident from the figure, millet consumption has been declining. The literature reveals that it had been declining in both urban and rural households, though per capita consumption was notably higher in rural areas between 1977–78 and 2011–12. In rural areas, jowar is consumed in larger quantities, followed by bajra, ragi, and small millets (Sukumaran Sreekala et al 2023). With rice and wheat being the highest consumed cereals, the total number of households consuming coarse grains (which includes millets) has declined between 1993–94 and 2011–12 (NITI Aayog, 2024). Rao et al (2021a) have identified demand- and supply-side factors that led to decline in the consumption of millets. The supply-side factors include relatively less profitable cultivation due to lower yields, fall in prices

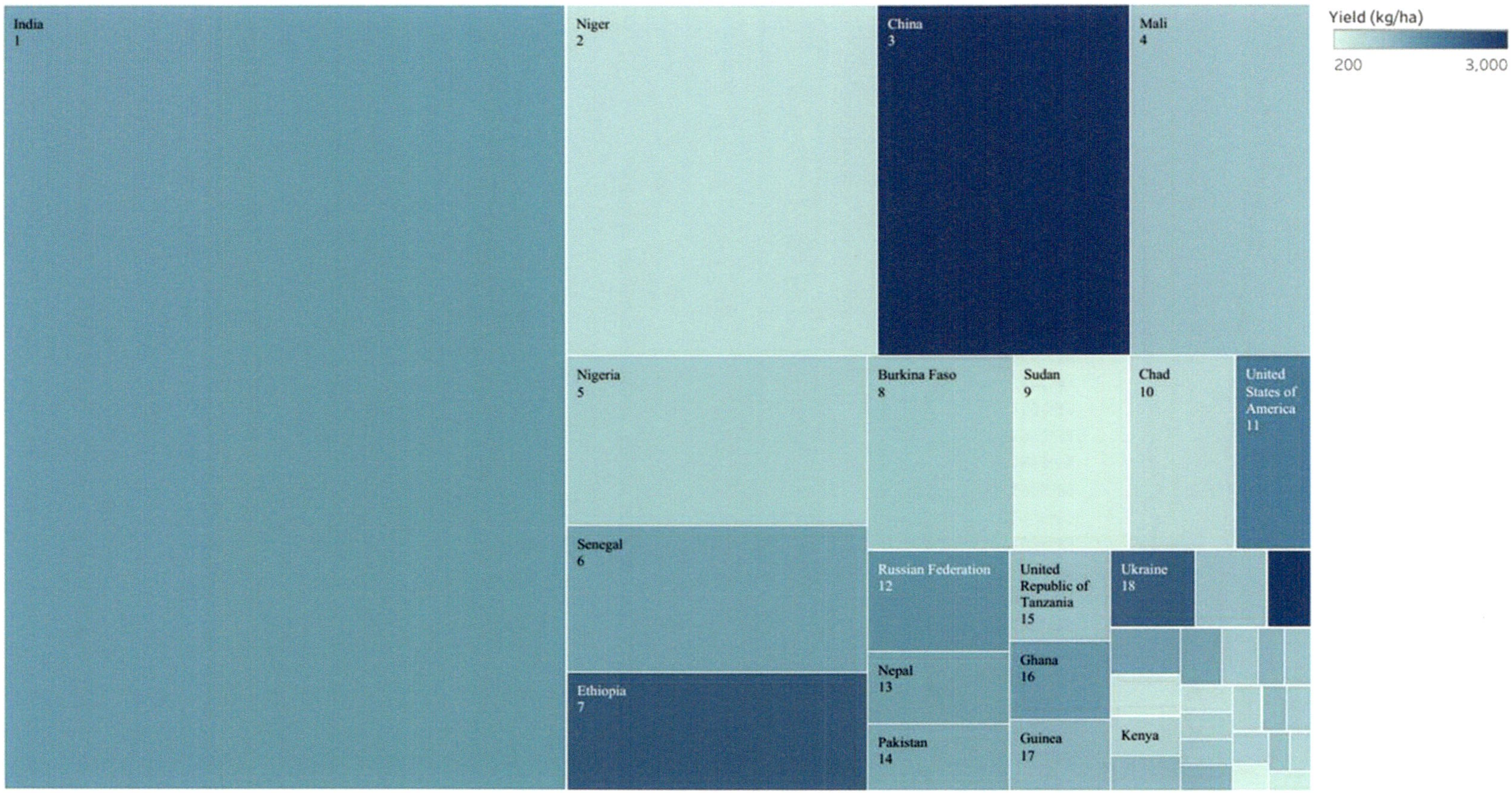

FIGURE 4.2 Millet production vs. yield of millet-producing countries. (Data Source: Authors' computation based on FAO (2023).)

Note: Ranks of countries in millet production are mentioned as numbers in the cells and millet yield is indicated in the colour legend for the year 2023. The size of the cell indicates millet production.

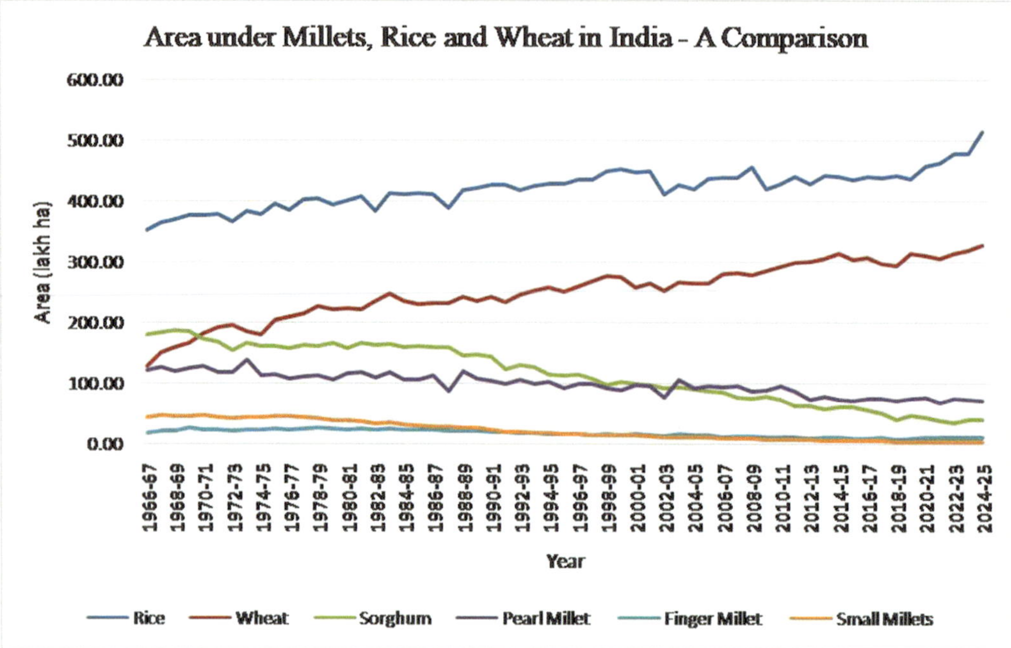

FIGURE 4.3 Area under millets, rice, and wheat in India. (Data source: Authors' computation based on GoI (2025).)

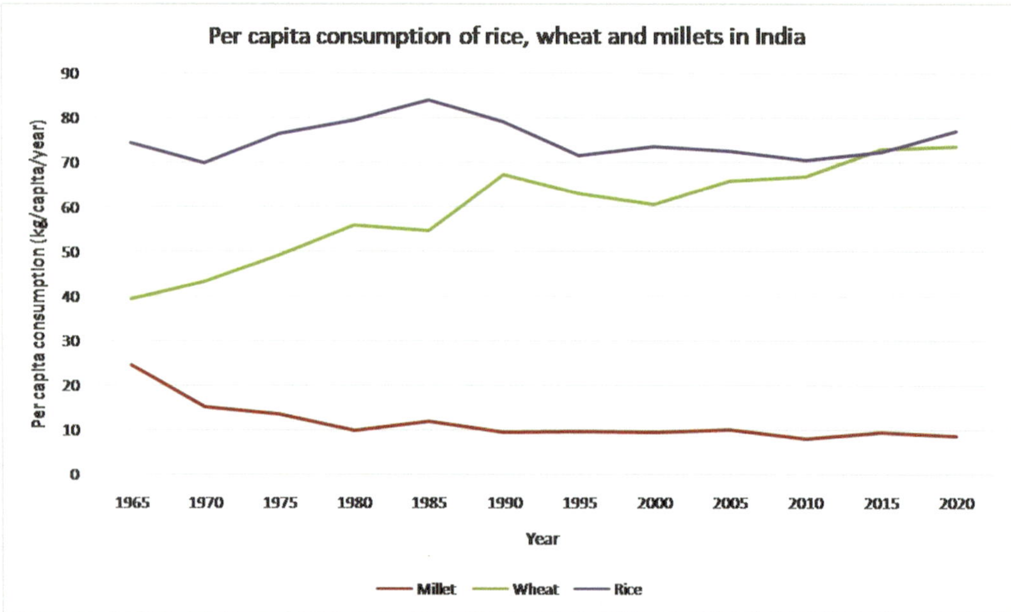

FIGURE 4.4 Annual per capita millet consumption (kg/capita/year) in India. (Data Source: Singh and Singh (2024).)

because of susceptibility to environmental conditions, as seen with kharif sorghum, reduced profitability and insufficient commercialization, lack of incentivization and government policies inclining to support irrigated crops with subsidies for inputs like irrigation and fertilisers. On the other hand, the demand-side factors include the challenging process of millet preparation due to lack of gluten, time-consuming millet preparation in contrast to the easily accessible fine cereal alternatives, evolution of consumer tastes and preferences towards tastier and more convenient foods, availability of fine cereals at subsidized prices, etc. Another demand-side factor is the limited awareness of the nutritional benefits of millets, although this is gradually improving through targeted campaigns and policy initiatives. With the scaling up of various initiatives (Annexure A1), availability of millets has shown improvement. However, an increase in their consumption remains a challenge.

4.3.1 Performance of Various Millets in India

This section discusses the decadal average of area, production, and yield of various millets in India for the post-Green Revolution period to the recent decade (1970–2019).

Figure 4.5 shows the scenario of millets during 1970–2019. The area under all the millets viz., sorghum, pearl millet, finger millet, and small millet decreased over the past five decades. Area under foodgrains which includes millets was gradually substituted by commercial crops as the importance of millets was diminishing. Meanwhile, the proportion of oilseeds and fruits and vegetables have risen during the same timeframe. This trend suggests that farmers are increasingly shifting towards more commercial crops like oilseeds, fruits, vegetables, and spices, from traditional staples (Majhi and Kumar 2018; Gulati and Juneja 2022). Particularly, in the post-Green Revolution period, the area under cultivation of nutri-cereals declined by 41.65% between 1950–51 and 2018–19 (Sukumaran Sreekala et al 2023).

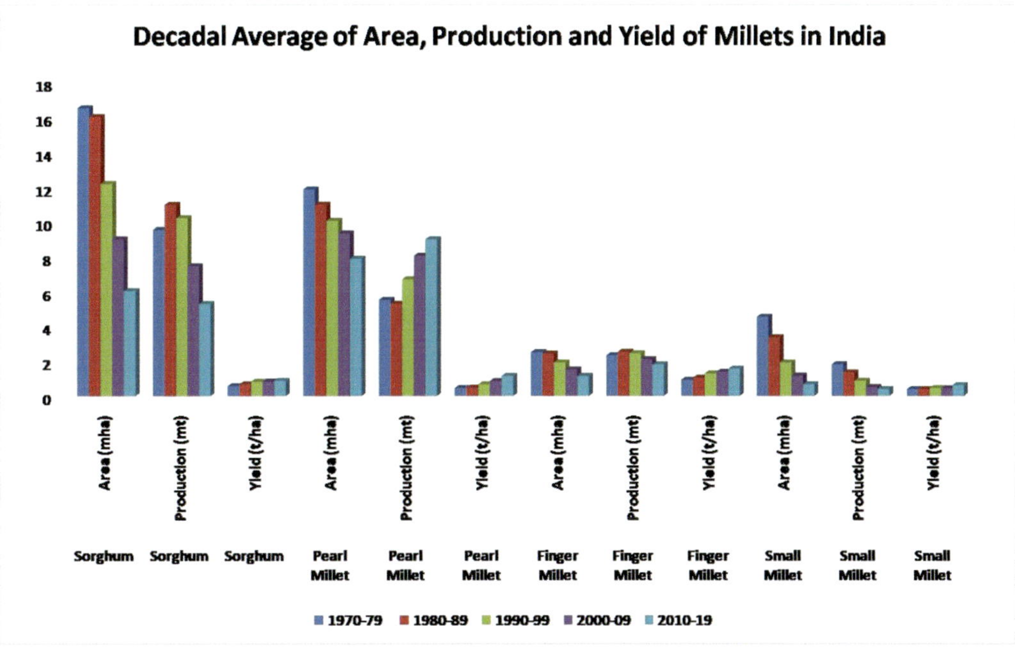

FIGURE 4.5 Decadal average of area, production, and yield of millets in India from 1970–79 to 2010–19. (Data Source: Authors' computation based on GoI (2025).)

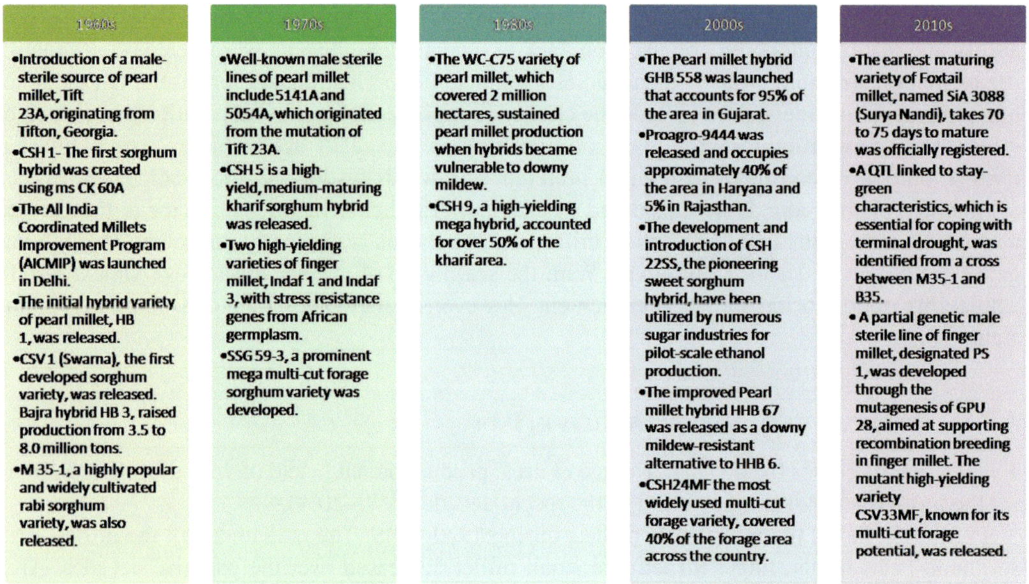

FIGURE 4.6 Key milestones in millet improvement. (Information source: Pathak et al (2022).)

Figure 4.5 also demonstrates the improvement in millet yield over the past five decades which may be attributed to the millet breeding initiatives. The milestones in the millet improvement are shown in Figure 4.6. Among the different types of millets, pearl millet has seen the highest number of varieties released. A total of 167 hybrids and 61 varieties have been identified and made available for cultivation through the ICAR-All India Co-ordinated Research Project (AICRP) on pearl millet. Regarding sorghum, 66 cultivars for grain production have been introduced since the launch of AICRP on sorghum. Between 1986 and 2016, approximately 54 ragi varieties were launched, while only 34 varieties of small millets were developed from 1999 to 2014 (including 9 for kodo millet, 6 for little millet, 5 for foxtail millet, 6 for barnyard millet, and 8 for proso millet) (Sukumaran Sreekala et al 2023; Aruna et al 2020; GoI 2014; Satyavathi et al 2018).

The introduced varieties show great potential for high yields. Nevertheless, their acceptance still poses a challenge, which is reflected in the declining trends of the acreage under most millets (Figure 4.6) and underlines importance of other initiatives aimed at increasing production of and demand for millets.

4.3.2 State-Wise Millets Scenario in India

In this section, we examine the current status of performance of millets in various states of India.

Small millets which include foxtail millet, proso millet, barnyard millet, kodo millet, and little millet show a more distributed cultivation pattern, with Madhya Pradesh emerging as the leader in recent years. The cultivation area in Madhya Pradesh grew significantly from 0.78 lakh ha in 2020–21 to peak at 1.45 lakh ha in 2022–23, before moderating to 1.06 lakh ha in 2024–25. Chhattisgarh shows a declining trend from 0.85 to 0.37 lakh ha.

Inefficiencies in millet cultivation distort input demand and cultivation costs, thereby discouraging millet cultivation. Technical efficiency which reflects a farming system's capacity to generate the highest possible output with a defined set of inputs or resources was reported to be a major challenge to attain with pearl millet farmers in Haryana, Gujarat, Rajasthan, Maharashtra, and Uttar Pradesh. The sorghum farmers have been found to face major inefficiencies especially in the states of Andhra Pradesh, Karnataka, Madhya Pradesh, Maharashtra, Rajasthan, and Tamil Nadu. On

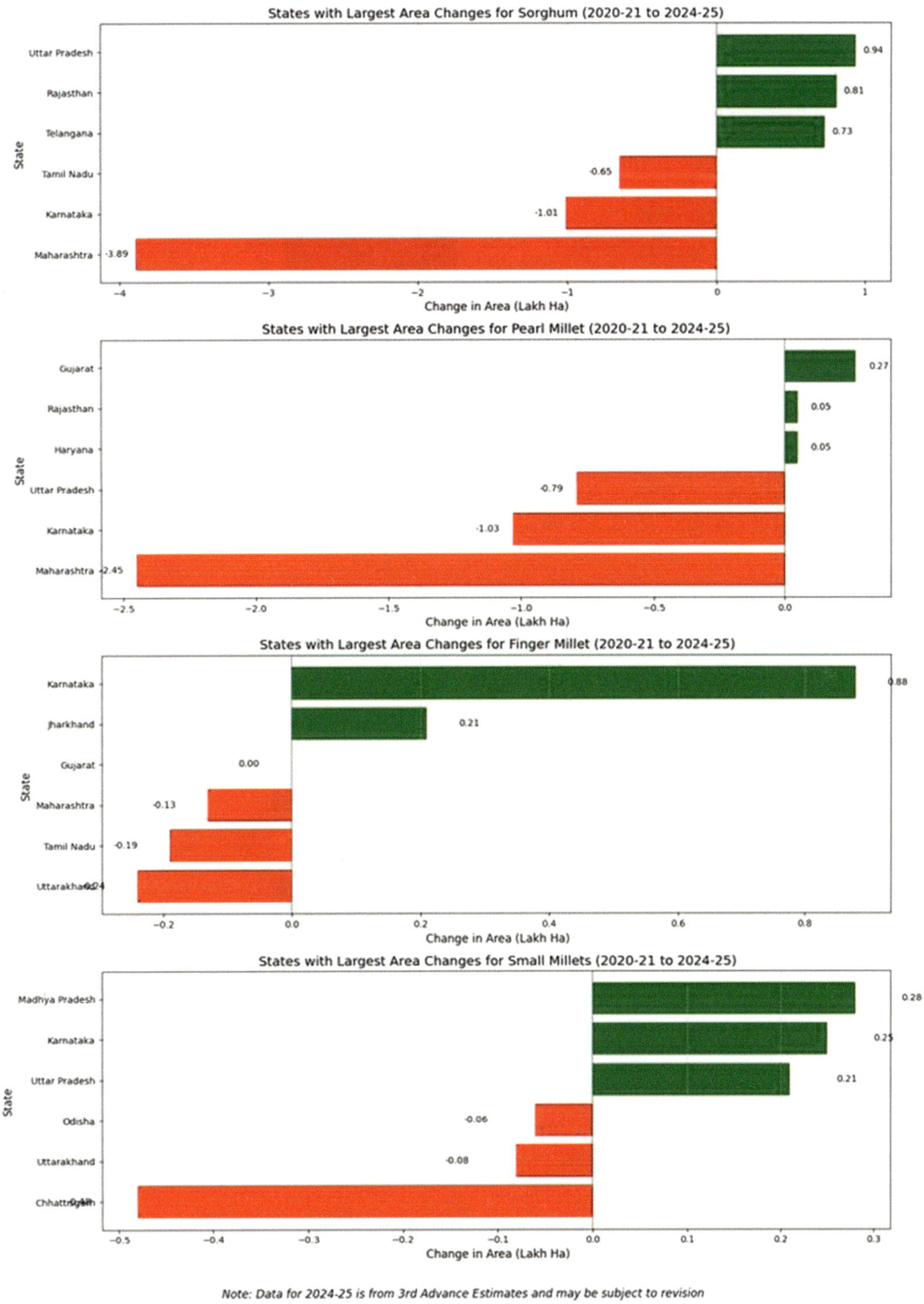

FIGURE 4.7 States with the largest absolute increases and decreases in millets area under the current scenario (2020–21 to 2024–25).

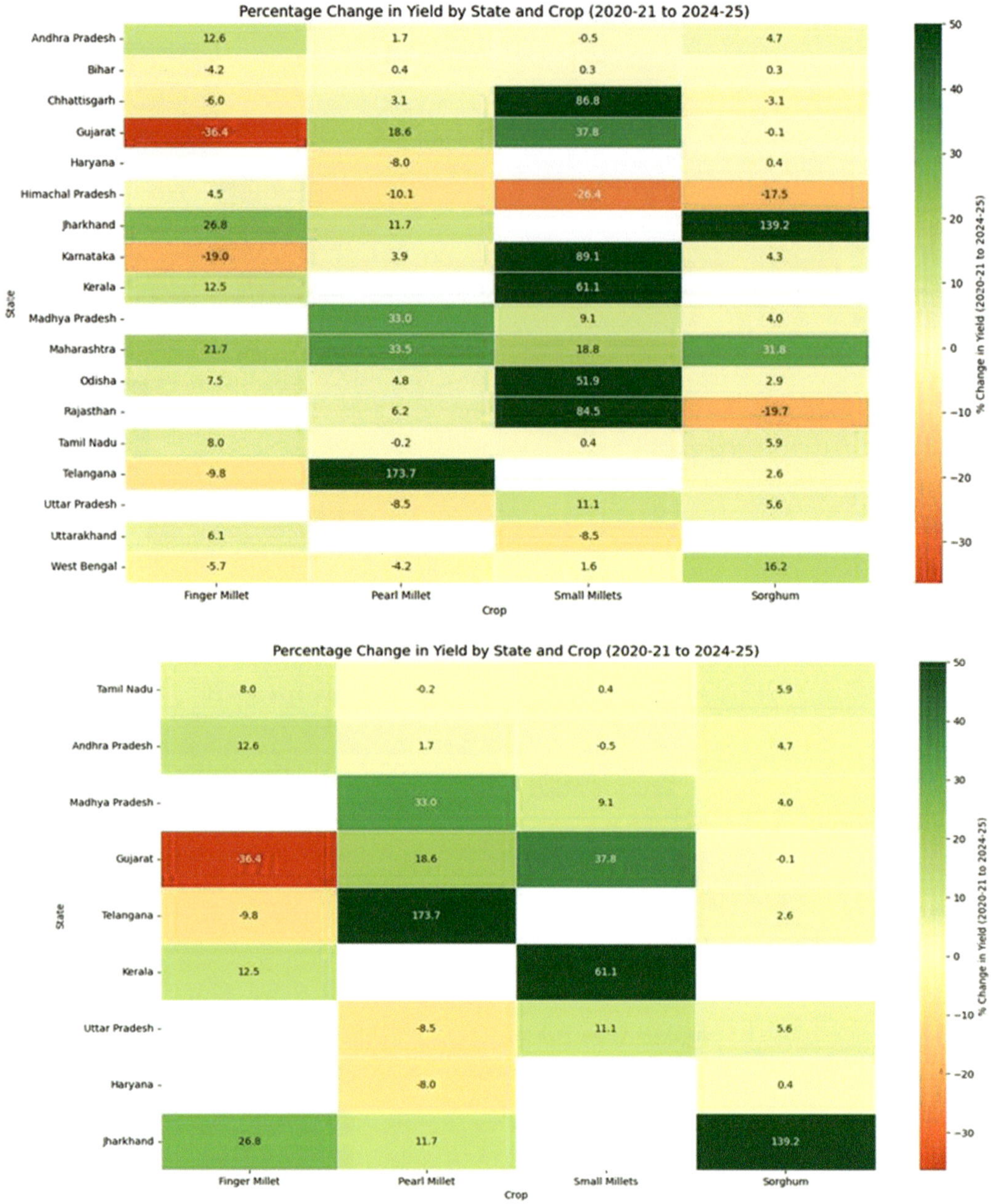

FIGURE 4.8 Percentage change in millet yield in various states under the current scenario (2020–21 to 2024–25).

the other hand, Karnataka and Odisha efficiently produce ragi (Felix et al 2024). As perceived by farmers participating in the historic Odisha Millets Mission, production and marketed surplus of millets increased as a result of area expansion and agronomic interventions and knowledge received through extension training (Jena and Mishra, 2025). Allocative efficiency which refers to the optimal distribution of resources across various production activities to maximize output remains a challenge to attain as animal, machine labour and fertilisers are over-utilized in pearl millet cultivation, while the same inputs are under-utilized in sorghum and finger millet cultivation (Felix et al 2024).

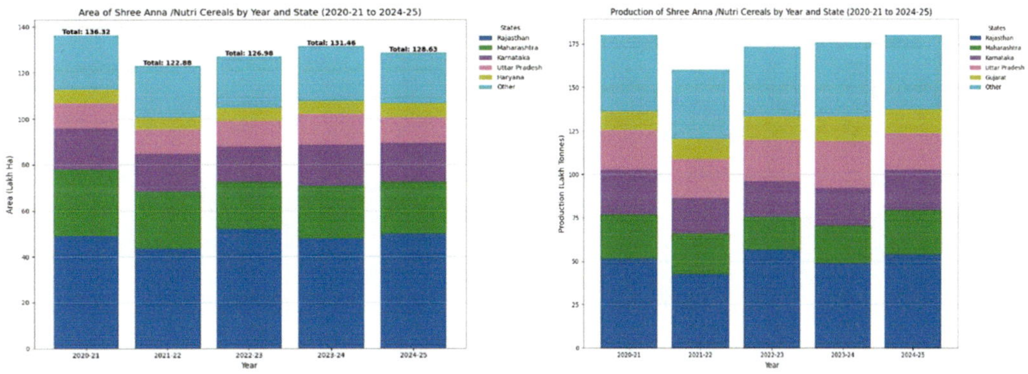

FIGURE 4.9 Area and production of nutri cereals in major states under the current scenario (2020–21 to 2024–25).

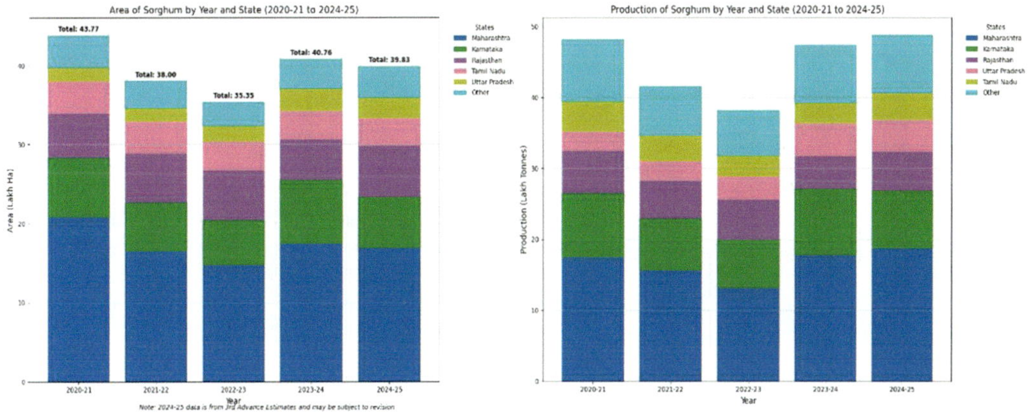

FIGURE 4.10 Area and production of sorghum in major states under the current scenario (2020–21 to 2024–25).

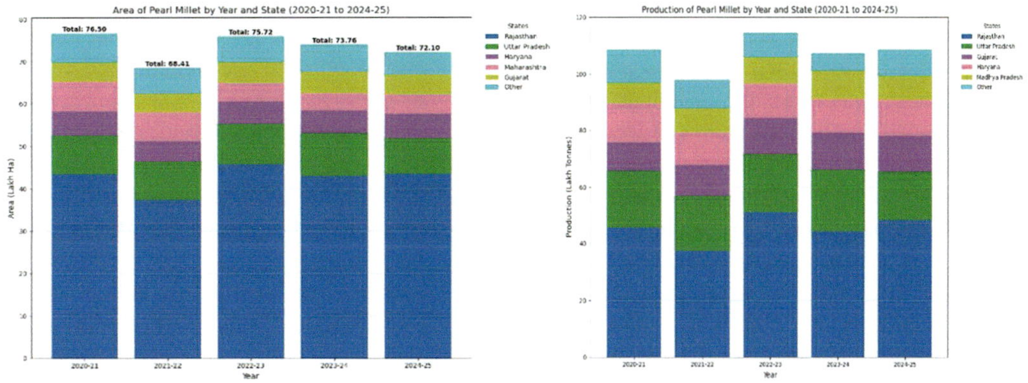

FIGURE 4.11 Area and production of pearl millet in major states under the current scenario (2020–21 to 2024–25).

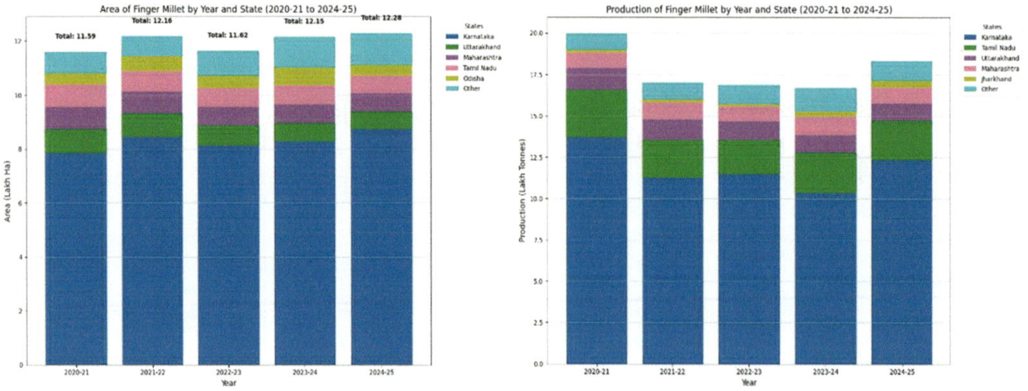

FIGURE 4.12 Area and production of finger millet in major states under the current scenario (2020–21 to 2024–25).

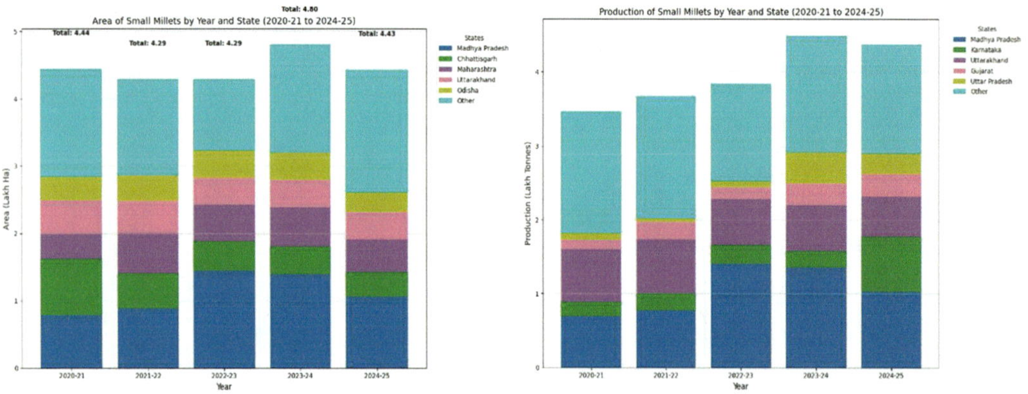

FIGURE 4.13 Area and production of small millet in major states under the current scenario (2020–21 to 2024–25). (Data Source: Authors' computation based on GoI (2025).)

4.4 MILLET VALUE CHAINS: ISSUES AND CHALLENGES

A value chain is a sequence of business operations that accounts for and displays the value created in a product or service from a specific input until it reaches the final consumption. The analysis of the value chain, which examines the journey from input to finished product through various intermediaries, is known as value chain analysis (McKay et al 1997). Value chain analysis consists of identifying and outlining the connections among four categories of characteristics: (1) the tasks carried out at each stage of the processing or product flow; (2) the value of inputs, time taken for processing, outputs, and the subsequent value addition; (3) the spatial dynamics, such as distances and logistics associated with the activities; and (4) the composition of economic agents, including suppliers, producers, and wholesalers (Rao 2019; Rao et al 2021b).

The millet value chains in India have several gaps such as the lack of dedicated supply chains connecting smallholders to market outlets, which necessitates enhancements in logistics infrastructure and supply chain management practices. There is a deficiency in both backward and forward linkages from conservation and production to consumption of millets. Despite the traditional recognition of millets for various end uses, there is a shortfall in efforts to specify end use–specific genotypes. In addition, the unavailability of efficient machinery for the primary processing of millets is leading to increased processing costs and inferior quality end products.

There is a shortage of suitable technologies for value addition in millets, and due to the absence of gluten, processing millets poses challenges. Acceptable value-added health food products made from millets are lacking in both domestic and international markets for enhancing the quality of life. Furthermore, there is no established processing protocol or machinery designed to enhance nutraceuticals for health benefits. The lack of standard guidelines for grains, their products, and processing technologies is also evident (Rao et al 2021a).

Moreover, there is a scarcity of sustainable and profitable business opportunities in the millet sector. There is a paucity of suitable market strategies aimed at generating demand for value-added products for startups in this area. This calls for greater policy support for millets, addressing both supply-side and demand-side challenges (Rao et al 2021a).

The millet value chain demonstrates strengths, weaknesses, opportunities, as well as challenges (Muskan et al 2025; Banu et al 2022; Poshadri et al 2023; Gupta et al 2024). The strengths lie in the nutritional benefits of millets and resilience to drought. However, it also faces weaknesses such as limitations in processing capabilities, unreliable supply, and weak market connections. There are opportunities arising from the increasing global demand and government initiatives promoting climate-resilient crops. On the other hand, challenges include competition from conventional cereals and insufficient infrastructure. To unlock the potential of the millet value chain, particularly in boosting farmers' income through value addition, it is crucial to tackle the weaknesses and capitalize on opportunities.

4.5 INITIATIVES TO STRENGTHEN DEMAND AND SUPPLY SIDES OF MILLET VALUE CHAINS

Acknowledging the challenges associated with demand and supply of millets, current policy conversations highlight the critical need to reinstate millets into the public procurement process and strengthen the supply chains (Figure 4.14). By implementing structured incentives, it is anticipated that farmers will alter their cropping patterns to support a more balanced food system. An examination of the reports of the Commission for Agricultural Costs and Prices (CACP) shows that the net returns over and above costs incurred in the case of jowar, bajra, and ragi were substantially lower than other kharif crops such as not only rice and wheat but also pulses and oilseeds in the last two

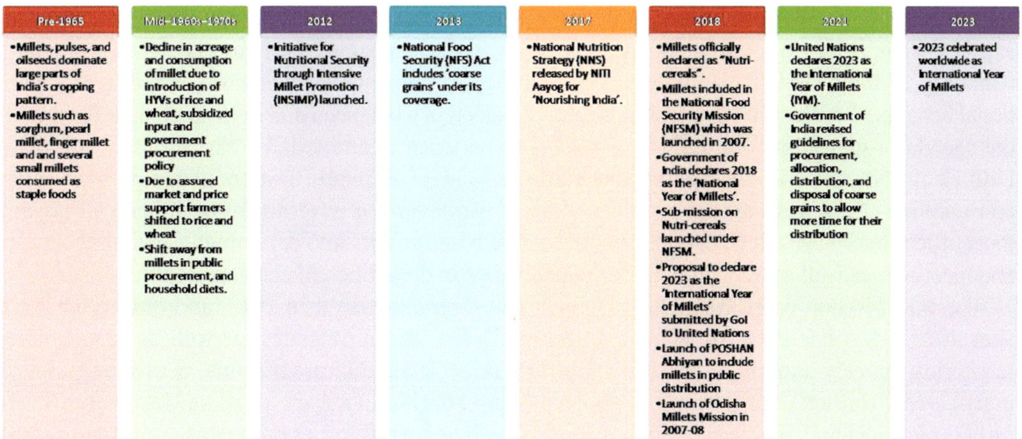

FIGURE 4.14 Timeline of historical events relevant to millet production and consumption in India. (Information source: Based on information provided in Shah and Vijayshankar (2022) and NITI Aayog (2023).)

to three years. This, therefore, underlines the need to reduce costs of production and ensure a higher relative price for these crops, which would encourage the producers to increase their supply.

A significant use for the procured millets could be within the Integrated Child Development Services (ICDS) and the Pradhan Mantri Poshan Shakti Nirman Yojana (PM POSHAN Scheme), as well as through the Public Distribution System (PDS), in accordance with the Government of India's POSHAN Abhiyaan nutrition initiative (Shah and Vijayshankar 2022).

In light of the potential nutritional benefits of millets for public health, the Government of India designated millets as nutri-cereals and recognized the year 2018 as the National Year of Millets. India also submitted a proposal to the United Nations General Assembly (UNGA) to declare an International Year of Millets (IYM), receiving support from approximately 70 countries, which led to the UNGA passing a resolution to commemorate 2023 as the IYM.

According to PIB (2024), under IYM, 2023, the Government of India adopted a multi-stakeholder engagement approach for enhancing production and productivity, consumption, export, strengthening of the millet value chain, branding and creating awareness for health benefits. The multi-stakeholder engagement involved various stakeholders such as various ministries/departments of the central government, governments of states/UTs, farmers, startups, exporters, retail businesses, hotels, Indian embassies, etc.

Under IYM, the Government of India organized a people's movement to promote Indian millets, recipes, and value-added products internationally. Millets were promoted globally during the G20 Presidency in India, the ASEAN India Millet Festival in Indonesia and Delhi, the Millet Culinary Carnival, International Trade Events, the Chef's Conference, the Farmers Producer Organizations (FPO) exhibition, road shows, kisan melas, and chef training for paramilitary forces, among other events. Notable events during IYM included Global Millets (Shree Anna Conference), the declaration of the Indian Institute of Millets Research (IIMR), Hyderabad as the Global Centre of Excellence for sharing research, technology, and best practices at national and international levels, the inauguration of the Regional Research Centre for Bajra at Gudamalani, Rajasthan, and the adoption of the Millets and Other Ancient Grains International Research Initiative (MAHARISHI) to strengthen research collaboration and public awareness of millets during the G20 Presidency. Besides these initiatives, Production Linked Incentive Scheme for Food Processing Industry for Millet-Based Products (PLISMBP) is also introduced for the period 2022–23 to 2026–27. Millets are now included under Poshan Abhiyan of the Ministry of Women and Child Development and procurement of millets is increased under the Targeted PDS (TPDS), ICDS, and Mid-Day Meal Scheme.

An Export Promotion Forum, specifically dedicated to enhancing the international market presence of millets, has been established with the objective of facilitating their promotion, marketing, and export development from India. As part of the Eat Right campaign, the Food Safety and Standards Authority of India (FSSAI) is undertaking initiatives to raise public awareness regarding the nutritional benefits of millets and to encourage their inclusion in a balanced and diversified diet. Furthering the agenda of mainstreaming millets, a Millets Experience Centre (MEC) has been inaugurated at Dilli Haat, INA, New Delhi, serving as a platform to increase public awareness and promote millet consumption. Also, to foster the adoption of Shree Anna among government personnel, all government offices have been advised to incorporate millet-based snacks into departmental training sessions and meetings, as well as to include millet-based dishes in departmental canteen menus.

The Sub-Mission on NFSM–Nutri Cereals was operationalized in 2018, and during the fiscal year 2023–24, it has been implemented across all districts in 28 states, as well as in two union territories, namely Jammu & Kashmir and Ladakh. Under this programme, a diverse range of nutri-cereals (millets) are promoted, encompassing sorghum (jowar), pearl millet (bajra), finger millet (ragi/mandua), and various minor millets such as foxtail millet (kangani/kakun), proso millet (cheena), kodo millet (kodo), barnyard millet (sawa/sanwa/jhangora), and little millet (kutki). In addition to it, two pseudo-millets—buckwheat (kuttu) and Amaranthus (chaulai)—are included under the ambit of the NFSM initiative.

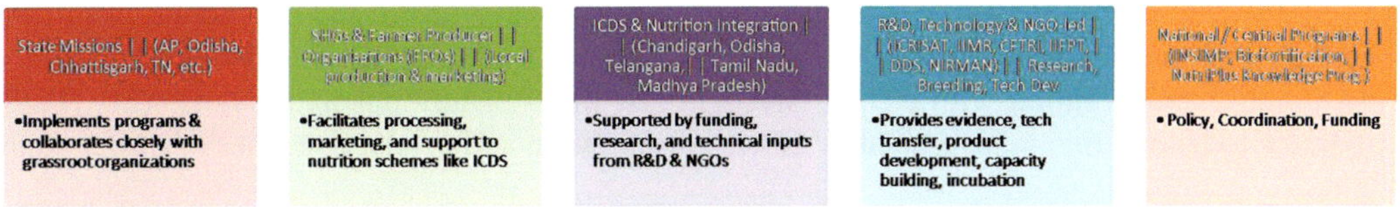

FIGURE 4.15 Roles of various constituent organizations in millet initiative. (Information Source: NITI Aayog (2023).)

Under the NFSM–Nutri Cereals initiative, incentives are offered to farmers via the states/UTs focusing on crop production and protection technologies, demonstrations based on cropping systems, the production and distribution of certified seeds from newly released varieties or hybrids, Integrated Nutrient and Pest Management practices, enhanced agricultural tools and equipment, water conservation devices, and the capacity building of farmers through training during the cropping season. In addition, events and workshops are organized, seed minikits are distributed, and publicity is conducted through print and electronic media, among other activities.

States can promote millet cultivation under the Rashtriya Krishi Vikas Yojana (RKVY) to address state-specific needs and priorities. Several states, including Assam, Bihar, Chhattisgarh, Karnataka, Madhya Pradesh, Maharashtra, Odisha, Rajasthan, Tamil Nadu, Uttarakhand, and Uttar Pradesh, have launched millet missions to promote the production and consumption of millets (PIB 2024).

Various state governments have launched state-level millet missions to boost acreage, production, and yield of millets in collaboration with R&D institutions, NGOs, self-help groups (SHGs)/FPOs (Figure 4.15). State missions implement programmes and collaborate with SHGs/FPOs. SHGs and FPOs facilitate millet production, processing, marketing, and support nutrition schemes. ICDS and Nutrition Integration programmes work closely with SHGs/FPOs and are supported by R&D/national programmes. R&D, technology, and NGOs provide scientific research, breeding, technology, incubation, and capacity building. National/central programmes provide policy framework, funding, and coordination. A summary of initiatives (state or central) is given in Annexure A1. The missions have been instrumental in increasing area, production, and yield of millets across various states as well as in improving food security status as mentioned in Annexure A1. Odisha Millets Mission launched in 2017 served as a flag bearer as it focused simultaneously on production, processing, marketing, consumption, and inclusion of millets in government schemes. Its success called for a nation-wide "policy for millets" to replicate the decentralized and historically successful Odisha Millets Mission in all the states (Raina et al 2022). The millet-related interventions led to an increase in the millet production and consumption, notably, in the tribal areas of Andhra Pradesh and Madhya Pradesh. Specifically, in Nagaland, the millet initiatives led to increased awareness, resulting in the adoption of improved millet production practices and the conservation of millet seeds. Especially in Odisha, more than 250 SHGs were trained in millet recipes that eventually led to an increase in the millet demand. In Tamil Nadu, the millet initiatives led to a doubling of the area under millets. In Chhattisgarh, the initiatives led to improvement in the malnutrition status.

4.6 CONCLUSION

Millets are recognized as Shree Anna/nutri-cereals because of their multifarious benefits and historical significance. The chapter explored strengths and weaknesses of demand and supply sides of millet value chains. With the advent of the Green Revolution, millets were obscured as the area under rice and wheat increased due to preferential policy initiatives and incentivization for the area expansion under rice and paddy. This was accompanied by assured procurement, as rice and wheat were included in the PDS. Recently, as 2018 was recognized as the National Year of Millets and 2023 as the IYM, the policies were reshaped to favour the production of millets and their inclusion in diets. Various initiatives, which involved national mission, state missions, and regional collaboration with NGOs, SHGs/FPOs, R&D institutions and inclusion in TPDS, are likely to lead to the improvement in millet consumption and production sides of millet value chains.

REFERENCES

Aggarwal, P., Roy, J., Pathak, H., Kumar, S. N., Venkateswarlu, B., & Ghosh, A. 2022. Managing climatic risks in agriculture. *Indian agriculture towards 2030: Pathways for enhancing Farmers' income, nutritional security and sustainable food and farm systems.* 83–108. https://doi.org/10.1007/978-981-19-0763-0

Aruna, C., Deepika, C., Raghavendra Rao, K. V., & Vilas, A. T. 2020. Golden Jubilee Publication: 50 years of Sorghum Research: Contribution of AICRP-Sorghum Centres, ICAR-Indian Institute of Millets Research, Hyderabad-500 030, Telangana, India. https://www.millets.res.in/pub/2020/GoldenJubileePublication_50Years_of_Publication.pdf

Arya, C., & Bisht, A. 2022. Nutritional profile of small millets. In *Small Millet Grains: The Superfoods in Human Diet.* Singapore: Springer Nature Singapore. 15–47. https://doi.org/10.1007/978-981-16-9306-9

Banu, A., Ganapathy, M. S., Govinda Gowda, V., Girish, M., Begum, S., & Kumar, T. M. 2022. Value chain analysis of minor millets for improving economic status of farmers in Tumakuru district of Karnataka. *Mysore Journal of Agricultural Sciences*, *56*(4).

Bisht, A., Joshi, S., & Srivastava, S. 2022. Small millets: An overview. *Small Millet Grains: The Superfoods in Human Diet*, 1–13. https://doi.org/10.1007/978-981-16-9306-9

Brown, R. H. 1999. Agronomic implications of C4 photosynthesis. *C4 Plant Biology*, *1*, 473–507.

FAO (Food and Agriculture Organization). 2023. www.fao.org/faostat/. Accessed on 3 August 2025.

Felix, K. T., Ramappa, K. B., & Govindarajan, P. L. 2024. Strategies to scale up the technical, allocative and economic efficiency of major millet growing farmers in India–A primal system approach. *Environmental and Sustainability Indicators*, 24, 100493. https://www.sciencedirect.com/science/article/pii/S2665972724001612

GoI (Government of India). 2014. Status paper on coarse cereals (Sorghum, Pearl Millet, Finger Millet, Small Millets, Maize and Barley). Directorate of millets development, Department of Agriculture and Cooperation, Ministry of Agriculture, Government of India. https://www.nfsm.gov.in/StatusPaper/StatusMillets2016.pdf. Accessed 3 September 2021.

GoI (Government of India). 2025. Unified Portal for Agricultural Statistics (UPAg) dataset. www.upag.gov.in. Accessed on 1 September 2025.

Gulati, A., & Juneja, R. 2022. Transforming Indian agriculture. *Indian agriculture towards 2030: Pathways for enhancing Farmers' income, nutritional security and sustainable food and farm systems.* 9–37. https://doi.org/10.1007/978-981-19-0763-0

Gupta, H., Panigrahi, T., Patle, U., Pandre, E., Singh, T., & Shweta, K. 2024. Revitalizing millets for nutritional security & fortifying food and uplifting small and marginal farmers in India: A review. *International Journal of Environment and Climate Change*, *14*(1): 14–26. https://journalijecc.com/index.php/IJECC/article/view/3789

Jena, D., & Mishra, S. 2025. Production gains and marketed surplus of finger millet: Sustainable lessons for the Global South. *International Social Science Journal.* https://doi.org/10.1111/issj.12584

Majhi, B., & Kumar, A. 2018. Changing cropping pattern in Indian agriculture. *Journal of Economic and Social Development*, *14*(1), 37–45.

McKay, A., Morrissey, O., & Vaillant, C. 1997. Trade liberalisation and agricultural supply response: Issues and some lessons. *The European Journal of Development Research*, *9*(2), 129–147. https://doi.org/10.1080/09578819708426693

Muskan, F., Redhu, M., Redhu, S., & Rahimi, M. 2025. Millets in the global market: A critical review of challenges and opportunities. *Food Production, Processing and Nutrition*, *7*(1), 37. https://doi.org/10.1186/s43014-025-00316-1

NITI Aayog. 2023. Promoting millets in diets: Best practices across states/UTs of India. *National Institution for Transforming India, New Delhi.* https://www.niti.gov.in/sites/default/files/2024-07/Report-on-Promoting-Best-practices-on-Millet-26_4_23.pdf

NITI Aayog. 2024. Working group report on crop husbandry, agriculture inputs, demand and supply. *National Institution for Transforming India (NITI Aayog), Government of India, New Delhi.* https://www.niti.gov.in/sites/default/files/2024-02/Working%20Group%20Report%20on%20Demand%20%26%20Supply%20Final_V9.pdf

Pathak, H., Mishra, J. P., & Mohapatra, T. 2022. Indian agriculture after independence. *Indian Council of Agricultural Research, New Delhi, 110*(001), 426. https://www.icar.org.in/sites/default/files/2023-02/Indian-Agriculture-after-Independence.pdf

Piara Singh, P., Boote, K. J., Kadiyala, M. D. M., Nedumaran, S., Gupta, S. K., Srinivas, K., & Bantilan, M. C. S. 2017. An assessment of yield gains under climate change due to genetic modification of pearl millet. *Science of the Total Environment, 601*, 1226–1237. https://doi.org/10.1016/j.scitotenv.2017.06.002

PIB. 2024. Cultivation of different types of millets. *Press Information Bureau (PIB), Delhi.* https://www.pib.gov.in/PressReleaseIframePage.aspx?PRID=2004510)

Poshadri, A., Deshpande, H. W., & Kshirsagar, R. B. 2023. The international year of millets-2023, millets as nutri-cereals of 21st centenary for health and wellness. *Agriculture Association of Textile Chemical and Critical Reviews Journal, 7.*

Raina, R., Mishra, S., Ravindra, A., Balam, D., & Gunturu, A. 2022. Reorienting India's agricultural policy: Millets and institutional change for sustainability. *Journal of Ecological Society, 34*(1), 1–15. https://doi.org/10.54081/JES.028/01

Rao, B. D. 2019. Sorghum value chain for food and fodder security. In *Breeding Sorghum for Diverse End Uses.* Woodhead Publishing. 409–419. https://doi.org/10.1016/B978-0-08-101879-8.00023-1

Rao, B. D., Bhandari, R., & Tonapi, V. A. 2021a. White paper on millets–A policy note on mainstreaming millets for nutrition security. *ICAR-Indian Institute of Millets Research (IIMR)*, Rajendranagar, Hyderabad. https://www.nutrihubiimr.com/_files/ugd/364c6c_0a449b26cbdc423b80f5b0d8ea23bc65.pdf

Rao, D. B., Bhat, V., Niranjan, T., Sujatha, M., & Tonapi, V. A. 2021b. Demand creation measures and value chain model on millets in India. In *Millets and Millet Technology.* Singapore: Springer Singapore. 381–411. https://doi.org/10.1007/978-981-16-0676-2_20

Satyavathi, C. T., Khandelwal, V., Rajpurohit, B. S., Supriya, A., Beniwal, B. R., Kamlesh, K., Sushila, B., Shripal, S., Mahesh, C. K., & Yadav, S. L. 2018. Pearl millet-hybrids and varieties. *ICAR-All India Coordinated Project on Pearl millet, Mandor, Jodhpur India, 142.* https://www.millets.res.in/technologies/finger_millets_varieties.pdf Accessed 2 May 2025.

Shah, M., & Vijayshankar, P. S. 2022. Symbiosis of water and agricultural transformation in India. *Indian agriculture towards 2030: Pathways for enhancing Farmers' income, nutritional security and sustainable food and farm systems.* 109–152. https://doi.org/10.1007/978-981-19-0763-0

Singh, B., Rastogi, R., Singh, B., Kaur, H., Singh, R., Dubey, R., Jagriti, & Tyagi, T. 2025. Shri-Anna (millets), super food for present epoch: A thoughtful study in diverse dimensions. *International Journal of Bioinformatics Research and Applications, 21*(2), 185–217. https://doi.org/10.1504/IJBRA.2025.145110

Singh, O. P., & Singh, P. K. 2024. Trends in millets production, consumption and export from India. *The Journal of Research ANGRAU, 52*(1). 121–133. https://doi.org/10.58537/jorangrau.2024.52.1.14

Sukumaran Sreekala, A. D., Anbukkani, P., Singh, A., Dayakar Rao, B., & Jha, G. K., 2023. Millet production and consumption in India: Where do we stand and where do we go?. *National Academy Science Letters, 46*(1). 65–70. https://doi.org/10.1007/s40009-022-01164-0

Vidhya, R., & Pragasan, L. A. 2022. Age effects of millet crops on phytolith carbon sequestration. *Applied Ecology and Environmental Sciences, 10*(12), 747–753. https://doi.org/10.12691/aees-10-12-7

Annexure A

TABLE A1
Summary of Initiatives to Increase Production/Consumption of Millets in Various States of India

S. No.	Initiative Name	State/Org and Type of Initiative	Type	Summary of the Initiative	Key Impact(s)
1	Comprehensive Revival of Millets Cultivation by Tribals in North Coastal Areas and Parts of Rayalaseema, Andhra Pradesh	Implemented by the State Government of Andhra Pradesh	State Mission	End-to-end millet revival in North Coastal and Rayalaseema tribal areas through establishment of Millet Hubs	Production increased to 2.35 lakh quintals; 28,000 acres under millet; 1 lakh households improved millet consumption
2	Andhra Pradesh Drought Mitigation Project (APDMP)	Andhra Pradesh Government and IFAD-funded programme with involvement of FPOs	State Mission	Strengthen drought resilience in 315 Gram Panchayats, crop diversification to millets, introduction of improved Package of Practices (PoPs) for foxtail/brown top/little millet	Millet area increased by 44%; local processing units; market linkages with buyers
3	Chhattisgarh Millet Mission	State Mission by the Government of Chhattisgarh	State Mission	Make state "Millet Hub"; focus on kodo, little millet, finger millet with MSP, processing units, inclusion in PDS/MDM/ICDS	Target to triple millet area; centre of excellence establishment, MSP: Rs. 30–33/kg
4	Bhavantar Bharpayee Yojana	Haryana: A scheme for Price Support	Price Support	Price deficiency payment up to Rs. 600/q for bajra if private buyers pay less than MSP.	Protected farmer incomes; encouraged bajra cultivation
5	INSIMP (Initiative for Nutritional Security through Intensive Millets Promotion): National Initiative by the Ministry of Agriculture and Farmers Welfare	MoA&FW (16 states)	National Mission	Seed production, processing units, demos, awareness	7.7 lakh ha covered; Increased productivity; centres of excellence established under this project
6	Promoting Kodo and Little Millets	Madhya Pradesh Government and a non-profit organization, Action for Social Advancement (ASA)	State + NGO	Support tribal women in Mandla/Dindori via dehulling units, etc.	Consumption and production of little millets improved in the tribal districts of Mandla and Dindori

(Continued)

TABLE A1 (Continued)
Summary of Initiatives to Increase Production/Consumption of Millets in Various States of India

S. No.	Initiative Name	State/Org and Type of Initiative	Type	Summary of the Initiative	Key Impact(s)
7	NFSM–Nutri Cereals Mission	Nagaland	State/NFSM	Foxtail millet promotion with training, seed prod., INM/IPM	Increased awareness; adoption of improved practices and seed conservation
8	Odisha Millets Mission (OMM)	Odisha	State Mission	Revive millets on farms/ plates; production, processing, marketing, govt. scheme inclusion	54 k/ha covered; doubled yields and incomes; ragi in PDS/ICDS; millet cafés, FPOs
9	Taptapani FPO	Odisha (Gajapati)	FPO	Strengthen marketing, inputs, reduce distress migration	699 members, 1400 qtl ragi procured; best FPO award
10	OMM–SHG Mission Shakti Convergence	Odisha	Convergence	SHGs trained in modern millet recipes; cafés, tiffin centres	262 SHGs trained; urban/rural millet demand increased
11	Tamil Nadu Millets Mission	Tamil Nadu	State Mission	Demo farms, input kits, training, mini mills	Doubled millet area; soil health increased; coarse cereals award
12	Mission on Sustainable Dry Land Agriculture (MSDA)	Tamil Nadu	State Mission	25 lakh acre dryland dev., millet/pulses/oilseed focus	Area increased; 174 value-added units; 801 custom hiring centres
13	Organic Production and Certification of Millets	Uttarakhand	Organic Farming	Cluster-based organic millet cultivation and certification	1.16 lakh/ha organic; 20–30% premium prices; 430 outlets planned
14	Procurement and Processing for Value Addition	Uttarakhand (UCF)	Procurement + Processing	Collection centres, assured buyback, multigrain processing unit	131.2 MT procured in pilot; better market reach
15	Inclusion of Millets in Take Home Ration	Chandigarh	ICDS Inclusion	Bajra/jowar in THR for 450 AWCs	Increased awareness and millet consumption among beneficiaries
16	Ragi in Supplementary Nutrition Prog.	Chhattisgarh	ICDS Inclusion	Ragi halwa/kodo-kutki khichdi for children, women	Awareness increased; improved malnutrition convergence
17	Kodo-Kutki in ICDS (Tejaswini Prog.)	Madhya Pradesh	ICDS Inclusion	Millet snacks and THR by SHGs in Dindori/ Mandla	Net income per farmer increased by 9 times; 16,289 farmers involved
18	Ragi Laddu in ICDS	Odisha (Keonjhar, Sundargarh)	ICDS Inclusion	Ragi laddus by SHGs as morning snack	1.4 lakh children reached; community acceptance high

(Continued)

TABLE A1 *(Continued)*
Summary of Initiatives to Increase Production/Consumption of Millets in Various States of India

S. No.	Initiative Name	State/Org and Type of Initiative	Type	Summary of the Initiative	Key Impact(s)
19	Local Traditional Recipes in ICDS	Tamil Nadu	ICDS Inclusion	Weaning food with malted/roasted ragi	3.27M beneficiaries; women-run coops produce food
20	Millets in ICDS	Telangana (Vikarabad, Adilabad)	ICDS Inclusion	Community-selected millet recipes, training	Regular millet meals; market ecosystem created
21	Giri Poshana/ Nutri-Food Basket	Telangana + ICRISAT	ICDS Inclusion	Sorghum/millet products for tribal ITDA areas	Decrease in stunting by 39%, wasting by 16%, anaemia by 41%
22	Decentralized Millet Meals in ICDS	Telangana (3 districts) + NITI Aayog	ICDS Inclusion	Local procurement, SHG/ FPO processing	94k beneficiaries; millets back in 1000 acres
23	Sorghum in Rice Fallows	ICAR-IIMR	R&D	PoP for sorghum under zero till in rice fallows	Yields increased to 7.7–8.6 MT/ha; 77% higher net returns
24	Nutrihub-TBI	ICAR-IIMR	Incubation	Millet startup incubation, tech transfer	185 startups; 170 tech transfers; 60+ products
25	Sweet Sorghum for Ethanol	ICRISAT + IIMR	R&D	Use sweet sorghum for ethanol blending	Varieties identified; mill tests successful
26	IIFPT Millet Mission	IIFPT	R&D + Product Dev	Millet-based foods, processing tech	120 trainings, 20+ entrepreneurs; 900 trainees
27	NutriPlus Knowledge Prog.	ICRISAT-AIP	R&D + Product Dev	Millet RTC/RTE tech, value-added products	20 millet product techs commercialized
28	Pearl Millet Hybrid Parents Consortium	ICRISAT	Breeding	Public–private improved parent lines	India's Pearl millet yield increased by 73%; hybrids based on consortium lines
29	Bio-fortified Millet and Sorghum	ICRISAT + ICAR-IIMR	Breeding	High Fe/Zn cultivars and value chains	100k+ farmers; school meal growth (50%)
30	Science-based Evidence on Millets	ICRISAT and partners	Research	Meta-analyses on health benefits	Millets decrease blood glucose (12–15%), increase Hb (13%)
31	Community Gene Fund/Seed Bank	DDS	Community Conservation	Women-led indigenous millet seed banks	85 varieties conserved; 1500 households self-sufficient
32	Shelf-stable Sorghum Flour	CFTRI	Processing Tech	Extend jowar flour shelf-life to 6–8 month	Tech commercialized to 6 entrepreneurs
33	Mechanized Processing Unit	NIRMAN (Odisha)	Processing Tech	Solar-powered millet dehusking	50 villages served; millet rice fetches double price
34	Improved Milling for Small Millets	CSIR-CFTRI	Processing Tech	Replace abrasive w/ impact dehuller	Yield increased by 2–3%, breakage reduced

Source: Authors' presentation based on NITI Aayog (2023).

5 Millet-Based Nutrition for Infants

A Healthy Start

Surabhi Singh Yadav
Nutrition and Dietetics Program, Symbiosis School of Culinary Arts and Nutritional Sciences (SSCANS), Symbiosis International (Deemed University) (SIU), Pune, Maharashtra, India

5.1 INTRODUCTION TO MILLETS

Millets encompass a diverse group of ancient crops that thrive well in arid and semi-arid conditions as rain-fed crops, under marginal conditions of soil fertility and water scarcity (Sabuz et al 2023). Millets are deeply rooted in ancient cultures and have contributed to the food security and nutrition of vulnerable populations such as infants. Millets rightly dignified as "nutri-cereals" are small-seeded annual grasses belonging to the Poaceae family (Sabuz et al 2023; Amadou et al 2013). They are popularly known as "mota annaj," "nutri-cereals," "coarse cereals," "cereals of the poor" and most recently as "Shree Ann – the mother of all grains" (Jain et al 2024).

Infancy is defined as a developmental stage from birth to two years of life marked with rapid physical and cognitive development. The nutrient demands of infants are very high; thus, nutrient-rich foods should be provided to support their growth and development (Bornstein 2002). Millets rightly called as miracle grains are highly nutritious and offer multiple health benefits and can be utilized as healthy infant foods compared to their conventional counterparts wheat and rice (Sabuz et al 2023; Rathore et al 2016). Owing to the sustainability of millets in adverse agro-climatic conditions, millets are depicted as crops that support food security (Sruthi and Rao 2021). Millets play a vital role in providing nutrition as they are a good source of energy and rich in nutrients viz. protein, dietary fiber, fatty acids, minerals, vitamins, phytonutrients especially polyphenols (Samtiya et al 2023; Sood et al 2016). "Shree Anna" or millets have a multifaceted role right from addressing contemporary challenges in food production and combating malnutrition in vulnerable populations to promoting sustainable farming practices and empowering smallholder farmers. The integration of millets into modern agricultural strategies and diets is advocated by governments, international organizations and health communities (Devi et al 2024). Millets prove to be health-promoting cereals as they possess antioxidant, antihypertensive, anti-inflammatory, antimicrobial, hypocholesterolemic, hypoglycemic and anti-carcinogenic potential (Samtiya et al 2023). Millets also support good gut health as they are gluten-free, easy to digest with a low glycemic index and non-acid-forming (Samtiya et al 2023; Ramashia et al 2019).

Millets are integrated into the traditional diets as staple foods due to their high nutritional content compared to other cereals such as wheat and rice (Amadou et al 2013). Millets – classified as major millet and minor millet – are rich in various nutrients (Tripathi et al 2023). Millets can be consumed as complementary food by infants in various forms such as steam-cooked food products, thick and thin porridges (Saleh et al 2013). Millets such as pearl millet, finger millet, foxtail millet, little millet, sorghum and kodo millet are promising candidates for nutritional interventions as they support good human health (Sabuz et al 2023; Samtiya et al 2023). Millets are rich in micronutrients; therefore, they are often processed and used to prepare healthy, nutritious food blends, infant weaning foods and complementary foods such as sorghum flakes, grains malt, puffed and popped

DOI: 10.1201/9781003686668-5

millets (Rathore et al 2016). Several value-added products prepared from millets have prebiotic and probiotic potential that possess significant health benefits (Das et al 2019).

Globally, shifting dietary patterns have led to a decline in millet consumption, contributing to the current nutritional paradox where undernutrition and micronutrient deficiencies coexist (Konapur et al 2014). Recently millets regained their lost value with the declaration of the year 2023 as the International Year of Millets (IYM) by the United Nations (UN) (FAO 2024). The inclusion of value-added millet foods in the daily diets is the promising strategy to address the rising global challenges of malnutrition, poverty and hunger (FAO 2024).The introduction of various processing techniques has led to the production of various ready-to-use, ready-to-cook and ready-to-eat millet food products that has increased millet consumption, leading to improved health status of infants (Mishra et al 2021).

Millets are versatile to be used in the preparation of a variety of infant weaning foods such as finger millet (ragi) porridge, pancakes and khichdi. Millet food products are rich in iron, calcium and fiber in addition to other health benefits such as improved digestion, better immune function and overall nutrition. Millets can be gradually introduced to an infant's diet as per their nutritional needs. Use of proper preparation methods, such as soaking and cooking, can enhance the digestibility and nutrient availability of millets for infants. Evidence suggests that consumption of millet-based diet improved the growth (height, weight, mid-upper arm circumference and chest circumference) of children (Anitha et al 2019).

5.2 HISTORICAL AND CULTURAL IMPORTANCE OF VARIOUS MILLETS IN THE DIET OF INFANTS

Millets, as staple crops, have been fundamental to traditional meals in numerous civilizations for generations. Their contribution to infant nutrition is notably tied not only to nutritional benefits but also has cultural significance in several communities. Millets, such as finger millet (ragi), pearl millet (bajra) and sorghum (jowar), have been staple grains for centuries and are grown for millennia, with archeological evidence indicating their origins in Africa and Asia more than 7,000 years ago (National Research Council (NRC) 1996). Traditionally, millets are among the first foods introduced to infants after breast milk. In India, finger millet porridge serves as a prevalent weaning dish, exemplifying longstanding traditions of integrating locally cultivated, nutrient-dense grains into newborn nutrition. In African societies, sorghum and pearl millet porridge serve as essential first feeds for infants, highlighting their suitability for local climates and their significance in food security (Musidzaramba et al 2025). The cultural inclination for millets in newborn nutrition is linked to their digestibility and appropriateness for immature digestive systems. Millets are integral to various feeding practices especially in rural parts of India. In South India foxtail millet porridge is given to infants as it supports easy digestion.

Recently, there has been a renewed interest in millets owing to their nutritional and ecological advantages. Governments and international organizations, including the UN Food and Agriculture Organization, promote millet consumption as a component of a diverse diet, particularly for at-risk groups such as infants. Health organizations and governments in millet-producing areas are reintegrating millet-based foods into public nutrition initiatives. The Government of India's Poshan Abhiyaan incorporates millet-based recipes to improve infant and child nutrition in both rural and urban regions (POSHAN Abhiyaan 2024).

5.3 HEALTH BENEFITS OF MILLETS FOR INFANTS

Millets are recognized globally for their nutritional richness and resilience toward adverse climatic conditions thus having the potential to enhance food security and nutrition (Mohod et al 2023). Millets are a nutrient-dense food source, offering several health benefits tailored for the growth and development of infants (Figure 5.1).

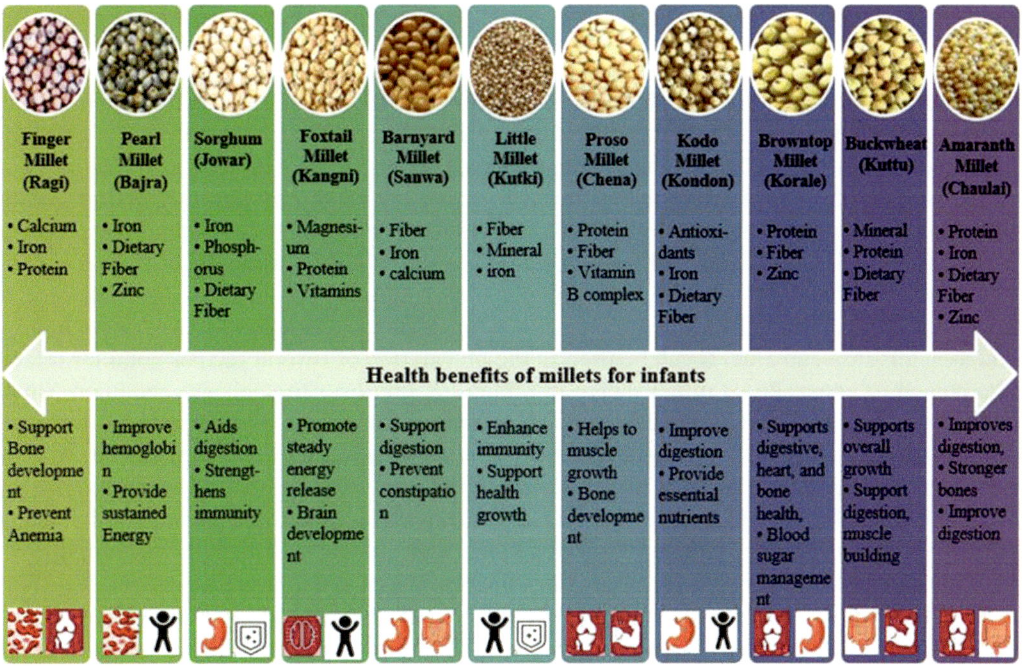

FIGURE 5.1 Health benefits of millets for infants.

Finger millet (ragi) is a promising source of multiple nutrients especially calcium, iron and fiber. Addressing the deficiency of the nutrients through diet is a key to supporting the infant's development. A recent systematic review ascertained that consumption of 100 g of finger millet would provide 122% of the calcium recommended dietary allowance for infants (Anitha et al 2021). The inclusion of finger millet in the daily diet of the infants can help in addressing several adverse health conditions in infants, such as anemia, disorders of teeth and bones due to calcium deficiency. Fiber in ragi aids in maintaining healthy gastrointestinal function, enhances the bioavailability of calcium and supports the development of a strong immune system (Jagati et al 2021). The malted ragi grain flour being rich in several nutrients is often termed nourishing and wholesome food for infants (Patel et al 2016).

Pearl millet is an important nutri-cereal that provides protein, iron and several B complex vitamins in addition to providing fiber, minerals (phosphorous, calcium, magnesium and zinc) and fat-soluble vitamins (A, E and K) cereals (Nibhoria et al 2024). The evidence suggests improvement in the hemoglobin concentration of children upon consumption of complementary foods made from the biofortified pearl millet (FeZnPM, Dhanashakti, ICTP-8203 Fe). It is a promising sustainable and low-cost food that would improve the nutritional status of children through integration in the existing Integrated Child Services Development Program in India that caters to millions of children (Mehta et al 2022). Recently a study found that daily consumption (100 g) of a low-cost, homemade complementary food formulated with pearl millet, finger millet and soybean (30:35:35), plus sugar and milk powder, provided high protein, fat, calcium and iron that are major nutrients for infant growth (Prajapati et al 2017). Pearl millet-based complementary foods also help to prevent iron deficiency (Sihag et al 2016).

Sorghum is an important millet for infant nutrition. It has a good amount of minerals such as potassium and magnesium. The antioxidant compounds like phenols in sorghum improve gut health. Sorghum grain has been recently used to prepare several functional foods and beverages (Xiong et al 2019). Sorghum is an excellent source of several vitamins and minerals that help improve the blood hemoglobin levels and reduce inflammation in the body. Overall sorghum plays an important role in promoting good health in infants (Lokhande et al 2019).

Small millets are highly nutritious crops and are a rich source of macronutrients, micronutrients and phytochemicals (Arya and Bisht 2022). Foxtail millet is a low-cost, protein-rich food with excellent nutritional properties (Sachdev et al 2021). Foxtail millet is a reservoir of protein, minerals, fiber, antioxidants and phytochemicals (Mokal 2024). Its regular consumption reduces inflammation and improves digestion. The foxtail millet has antioxidant, low glycemic index and hypolipidemic properties (Sharma and Niranjan 2018).

Barnyard millet is a nutrient-rich grain and -dense source of protein, fiber and especially iron and magnesium (Renganathan et al 2020). It holds strong potential for improving food and nutritional security. Including barnyard millet in weaning foods by using methods like malting or fermentation could address undernutrition in children due to inadequate complementary feeding (Bisht 2022). Little millet is highly nutritious for infants and is a good source of B vitamins and minerals iron and zinc. It can be used in the preparation of several recipes good for infants like pongal or kheer. Proso millet intake in infant diet improves the pellagra condition, which is caused due to niacin (vitamin B3) deficiency. Proso millet contains phosphorous and other antioxidants. Kodo millet is rich in phytochemicals, antioxidants and fiber which helps in good digestion (Ambati and Sucharitha 2019).

Brown-top millet is a nutrient-dense cereal rich in protein, fiber, iron, calcium and essential micronutrients, surpassing many staple grains in nutritional quality. Its high mineral and dietary fiber content makes it suitable for improving infant nutrition and preventing deficiencies. With proper processing, it can be safely included in complementary feeding to support growth and immunity (Kamble and Karkannavar 2024; Singh et al 2022). Buckwheat, a gluten-free pseudo-cereal rich in protein, fiber, iron, zinc and antioxidants, supports infant growth, immunity and cognitive development when included in complementary feeding. Its high nutrient and bioactive content make it particularly valuable for preventing early-life deficiencies (Lițoiu et al 2025). Amaranth is a nutrient-dense, gluten-free seed rich in protein, iron, zinc, calcium, fiber and antioxidant compounds, making it highly suitable for infant complementary feeding after six months. Its nutritional composition supports healthy growth and immunity while addressing micronutrient deficiencies common in early childhood (Kayanda et al 2025).

5.4 TYPES OF MILLETS USED FOR INFANT NUTRITION

Millets have traditionally served as a vital weaning food to growing infants as they transition to consume solid foods after full dependence on mother's milk for the initial six months of life (FAO 2024). During infancy the nutrient requirements are high due to rapid physical and intellectual development. Millets such as finger millet, pearl millet, sorghum and foxtail millet are excellent alternatives to traditional cereal foods as they possess nutrient-rich profiles essential for infants during their critical growth period. Finger millet (ragi) is popular for its smooth texture and high nutrient content (calcium, iron and essential amino acids) (Mahajan et al 2021). Finger millets are rich in calcium, carbohydrates, proteins and dietary fiber that ensure good bone development and provide sustained high energy levels during infancy (Thapliyal and Singh 2015). Pearl millet (bajra) and finger millet have good iron reserves that help in the prevention of iron-deficiency anemia in infants (Jagati et al 2021). Pearl millet possesses anti-allergic properties, therefore, can be included in the infant diets (Dayakar Rao et al 2017). Millets offer a paradigm of nutrients that support the overall development of infants. Foxtail millet supports digestion, metabolism and overall well-being of children due to its richness in dietary fiber, B vitamins and minerals like magnesium and phosphorus(Jaiswal et al 2019; Zhu et al 2018). Pearl millet and sorghum, being rich in folate, can be incorporated into the diet of pregnant women and support fetal development (Krishnan and Meera 2018). Pregnancy is marked by high demand of iron and calcium which can be met by including ragi and bajra food items in the diet. Finger millet and pearl millet recipes help to regulate bowel movements and prevent constipation and anemia in addition to supporting the infant's bone and teeth development. Foxtail millet and barnyard millet consumption helps to attain good digestive health (Nesari 2023).

5.5 PREPARATION METHODS FOR COMPLEMENTARY FEEDING

Millets being small-grained cereals offer significant prospects for innovation in harvesting, processing and food technologies to create products attractive to consumers (FAO 2023b). Nutrition in early life years is important for the growth and development of individuals. Mother's milk is insufficient to cater to the nutritional needs of infants after six months of age; therefore, complementary or weaning foods should be introduced to fulfill the increasing nutrient needs of infants. Complementary foods are soft digestible baby foods prepared from locally available cereal grains and fruits. Millets are recommended for infants' diet because their waxy phenotype contains 0% amylose and 100% amylopectin that is glutinous in nature and easily digestible (Vinoth and Ravindhran 2017; Englyst et al 1992; Dreher et al 1984). Millets fit as an essential component of complementary feeding as they possess a mild taste, semi-solid texture and consistency which facilitates transition from milk to acceptance of solid foods. Additionally, pseudo-cereals such as amaranth, quinoa and buckwheat are often incorporated in infants' diet to enhance nutritional diversity (Klerks et al 2019). Complementary food prepared from iron- and zinc-biofortified pearl millet improved the hemoglobin concentration in male infants (Mehta et al 2026). Milk–cereal-based complementary foods are rich in minerals and vitamins; however, exogenous factors such as packaging materials, headspace air quality, storage temperature, humidity and handling are some of the reported factors that can alter the quality of foods (Raju et al 2015). Pearl millet starch is employed as a cost-effective ingredient in infant foods and functional food products like beverages and soup mixes (Aruna and Parimalavalli 2017). Pearl millet can be effectively utilized in the preparation of bread, cookies or breakfast items such as upma and khichdi (Aruna and Parimalavalli 2017). Koko is a popular low-viscosity porridge used as a complementary food for infants in West Africa. It is prepared from fermented sorghum or millet dough (Saalia et al 2012).The infant food premix (100 g on dry weight) comprising pearl millet, finger millet, roasted Bengal gram, pumpkin powder, milk powder and niger seeds had high protein (17.4 g), energy (406 kcal), fat (9.65 g), iron (7.78 mg), calcium (481.83 mg), carbohydrate (62.40 g) and beta-carotene (1251 μg) content that had potential to improve infants' (6–24 months) nutritional status (Singh and Dunkwal 2020). Roasting millets and grinding them into fine flour is a simple method to prepare nutritious complementary foods for infants. Finger millet foods such as ragi bites and millet pasta are nutritionally rich and support growth and development in older infants (Figure 5.2).

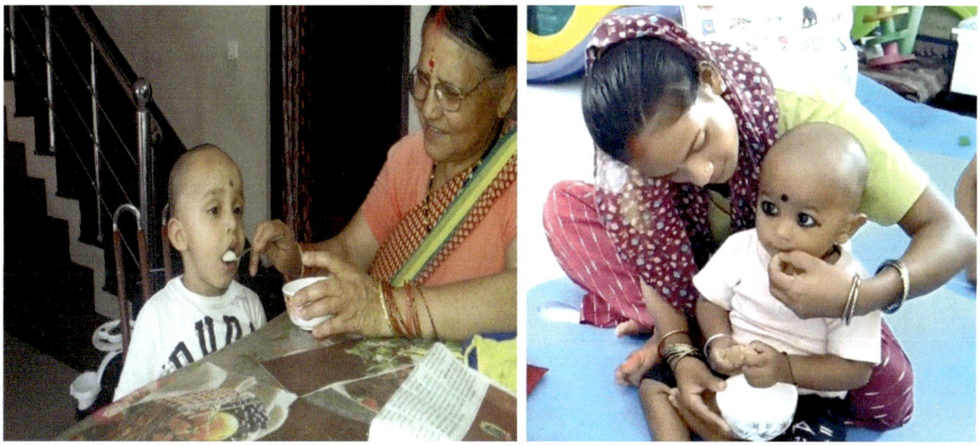

FIGURE 5.2 Feeding babies' millet-based gruel and laddu.

5.6 PROCESSING METHODS TO IMPROVE THE SHELF LIFE OF MILLET-BASED FOODS

Millets hold significant potential for enhancing food security as they showcase rich nutritional profile, drought tolerance, adaptability to local farming conditions, pest and disease resistance and resilience to environmental encounters (Latha Ravi and Rana 2024). Maximizing the nutritional value and shelf life of millets can be attained through processing and thereby reducing the food wastage. Challenges such as rapid rancidity due to enzymatic activity of lipase, lipoxygenase, peroxidases and polyphenol oxidase highlight the need for advanced processing methods. To stabilize millet-based food products, various food processing techniques have gained attention as they promise minimum nutrient loss, decrease antinutritional factors and energy-saving benefits. These food processing techniques include thermal methods such as microwave, radiofrequency, infrared and ohmic heating, as well as non-thermal approaches like pulsed electric fields, cold plasma, irradiation, high-pressure processing, ozonation and ultrasound treatment (Latha Ravi and Rana 2024). Processing methods like drying, roasting or puffing decrease moisture levels, reducing the risk of microbial growth, contamination and spoilage. Processing of millets allows commercial viability and accessibility that helps them to reach the distant markets. In urban settings, convenience foods are more preferred over the traditional recipes that need more preparation time; therefore, extrusion processing technology and packaging create way for ready-to-cook or ready-to-eat options. Unprocessed millets are susceptible to infestation by pests and insects during storage. Milling, drying or coating with edible films protect the grains from pest infestation and reduce storage losses. Processing techniques such as freeze-drying and vacuum packaging help to retain millet's nutrients during storage and preserve their original nutritional profile. The combination of advanced processing technologies with targeted breeding techniques, such as marker-assisted selection and genome editing, led to the development of low-rancidity pearl millet varieties with improved flour shelf life and better keeping quality (Padmaja et al 2024). Millets are high in antinutrients such as phytates and tannins that hamper the bioavailability of nutrients. Traditional processing methods like soaking, sprouting, fermentation, malting and germination improve the nutrient quality and storage stability in millet products (Sruthi and Rao 2021). Sprouted finger millet grains are good for infants. Supplementing infants' diet with the germinated finger millet-based food showed improved hemoglobin status in infants (Dayakar Rao et al 2017). Innovative thermal and non-thermal techniques have demonstrated effectiveness in microbial decontamination and enzyme inactivation in millets. Despite this, their use in millet flour production remains underutilized. As millets have gained renewed popularity and become a staple food among health-conscious consumers, these methods hold significant potential for further research and development (Sruthi and Rao 2021). Processed pearl millet flour stored in laminated packaging and the modified atmosphere was effective in extending shelf life (Padmaja et al 2024). The limited consumer appeal and restricted use of pearl millet in the food industry is largely attributed to its poor shelf life and suboptimal dough quality. Researchers recommend various heat treatment methods (hydrothermal, near-infrared, microwave and ohmic heating), decortication, malting, germination and fermentation to extend the shelf life of pearl millet flour. In addition, inclusion of vital wheat gluten into pearl millet flour can be an alternative method to improve the pearl millet dough quality (Goswami et al 2023).

5.7 ROLE OF MILLETS IN PREVENTING MALNUTRITION

Millets being a rich reservoir of macro- and micronutrients are recommended for the growth and well-being of the infants. Poor dietary quality and infant feeding practices are responsible for malnutrition in infants where millets can act as the savior (Nnam et al 2024). The newly introduced hybrid millet varieties such as pearl millet – MH 2417 (PUSA 1801), finger millet – VL

Mandura 402, sorghum – DSH-6 (CSH-49), (SPH-1943) and proso millet – CPRMV-1 (DHPM-60-4/PMV 466) contain a whooping amount of iron and zinc compared to their conventional counterparts which makes them suitable to tackle nutritional challenges especially malnutrition (ICAR 2024). Pearl millet is rich in iron, zinc and lysine; hence, consumption of value-added foods prepared from pearl millet can help to address protein and micronutrient malnutrition (Hadimani et al 2001; McDonough et al 2000). Finger millets contain a high amount of calcium, magnesium and potassium that aids in good bone health and helps in the prevention of rickets (Devi et al 2024; Saleh et al 2013; Pettifor 2004). Finger millets are a reservoir for amino acids like methionine, lysine and tryptophan responsible for the development of tissues and organs in early life years (Bhatt et al 2011). Polyphenols in finger millets support good immunity (Devi et al 2014). Common millet, with a protein content of 12.5%, and barnyard millet, containing 13.6% crude fiber, are excellent for meeting the increased protein and energy requirements during infancy (Saleh et al 2013). A recent study supported the inclusion of millets and orange-flesh sweet potatoes in infant complementary foods to address the deficiency of essential amino acids and micronutrients (Nnam et al 2024). The protein content of the biscuits prepared by combination of various millets (sorghum and pearl millet) and pulses (chickpea and green gram) had higher digestibility and net protein digestibility, suggesting that millet biscuits had good protein quality (Geervani et al 1996). Consumption of protein-rich millet biscuits is good for infant growth thus preparing a base for coming years in life. Recently, the cereal-based composite weaning mixes have been replaced by the millet (kodo, foxtail, finger and little millets) mixes for better nutritional status as they are rich in protein, ash, crude fiber and calcium content (Prasanna et al 2020). Millets such as finger millet, barnyard millet, foxtail millet, kodo millet, little millet, proso millet and brown-top millet contain dietary carbohydrates (60–70%), protein (6–10%), fat (1.5–5%), dietary fiber (12–20%), minerals (2–4%) and phytochemicals (phenolics, flavonoids, tocopherols and carotenoids) (Hadimani et al 1995). The nutrient-dense profile of small millets makes them suitable to be included in various value-added products that would help in the proper growth and development of infants (Banerjee and Maitra 2020). Ready-to-use therapeutic foods (RUTF) prepared from soya, millet, rice, maize and sugar met the nutritional and microbiological needs of children (6–59 months) suffering with moderate acute malnutrition, thus suggesting that millets can help in combating malnutrition (N'guessan et al 2024). Weaning food prepared from malted flour of pearl millet, malted barley and soybean in the ratio of 50:25:25 had a good percentage of protein (28%), carbohydrate (67%), calcium (108 ppm) and iron (18.6 ppm). The inclusion of weaning foods in the infant diets would be adequate to meet the growing infants' needs and also combat against both macronutrient and micronutrient malnutrition (Palukurty 2019). Overall, millets prove to be good solution to address "hidden hunger" by providing vital micronutrients such as iron and zinc and minerals like calcium that are often absent in traditional infant diets, reducing risks of stunting, and related developmental delays. Being rich in antioxidants and phytochemicals, millets strengthen the infant's immune system and help them to fight against infections. Evidence suggests that millets are rich in fibers, thus promoting good digestion and protection from constipation. Millets are versatile and offer variety in taste and textures of millet-based food items. Millet-based foods are proven to have good overall acceptability. Millets are a good source of complex carbohydrates, providing sustained energy essential for active infants.

5.8 MILLET-BASED FOODS IN TRADITIONAL CULTURES (TRADITIONAL RECIPES)

Millets show a wide range of culinary possibilities, as they possess a mildly nutty flavor that pairs well with savory and sweet ingredients, providing great combination options to invent creative recipes (FAO 2023a). Millet-based recipes are rich in essential nutrients such as protein, dietary fiber, vitamins, minerals and antioxidants that aid infants with good digestion, prevent constipation, support good gut health, promote satiety, reduce oxidative stress and inflammation (Maurya et al 2023). Recipes such as pearl millet mudde (ball), pearl millet and sweet potato pulao and pearl millet porridge are rated as highly acceptable when consumed by the infants (6–24 months), suggesting that inclusion of millets into traditional recipes could help to combat micronutrient (iron, zinc and vitamin A) deficiencies (Gannon et al 2019). Foxtail millet and barnyard millet exhibit the prebiotic properties that support healthy gut microbiota comprising *Bifidobacteria* and *Lactobacilli* bacteria and inhibit the harmful bacterial growth (Balasubramanian et al 2021; Oh and Jung 2015). Incorporating small millets as a staple food could help in the prevention of nutritional deficiency diseases and reduce the risk of non-communicable diseases (Bisht 2022). Millet-based recipes such as finger millet porridge and pearl millet khichdi are a gluten-free alternative to individuals diagnosed with gluten sensitivities or celiac disease (Maurya et al 2023; Jeelani et al 2020). The millet-based recipes that can be included in the diet of the infants are shown in Table 5.1.

5.9 CHALLENGES IN PROMOTING MILLET-BASED INFANT NUTRITION

Even though millets are nutritionally superior to other cereals and promise several health benefits to infants, their promotion and adoption remain a challenge in recent times. Leveraging millets holds the potential to significantly alleviate the challenges of food insecurity and malnutrition amongst different populations. Addressing these challenges is pivotal to integrating millet-based foods effectively into infant diets and nutrition programs. Limited awareness among the caregivers about nutritional superiority of millets over conventional staples like wheat and rice poses a threat to the adoption of millets in infant food. Millets are less favored and adopted in some societies as they are perceived as "poor man's crop" or "a famine food" or "food for the poor" (Mohod et al 2023). Such negative perceptions discourage their inclusion in modern diets especially for infants. Traditional knowledge about the millet processing and cooking methods is meager in today's times due to urbanization, communication gap across generations and shift of dietary choices toward convenience foods (Jayashree and Aram 2019). Limited knowledge about the diverse millet-based recipes by the caregivers could be the reason behind underutilization of millets in infant diets (Mohod et al 2023). More processing and preparation time required to prepare millet-based recipes could force the caregivers to opt for the less healthy recipe options. Millet-based infant products are often priced high compared to their less nutritious alternatives, thus making them unaffordable for many low-income households (Harish et al 2024). In addition, literature on food choice and adoption behavior for millet consumption is scanty in contrast to other wheat and rice alternatives such as organic and ready-to-eat foods (Shah et al 2024). Insufficient inclusion of millets in national nutrition programs, such as Public Distribution System (PDS) and Integrated Child Development Services (ICDS) schemes also adds on to the missed opportunity by policy makers to popularize millets through government-supportive initiatives (Harish et al 2024). Due to urbanization and shift toward convenience foods, millets are often overlooked and have lost their space in human diets (Mohod et al 2023). Millets supply chain is often disrupted due to dwindling supply and demand of millets, thus affecting their commercial viability. Ensuring the quality assurance of millet products is a challenge as they have poor shelf life due to their intrinsic enzyme activity and water activity. The quality assurance of millet products greatly depends on the pre-treatment and storage conditions of millets (Harish et al 2024). Overcoming such barriers through multi-pronged strategies such as creating awareness campaigns about nutritional benefits of millets, conducting workshops on various millet-based nutritious recipes, inclusion of millets in public nutrition programs, development of traditional feeding practices, promotion of long-shelf-life millet-based products, cultural integration of millet promotion and advancement in the millet processing technologies could promote the inclusion of millets as infant foods (Mohod et al 2023).

TABLE 5.1
Millet-Based Recipes for Infants

S. No.	Category	Recipe	List of Ingredients: Quantity	Cooking Steps	Cooking Time	Reference
1	Breakfast/snacks	Pearl millet upma	*Pearl millet rawa*: 1 cup *For seasoning*: chopped onions, green chilies, carrot, beans, potato, ginger, mustard seeds, black gram dal, Bengal gram dal, curry leaves *Oil*: 1 tbsp *Salt*: to taste *Water*: as required	1. Roast pearl millet rawa until light brown color appears. 2. In a pan add seasonings such as mustard seeds, curry leaves, green chilies, black gram dal, Bengal gram dal and onions. 3. Add finely diced carrots, beans, potatoes and sauté for 2–3 min. 4. Add water to the mixture and then add roasted pearl millet rawa. 5. Cook well till it becomes soft and serve hot.	25–30 min	Dayakar Rao et al (2016)
2	Breakfast/snacks	Proso millet rawa` idli	*Proso millet idli rawa*: 1 cup *Urad dal*: 1 cup *Water*: 2 cups *Salt*: to taste	1. Soak dal for 4–6 h in water, remove excess water and grind it into a smooth batter. 2. Add one cup of proso millet idli rawa to smooth dal batter and add salt. Allow it to ferment for overnight. 3. Add the fermented batter into idli molds and cook in an idli cooker for 7–10 min. 4. Serve hot idli with coconut chutney or sambar.	20–25 min	Dayakar Rao et al (2016)
3	Snacks/breakfast	Foxtail millet bread	*Foxtail millet flour*: 1 cup *Refined wheat flour*: 1 cup *Milk*: 15 ml *Salt*: 1 g *Yeast*: 2 g *Sugar*: 5 g *Water*: 30 ml *Egg*: 1 *Oil*: for greasing	1. Dissolve yeast in warm water in a small glass bowl. Combine sugar, salt, oil and keep aside and let it rest for 2 min. 2. Combine foxtail millet flour, maida, milk and mix them to a smooth dough. 3. Prepare the dough for about 8–10 min until it becomes smooth and elastic. Put the dough in a greased bowl. 4. Cover the bowl and let the dough rise in a warm place for 1½ h. Preheat the oven to 190°C temperature. 5. After 1½ h, punch down the dough onto a floured surface. 6. Shape the dough into a loaf and keep it on a greased loaf pan, and bake them at 190°C for 15–20 min. 7. Remove the loaf from the pan and allow it to cool for some time. Slice it into desired loaves and pack.	40–60 min	Dayakar Rao et al (2016)

(Continued)

TABLE 5.1 *(Continued)*
Millet-Based Recipes for Infants

S. No.	Category	Recipe	List of Ingredients: Quantity	Cooking Steps	Cooking Time	Reference
4	Breakfast/ snacks/main course	Kodo millet adai	*Kodo millet*: 1/2 cup *Toor dal*: ¼ cup *Channa dal*: ¼ cup *Moong dal*: 1 tsp *Urad dal*: 1 tsp For seasoning *Red chilies*: 2 number *Fennel seeds*: 1 tsp (optional) *Onion (small size)*: 1/4 cup chopped finely *Curry leaves*: a few crushed *Coriander leaves*: 1 tbsp *Mint leaves*: 1 tbsp finely chopped *Salt*: to taste	1. Soak all dals and millets for 4 h in water. Drain excess water. 2. Add red chilies, fennel seeds, mixed millet mixture, in a mixer and grind to a coarse mixture. 3. Add chopped onion, coriander leaves and salt to the grounded mixer. The batter consistency should be slightly runny (in between idli and dosa batter). 4. Heat the adai pan and apply little oil for greasing. Make round adai and cook until golden brown and crisp. 5. Add onion, mint leaves and salt. 6. Garnish with coriander leaves and serve hot.	30–45 min	Dayakar Rao et al (2016)
5	Main course	Sorghum khichdi	*Sorghum khichdi rawa*: 1 cup *Moong dal*: ½ cup *For seasoning*: mustard seeds, chopped onions, green chilies, tomato, curry leaves, ginger garlic paste and turmeric powder *Salt*: to taste *Water*: as required	1. Soak moong dal and sorghum rawa for 15 min. 2. Season with mustard seeds, onion, green chilies, ginger garlic paste, tomatoes, curry leaves and turmeric powder. 3. Add required water and salt, cook at low heat. Serve hot.	30 min	Dayakar Rao et al (2016)
6	Main course	Soft finger millet mudde/ragi mudde	*Finger millet (ragi) flour*: 1/4 cup *Water*: 1 cup	1. Mix 2 tsp of finger millet (ragi) flour with water to form a smooth mixture. 2. In a thick bottomed utensil boil the water and add salt. 3. Gradually, add finger millet mixture to boiling water and stir continuously to avoid lumps. 4. Add the remaining finger millet flour and simmer for 3–4 min. 5. Transfer half of the liquid to a separate utensil. 6. Stir the remaining mixture until it forms a uniform paste with no lumps, then add back the transferred liquid to the mixture. 7. Cover the utensil and cook on low heat mode for another 2–3 min. 8. Roll the paste into ball and serve hot with sambhar or chutney.	12–15 min	Dayakar Rao et al (2016)

7	Main course	Little millet curd rice	*Little millet*: 1/2 cup *Water*: 2 cups *Curd*: 3/4 cup *Milk*: 1/4 cup *Grated carrot*: 3 tbsp *Coriander leaves*: 2 tsp finely chopped *Salt*: to taste *For tempering*: *Oil*: 1 tsp *Mustard seeds*: 1/2 tsp *Split urad dal*: 1/2 tsp *Curry leaves*: few *Green chili*: 1 finely chopped *Ginger*: ¼ inch piece	1. Boil the water, add the millet and cook until it softens. 2. Transfer the millet to a mixing bowl, mash it and add curd, followed by milk and mix it thoroughly. 3. For tempering, heat oil in a tadka pan, add the seasoning and let it splutter. 4. Transfer the tempering to the little millet curd rice, add grated carrot, coriander leaves and required salt. Mix everything well. 5. Serve chilled and garnish with carrots and coriander leaves.	20–25 min	Dayakar Rao et al (2016)
8	Snacks	Millet bhel	*Sorghum*: ½ cup *Pearl millet*: ½ cup *Foxtail millet*: ½ cup *Finger millet*: ½ cup *Kabuli chana*: ¼ cup *Chat masala*: to taste Onion, tomatoes and green chili *Salt*: to taste *Roasted cumin powder*: as required	1. Wash and soak the millets and kabuli chana overnight in sufficient water. 2. Pressure cook on medium flame for two whistles. 3. Drain the excess water from the cooked millets and sauté them on a low flame in little oil by stirring frequently. 4. Combine chopped onion, tomatoes, green chili, salt, roasted cumin powder and chat masala and mix them thoroughly well. 5. Serve the bhel topped with lemon juice if needed and garnish with coriander leaves.	5–10 min	Dayakar Rao et al (2016)
9	Beverage	Finger millet smoothie	*Finger millet*: 2 tbsp *Banana*: half medium *Dates*: 2 number *Yoghurt/thick curd*: 2 tbsp *Water*: 120 ml *Vanilla extract*: ¼ tsp *For garnishing*: 1 tsp chopped almonds	1. In a saucepan, add the finger millet and water. Cook over low heat, stirring continuously until it thickens to a smooth glossy paste. 2. Remove the cooked millet from heat and allow it to cool down to room temperature. 3. Blend the cooked millet, banana, dates, yoghurt, water and vanilla extract in a blender, till it becomes smoother and creamier. 4. Pour the blended finger millet smoothie into a glass, garnish with chopped almonds and serve chilled	7–8 min	FAO (2023a)

(Continued)

TABLE 5.1 *(Continued)*
Millet-Based Recipes for Infants

S. No.	Category	Recipe	List of Ingredients: Quantity	Cooking Steps	Cooking Time	Reference
10	Dessert/sweets	Finger millet laddu	*Finger millet flour (ragi)*: 1 cup *Powdered sugar*: 1/2 cup *Ghee*: 3 tsp *Milk*: 1/4 cup *Cardamom powder*: 1 tsp *For garnishing*: grated coconut and dry fruits (finely diced)	1. Roast finger millet flour till roasted aroma appears. 2. In a pan add ghee and roast dry fruits, heat the milk and melt the jaggery. 3. Combine all the roasted ingredients together and mix thoroughly. 4. Shape the ready mixture into round lemon-sized balls manually and serve.	25–30 min	Dayakar Rao et al (2016)
11	Dessert/sweets	Foxtail millet kheer	*Dehulled foxtail millet grain*: 1 cup *For garnishing*: dry fruits Ghee, water, sugar, milk *Cardamom powder*: as required	1. Cook the dehulled foxtail millet in boiling water for 5 min. 2. Roast the dry fruits in ghee until fragrant appears. 3. In a separate pan, boil the water and milk. Add the cooked millet and sugar, and stir gently for 10–15 min until it is cooked fully. 4. Add cardamon powder and decorate with cashew nuts and other dry fruits.	30–35 min	Dayakar Rao et al (2016)
12	Dessert	Barnyard millet payasam	*Barnyard millet*: 150 g *Sugar*: 250 g *Milk*: 250 ml *Saffron*: 4–5 strands *Dry fruits (cashew, almond and pista)*: 50 g *Ghee*: 30 ml	1. Put together barnyard millet, saffron and milk. Cook over low heat until the millet softens. 2. Add sugar to the cooked payasam and mix gently. 3. Heat ghee in a small pan and roast dry fruits until golden color. 4. Add roasted dry fruits to the prepared payasam. 5. Serve either hot or cold, as desired.	30–35 min	Dayakar Rao et al (2016)

5.10 GOVERNMENT AND GLOBAL INITIATIVES

Millets play a pivotal role in enhancing global food security; therefore, the cultivation and consumption of millets should be encouraged by the government through subsidies, research and market support (Devi et al 2024). Globally, nearly half of under-five children's deaths are linked to undernutrition and approximately 149 and 45 million under-five children are estimated to be stunted and wasted, respectively (WHO 2024). Various global initiatives are taken to face such a grave situation by creating sustainable, resilient food systems for healthy diets. The UN recognized the potential of millets as a reservoir of nutrients and a sustainable solution to challenges of food insecurity, nutrition insecurity and climate change and declared 2023 as the IYM (Harish et al 2024). India spearheaded international-, national- and state-level efforts to increase millet consumption globally and domestically. The Government of India declared 2018 as the "National Year of Millets" and also featured millets in several cross-border initiatives like the Adaptation of African Agriculture funded by the African Development Bank. In India, IYM 2023 was marked as "peoples movement" and India was positioned as the "Global Hub for Millets" (Nesari 2023). Furthermore, the efforts to include millets in government programs such as ICDS and Mid-Day Meal Scheme recently gained momentum to strategically combat malnutrition, support sustainable agriculture and improve dietary diversity. In Rajasthan and Karnataka, millet-based foods are included in school feeding programs to improve the nutritional status of children. The Indian government integrated millets such as jowar, bajra and ragi into the PDS to make them accessible to low-income families, benefiting child nutrition (Singh 2024). Karnataka and Tamil Nadu states in India provide millets by the PDS (Pingali et al 2019). The Poshan Abhiyaan (National Nutrition Mission) promotes dietary diversity and the inclusion of nutrient-rich foods, including millets, in the diets of under-five children (POSHAN Abhiyaan 2024). In India, Agricultural and Processed Food Products Export Development Authority (APEDA) promotes millets at global food fairs like Anuga Food Fair and organizes food sampling and tasting of millet-based products by customers at the local retail stores to create awareness and increase their acceptance. In addition, the government promotes millets by supporting the innovative start-ups of the "Ready to Eat" and "Ready to Serve" millet-based infant foods and cereal mixes (Harish et al 2024). The Food and Agriculture Organization (FAO) also collaborated with governments and policy makers to promote the production and trade of millets, emphasizing the nutritional benefits of millets in reducing child malnutrition (FAO 2024). Several international and national campaigns by the governing bodies are launched to promote millet consumption globally (Mishra et al 2022). A global biofortification initiative has been taken under the Consultative Group for International Agricultural Research (CGIAR) by developing nutrient-enriched millet varieties to combat iron deficiency in children (Birol and Bouis 2023). In India, a study reported that daily consumption of iron- and zinc-biofortified pearl millet-based complementary foods led to a significant increase in the hemoglobin concentrations of the male infants suggesting that incorporation of iron- and zinc- biofortified pearl millet-based complementary foods into the ICDS supplemental meal program could decrease the risk of anemia in children (Mehta et al 2022). Global Alliance for Improved Nutrition (GAIN) works with governments, policy makers and industry to tackle malnutrition through concerted action and effective policy change (GAIN 2024). UNICEF nutrition programs advocate the use of locally available nutrient-rich millets for complementary feeding in infants and young children, emphasizing their role in preventing stunting and wasting (UNICEF 2023). Millet-based value-added products could be the healthy alternative to fulfill the rising demand for health-benefiting food products.

5.11 COMMERCIAL MILLET-BASED INFANT NUTRITION

During infancy and early childhood proper nutrition is crucial as they are often predisposed to several micronutrient deficiencies due to increased nutrient demand. Early weaning is a leading contributor to child malnutrition, putting infants at high risk of morbidity and mortality. After six months, breast milk alone becomes inadequate to meet the optimal growth and developmental needs of babies; hence, cereal-based foods are gradually introduced to support the increasing nutritional needs of infants (Jeelani et al 2020). Millet-based infant foods are a rich source of essential nutrients such as calcium, iron, magnesium and vitamins (Jaybhaye et al 2014). With increasing awareness about millets' rich nutritional profile and suitability as weaning foods, the demand for minimally processed millet-based baby foods has increased (Jain et al 2024). The government should provide incentives and subsidies to new millet-based start-ups (Dudhagara et al 2022). Commercially many millet-based infant foods such as porridge or cereal mixes, millet biscuits, millet puffs, ready-to-cook millet mixes and millet-based infant formulas are available in the market as nutrient-dense convenience foods.

5.12 RECIPES AND PRACTICAL APPLICATIONS IN MILLETS

Millets are ideal for promoting infant health through complementary feeding. The mild flavor of millets makes them suitable to be included in a variety of recipes catering to the evolving needs of infants. Millet-based recipes such as finger millet pancakes, millet and vegetable khichdi, finger millet or pearl millet porridge etc. provide infants with the essential nutrients with diverse flavors and textures that would help to shape the eating habits of infants. The millets can be practically used to prepare commercially fortified complementary infant foods. Furthermore, through community nutrition workshops caregivers should be educated about the diverse benefits of millets and new millet recipe-preparation methods. The new millet recipes should be aligned with local traditions and community culture to increase their acceptance.

5.13 PUBLIC HEALTH AND POLICY IMPLICATIONS

Millets are gaining global recognition, and they offer a sustainable and health-promoting alternative to conventional cereal-based foods for infants. Millets, with their high nutritional profile and adaptability, are capable of addressing the challenges of high rates of malnutrition in infants. Recognizing the potential of millets, policy makers and public health advocates are increasingly focusing on their inclusion in national nutrition programs to improve child health outcomes and foster food security. Policy development and dietary guidelines for millet inclusion in daily diets play a crucial role in promoting millet consumption (Maurya et al 2023). Following are some recommendations for the government for better acceptance of millets:

i. The government should support various millet-based industries by providing incentives to promote the production of millet-based infant cereals, porridges and snacks.
ii. Awareness campaigns should be launched by stakeholders highlighting the benefits of inclusion of millets in infant diets and their role in improving infant health outcomes.
iii. Integration of millets into various national nutrition programs such as PDS and ICDS can improve access to nutrient-rich foods for infants from low-income households.
iv. Millets should be incorporated into maternal and child health program schemes to address malnutrition in mothers and their infants.
v. The government should provide subsidies and incentives to farmers to ensure consistent production and supply of millets for infant nutrition programs.
vi. Millet-based foods should be promoted by the government through nutritional programs targeting vulnerable populations, especially infants and young children.
vii. Encourage the public–private partnership to successfully include millets and millet-based foods in the mainstream.

By prioritizing the integration of millets into various national health programs and policies, nations can foster healthier generations, combat malnutrition and support sustainable agricultural practices.

5.14 CONCLUSION

Millets are magical nutrient-dense superfoods that provide a sustainable solution to combat malnutrition in infants and lay the foundation for healthier adults in future. The government and policy makers should ascertain to increase millet production through the provision of subsidies and incentives to millet farmers. Furthermore, efforts to increase millet consumption should focus on creating awareness about their nutritional benefits, commercializing millet-based products, integrating millets into the national nutrition programs, increasing their accessibility in local market, adopting advanced processing techniques to diversify millet-based products. A collaborative public–private partnership is essential to successfully integrate millets and millet-based foods into the mainstream and ensuring their wider acceptance and inclusion in infant diets. Thus, millets celebrated as "Shree Anna" ensure food and nutrition security for infants.

REFERENCES

Amadou, I., Gounga, M. E., and Le, G. W. 2013. Millets, nutritional composition, some health benefits and processing. *Emir J Food Agric* **25**, no. 7: 501–508. https://doi.org/10.9755/ejfa.v25i7.12045

Ambati, K., and Sucharitha, K. V. 2019. Millets-review on nutritional profiles and health benefits. *Int J Recent Sci Res* **10**, no. 7: 33943–33948. https://doi.org/10.24327/IJRSR

Anitha, S., Givens, D. I., Botha, R., et al. 2021. Calcium from finger millet – A systematic review and meta-analysis on calcium retention, bone resorption, and in vitro bioavailability. *Sustainability* **13**, no. 16: 8677. https://doi.org/10.3390/su13168677

Anitha, S., Kane-Potaka, J., Tsusaka, T. W., et al. 2019. Acceptance and impact of millet-based mid-day meal on the nutritional status of adolescent school going children in a peri urban region of Karnataka State in India. *Nutrients* **11**, no. 9: 2077. https://doi.org/10.3390/nu11092077

Aruna, M., and Parimalavalli, R. 2017. Properties of pearl millet: native and modified starch. *South Asia J Multidiscip Stud* **4**: 31–44. https://infosat.icrisat.org

Arya, C., and Bisht, A. 2022. Nutritional profile of small millets. In *Small millet grains: The superfoods in human diet*, 15–47. Singapore: Springer Nature Singapore. https://doi.org/10.1007/978-981-16-9306-9_2

Balasubramanian, B., Soundharrajan, I., Al-Dhabi, N. A., et al. 2021. Probiotic characteristics of Ligilactobacillus salivarius AS22 isolated from sheep dung and its application in corn-fox tail millet silage. *Appl Sci* **11**, no. 20: 9447. https://doi.org/10.3390/app11209447

Banerjee, P., Maitra, S., and Banerjee, P. 2020. The role of small millets as functional food to combat malnutrition in developing countries. *Indian J Nat Sci* **10**, no. 60: 20412–20417. https://www.researchgate.net/profile/Sagar-Maitra/publication/342153966

Bhatt, D., Negi, M., Sharma, P., Saxena, S. C., Dobriyal, A. K., and Arora, S. 2011. Responses to drought induced oxidative stress in five finger millet varieties differing in their geographical distribution. *Physiol Mol Biol Plants* **17**, no. 4: 347–353. https://doi.org/10.1007/s12298-011-0084-4

Birol, E., and Bouis, H. E. 2023. Role of socio-economic research in developing, delivering and scaling new crop varieties: The case of staple crop biofortification. *Front Plant Sci* **14**: 1099496. https://doi.org/10.3389/fpls.2023.1099496

Bisht, A. 2022. Small-millet-based baby food. In Srivastava, S. (eds) *Small millet grains. Cereals, pulses and oilseeds*. Singapore: Springer Singapore. https://doi.org/10.1007/978-981-16-9306-9_7

Bornstein, M. H. 2002. *Development in infancy: An introduction*. Psychology Press. https://doi.org/10.4324/9781410602596

Das, S., Khound, R., Santra, M., and Santra, D. 2019. Beyond bird feed: Proso millet for human health and environment. *Agriculture* **9**, no. 3: 64. https://doi.org/10.3390/agriculture9030064

Dayakar Rao, B., Vishala, A. D., Arlene Christina, G. D., and Tonapi, V. A. 2016. *Millet recipes a healthy choice*. ICAR – Indian Institute of Millets Research. https://www.millets.res.in/m_recipes/Millets_Recipes-A_Healthy_choice.pdf

Dayakar Rao, B., Bhaskarachary, K., Arlene Christina, G. D., Sudha Devi, G., and Vilas, A. T. 2017. *Nutritional and health benefits of millets*. 112. https://millets.res.in/m_recipes/Nutritional_health_benefits_millets.pdf

Devi, O. A., Saikia, A. R., Ghorband, A. S., et al. 2024. Shree Anna (Millets): A nutritional and agrarian solution to food production. *J Sci Res Rep* **30**, no. 5: 316–327. https://doi.org/10.9734/jsrr/2024/v30i51947

Devi, P. B., Vijayabharathi, R., Sathyabama, S., Malleshi, N. G., and Priyadarisini, V. B. 2014. Health benefits of finger millet (*Eleusine coracana* L.) polyphenols and dietary fiber: A review. *J Food Sci Technol* **51**, no. 6: 1021–1040. https://doi.org/10.1007/s13197-011-0584-9

Dreher, M. L., Dreher, C. J., Berry, J. W., and Fleming, S. E. 1984. Starch digestibility of foods: A nutritional perspective. *Crit Rev Food Sci Nutr* **20**, no. 1: 47–71. https://doi.org/10.1080/10408398409527383

Dudhagara, C., Mahera, A., Lokesh, K., Kumar M. S., and Patel, H. 2022. Millets: The future smart food. *Pharma Innov* **11**, no. 4: 75–84. https://www.thepharmajournal.com

Englyst, H. N., Kingman, S. M., and Cummings, J. H. 1992. Classification and measurement of nutritionally important starch fractions. *Eur J Clin Nutr* **46**, no. *Suppl 2*: S33–50. https://pubmed.ncbi.nlm.nih.gov

FAO. 2023a. Millets recipe book – *International Year of Millets*. Rome.

FAO. 2023b. Unleashing the potential of millets. https://openknowledge.fao.org/handle/20.500.14283/cc7484en

FAO. 2024. International year of millets 2023: Final report. https://openknowledge.fao.org/handle/20.500.14283/cd2103en

GAIN 2024. https://www.gainhealth.org/impact/countries/india (Accessed on 26 December 2024)

Gannon, B. M., Thakker, V., Bonam, V. S., et al. 2019. A randomized crossover study to evaluate recipe acceptability in breastfeeding mothers and young children in India targeted for a multiple biofortified food crop intervention. *Food Nutr Bull* **40**, no. 4: 1–11. https://doi.org/10.1177/0379572119855588

Geervani, P., Vimala, V., Pradeep, K. U., and Devi, M. R. 1996. Effect of processing on protein digestibility, biological value and net protein utilization of millet and legume based infant mixes and biscuits. *Plant Foods Hum Nutr* **49**, no. 3: 221–227. https://doi.org/10.1007/BF01093218

Goswami, S., Thimmegowda, V., Kumar, R., et al. 2023. Insights into recent techniques for improving shelf life and value addition in pearl millet flour: A mini review on recent advances. *Ann Arid Zone* **62**: 103–108. https://doi.org/10.59512/aaz.2023.62.2.1

Hadimani, N., Ali, S., and Malleshi, N. 1995. Physico-chemical composition and processing characteristics of pearl millet varieties. *J Food Sci Technol*: 193–198. http://ir.cftri.res.in/id/eprint/299

Hadimani, N. A., Muralikrishna, G., Tharanathan, R. N., and Malleshi, N. G. 2001. Nature of carbohydrates and proteins in three pearl millet varieties varying in processing characteristics and kernel texture. *J Cereal Sci* **33**, no. 1: 17–25. https://doi.org/10.1006/jcrs.2000.0342

Harish, M. S., Bhuker, A., and Chauhan, B. S. 2024. Millet production, challenges, and opportunities in the Asia-Pacific region: A comprehensive review. *Front Sustain Food Syst* **8**. https://doi.org/10.3389/fsufs.2024.1386469

ICAR. 2024. PM dedicates 109 climate-resilient and bio-fortified varieties of crops. https://www.pib.gov.in/PressReleasePage.aspx?PRID=2044302 (Accessed on 29 December 2024)

Jagati, P., Mahapatra, I., and Dash, D. 2021. Finger millet (ragi) as an essential dietary supplement with key health benefits: A review. *Int J Home Sci* **7**, no. 2: 94–100. https://doi.org/10.22271/23957476.2021.v7.i2b.1152

Jain, V., Agarwal, N., and Bhatia, V. 2024. Promoting millets: charting a journey from food security to health. *Indian J Community Med: Official Publication of Indian Association of Preventive* and *Social Medicine* **49**, no. 1: 5–10. https://doi.org/10.4103/ijcm.ijcm_107_23

Jaiswal, V., Bandyopadhyay, T., Gahlaut, V., et al. 2019. Genome-wide association study (GWAS) delineates genomic loci for ten nutritional elements in foxtail millet (*Setaria italica* L.). *J Cereal Sci* **85**: 48–55. https://doi.org/10.1016/j.jcs.2018.11.006

Jayashree, B., and Aram, I. 2019. Conservation of millets: The role of community leaders in Kolli Hills, South India. *Indian J Tradit Knowl* **19**, no. 1: 101–110.

Jaybhaye, R. V., Pardeshi, I. L., Vengaiah, P. C., and Srivastav, P. P. 2014. Processing and technology for millet based food products: A review. *J Ready Eat Food* **1**, no. 2: 32–48. https://www.academia.edu/64857844

Jeelani, P., Ghai, A., Saikia, N., et al. 2020. Baby foods based on cereals. In *Food science, technology and nutrition for babies and children*, 59–97. Cham: Springer International Publishing. https://doi.org/10.1007/978-3-030-35997-3_4

Kamble, V., and Karkannavar, S. 2024. Nutritional properties of browntop millet (*Brachiaria ramosa*) based ribbons. *Int J* **8**, no. 12S: 01–04. https://doi.org/10.33545/26174693.2024.v8.i12Sa.3053

Kayanda, R. A., Mogha, N. G., Makori, N., and Kassim, N. 2025. The potential of amaranth grain-based flour in complementary feeding: A community-based approach in Kongwa district, Tanzania. *Curr Res Nutr Food Sci* **13**, no. 2. https://dx.doi.org/10.12944/CRNFSJ.13.2.16

Klerks, M., Bernal, M. J., Roman, S., Bodenstab, S., Gil, A., and Sanchez-Siles, L. M. 2019. Infant cereals: current status, challenges, and future opportunities for whole grains. *Nutrients* **11**, no. 2: 473. https://doi.org/10.3390/nu11020473

Konapur, A., Gavaravarapu, S. R. M., Gupta, S., and Nair, K. M. 2014. Millets in meeting nutrition security: issues and way forward for India. *Indian J Nutr Diet* **51**, no. 3: 306–321. https://www.informaticsjournals.co.in/index.php/ijnd/article/view/2534

Krishnan, R., and Meera, M. S. 2018. Pearl millet minerals: effect of processing on bioaccessibility. *J Food Sci Technol* **55**, no. 9: 3362–3372. https://doi.org/10.1007/s13197-018-3305-9

Latha Ravi, J., and Rana, S. S. 2024. Maximizing the nutritional benefits and prolonging the shelf life of millets through effective processing techniques: A review. *ACS Omega* **9**, no. 37: 38327–38347. https://doi.org/10.1021/acsomega.4c03466

Lițoiu, A. A., Păucean, A., Lung, C., Zmuncilă, A., and Chiș, M. S. 2025. An overview of buckwheat – A superfood with applicability in human health and food packaging. *Plants* **14**, no. 14: 2200. https://doi.org/10.3390/plants14142200

Lokhande, P., Kharche, A., Wagh, S. G., Manithe, D., and Harke, S. 2019. Immune boosting super food supplement from natural resources. *J Pharmacogn Phytochem* **8**, no. 5: 2108–2113. https://www.phytojournal.com

Mahajan, P., Bera, M. B., Panesar, P. S., and Chauhan, A. 2021. Millet starch: A review. *Int J Biol Macromol* **180**: 61–79. https://doi.org/10.1016/j.ijbiomac.2021.03.063

Maurya, R., Boini, T., Misro, L., Radhakrishnan, T., Sreedharan, A. P., and Gaidhani, D. 2023. Comprehensive review on millets: nutritional values, effect of food processing and dietary aspects. *J Drug Res in Ayurvedic Sci* **8**: S82–S98. https://doi.org/10.4103/jdras.jdras_123_23

McDonough, C. M., Rooney, L. W., and Serna-Saldivar, S. O. 2000. The millets. In *Handbook of cereal science and technology*, 177–201. CRC Press. https://www.taylorfrancis.com

Mehta, S., Huey, S. L., Ghugre, P. S., Potdar, R. D., Venkatramanan, S., Krisher, J. T., et al. 2026. A randomized trial of iron-and zinc-biofortified pearl millet-based complementary feeding in children aged 12 to 18 months living in urban slums. *Clin Nutr* 59: 106517. https://doi.org/10.1016/j.clnu.2025.11.002.

Mishra, G. P., Dikshit, H. K., Kukreja, P., et al. 2022. Historical overview of biofortification in crop plants and its implications. In *Biofortification of staple crops*, 31–61. Singapore: Springer Singapore. https://doi.org/10.1007/978-981-16-3280-8_2

Mishra, P., Prakash, H. G., Devi, S., et al. 2021. Nutritional quality of millets and their value added products with the potential health benefits: A review. *Int J Curr Microbiol Appl Sci* **10**, no. 10: 163–175. https://doi.org/10.20546/ijcmas.2021.1010.019

Mohod, N. B., Ashoka, P., Borah, A., et al. 2023. The international year of millet 2023: A global initiative for sustainable food security and nutrition. *Int J Plant Soil Sci* **35**, no. 19: 1204–1211. https://doi.org/10.9734/IJPSS/2023/v35i193659

Mokal, A. 2024. Nutritional benefits of millets in early childhood: A review. *Asian J Dairy Food Res* **43**, no. 4. https://doi.org/10.18805/ajdfr.DR-2221

Musidzaramba, T. J., Mvumi, B. M., Nyanga, L. K., Kadzere, I., Kiboi, M., Mahlangu, M., et al. 2025. Nutritional profile and food safety of raw and value-added food products of sorghum and millets in sub–Saharan Africa and South Asia. Cogent Food & Agri 11, no. **1**: 2461628. https://doi.org/10.1080/23311932.2025.2461628

N'guessan, A., Aka, F., Yeboue, K., Gnonde, A., Ake-Tano, S., and Yapi, A. 2024. Preparation of ready-to-use therapeutic foods based on soy, millet, rice, corn, and sugar for the management of infant with moderate acute malnutrition. *J Food Nutr Sci* **12**, no. 6: 255–260. https://doi.org/10.11648/j.jfns.20241206.11

National Research Council (NRC). 1996. *Lost crops of Africa: Volume I: Grains.* Washington, DC: The National Academies Press. https://doi.org/10.17226/2305

Nesari, T. M. 2023. Celebrating international year of millets: way towards holistic well-being. *J Ayurveda Case Rep* **6**, no. 1: 1–4. https://doi.org/10.4103/jacr.jacr_14_23

Nibhoria, A., Kumar, M., Arya, R. K., and Siroha, A. K. 2024. Pearl millet for good health and nutrition – An overview. *CABI Rev* **19**, no. 1. https://doi.org/10.1079/cabireviews.2024.0041

Nnam, N. M., Orisa, C. A., and Okorie, I. 2024. Functional and sensory properties of infant complementary foods formulated from millets, orange-flesh sweet potatoes, carrots, periwinkle and oyster. *J Gene Engg Bio Res* **6**, no. 3: 01–07. https://doi.org/10.33140/JGEBR.06.03.01

Oh, Y. J., and Jung, D. S. 2015. Evaluation of probiotic properties of *Lactobacillus* and *Pediococcus* strains isolated from *Omegisool*, a traditionally fermented millet alcoholic beverage in Korea. *LWT – Food Sci Technol* **63**, no. 1: 437–444. https://doi.org/10.1016/j.lwt.2015.03.005

Padmaja, P. G., Venkateswarlu, R., Singh, S. P., and Tonapi, V. A. 2024. Enhancing shelf life of pearl millet flour. In *Pearl millet in the 21st century: Food-nutrition-climate resilience-improved livelihoods*, 549–566. Singapore: Springer Nature Singapore. https://doi.org/10.1007/978-981-99-5890-0_21

Palukurty, D. M. A. 2019. Formulation of weaning food to reduce malnutrition using pearl millets, barley and soya bean flour – A study. *Think India J* **22**, no. 14. https://doi.org/10.13140/RG.2.2.36698.08646

Patel, I., Patel, K., Pinto, S., and Patel, S. 2016. Ragi: A powerhouse of nutrients. *Res Rev J Dairy Sci Technol* **5**: 36–47.

Pettifor, J. M. 2004. Nutritional rickets: deficiency of vitamin D, calcium, or both? *Am J Clin Nutr* **80**, no. 6: 1725S–1729S. https://doi.org/10.1093/ajcn/80.6.1725S

Pingali, P., Aiyar, A., Abraham, M., and Rahman, A. 2019. The way forward: food systems for enabling rural prosperity and nutrition security. In *Transforming food systems for a rising India*, 277–311. Cham: Springer International Publishing. https://doi.org/10.1007/978-3-030-14409-8_11

POSHAN Abhiyaan. 2024. https://poshanabhiyaan.gov.in/ (Accessed on 26 December 2024)

Prajapati, M. R., Kamaliya, K. B. and Chawda, H. H. 2017. Optimization of millet based low cost weaning food formula and evaluation of its nutritional composition. *Guj J Ext Educ* **18**, no. 2: 2017. https://www.gjoee.org/papers/772.pdf

Prasanna, M. S., Sowjanya, V. S., Jaya, E., and Rajender, G. 2020. Development of millet based instant weaning mix. *J Pharmacogn Phytochem* **9**, no. 4: 1908–1913. https://www.phytojournal.com

Raju, P. N., Manoj Kumar, C. T., Singh, A. K., Ganguly, S., and Patel, M. M. 2015. Milk-cereal-based composite complementary foods and their storage stability: A mini review. *Res Rev J Dairy Sci Technol* **4**, no. 1: 1–9. https://dx.doi.org/10.22271/phyto

Ramashia, S. E., Anyasi, T. A., Gwata, E. T., Meddows-Taylor, S., and Jideani, A. I. O. 2019. Processing, nutritional composition and health benefits of finger millet in sub-saharan Africa. *Food Sci Technol* **39**: 253–266. https://doi.org/10.1590/fst.25017

Rathore, S., Singh, K., and Kumar, V. 2016. Millet grain processing, utilization and its role in health promotion: A review. *Int J Nutr Food Sci* **5**, no. 5: 318–329. https://doi.org/10.11648/j.ijnfs.20160505.12

Renganathan, V. G., Vanniarajan, C., Karthikeyan, A., and Ramalingam, J. 2020. Barnyard millet for food and nutritional security: current status and future research direction. *Front Genet* **11**: 500. https://doi.org/10.3389/fgene.2020.00500

Saalia, F. K., Ankamah, S., Otubuah, B., Barfi, N. K., and Tano-Debrah, K. 2012. Development and characterization of low viscosity porridge (koko). *Flour by Co-Fermenting with Millet Malt* **1**, no. 551: 2.

Sabuz, A. A., Rana, M. R., Ahmed, T., et al. 2023. Health-promoting potential of millet: A review. *Separations* **10**, no. 2: 80. https://doi.org/10.3390/separations10020080

Sachdev, N., Goomer, S., and Singh, L. R. 2021. Foxtail millet: A potential crop to meet future demand scenario for alternative sustainable protein. *J Sci Food Agric* **101**, no. 3: 831–842. https://doi.org/10.1002/jsfa.10716

Saleh, A. S., Zhang, Q., Chen, J., and Shen, Q. 2013. Millet grains: nutritional quality, processing, and potential health benefits. *Compr Rev Food Sci Food Saf* **12**, no. 3: 281–295. https://doi.org/10.1111/1541-4337.12012

Samtiya, M., Aluko, R. E., Dhaka, N., Dhewa, T., and Puniya, A. K. 2023. Nutritional and health-promoting attributes of millet: current and future perspectives. *Nutr Rev* **81**, no. 6: 684–704. https://doi.org/10.1093/nutrit/nuac081

Shah, P., Mehta, N., and Shah, S. 2024. Exploring the factors that drive millet consumption: insights from regular and occasional consumers. *J Retail Consum Serv* **76**: 103598. https://doi.org/10.1016/j.jretconser.2023.103598

Sharma, N., and Niranjan, K. 2018. Foxtail millet: properties, processing, health benefits, and uses. *Food Rev Int* **34**, no. 4: 329–363. https://doi.org/10.1080/87559129.2017.1290103

Sihag, M. K., Sharma, V., Goyal, A., Arora, S., and Kapila, R. 2016. In vivo assessment of iron bioavailability from fortified pearl millet based weaning food. *J Sci Food Agric* **96**, no. 13: 4410–4415. https://doi.org/10.1002/jsfa.7651

Singh, P. 2024. Celebrating International Year of Millet 2023: Analysing sustainable food security in India since independence to the amrit kaal from the lens of millets. *Indian J Pub Admin* **70**, no. 4: 788–800. https://doi.org/10.1177/00195561241251382

Singh, S., and Dunkwal, V. 2020. Development and nutritional evaluation of infant food premix to improve the nutritional status of the malnourished infants (06–24 months). *Indian J Nutr Diet* **57**, no. 4: 439–449. https://doi.org/10.21048/ijnd.2020.57.4.25430

Singh, S., Suri, S., and Singh, R. 2022. Potential and unrealized future possibilities of browntop millet in the food sector. *Front Sustain Food Syst* **6**: 974126. https://doi.org/10.3389/fsufs.2022.974126

Sood, S., Kumar, A., Babu, B. K., et al. 2016. Gene discovery and advances in finger millet [*Eleusine coracana* (L.) Gaertn.] genomics- an important nutri-cereal of future. *Front Plant Sci* **7**: 1634. https://doi.org/10.3389/fpls.2016.01634

Sruthi, N. U., and Rao, P. S. 2021. Effect of processing on storage stability of millet flour: A review. *Trends Food Sci Technol* **112**: 58–74. https://doi.org/10.1016/j.tifs.2021.03.043

Thapliyal, V., and Singh, K. 2015. Finger millet: potential millet for food security and power house of nutrients. *Int J Res Agric Forestry* **2**, no. 2: 22–33.

Tripathi, G., Jitendrakumar, P. H., Borah, A., et al. 2023. A review on nutritional and health benefits of millets. *Int J Plant Sci* **35**, no. 19: 1736–1743. https://doi.org/10.9734/IJPSS/2023/v35i193722

UNICEF. 2023. Everything about millets (POSHAN) power. Retrieved December 25, 2024, from https://knowledge.unicef.org/resource/everything-about-millets-poshan-power

Vinoth, A., and Ravindhran, R. 2017. Biofortification in millets: A sustainable approach for nutritional security. *Front Plant Sci* **8**: 29. https://doi.org/10.3389/fpls.2017.00029

WHO 2024. Retrieved December 25, 2024, from https://www.who.int/news-room/fact-sheets/detail/malnutrition

Xiong, Y., Zhang, P., Warner, R. D., and Fang, Z. 2019. Sorghum grain: From genotype, nutrition, and phenolic profile to its health benefits and food applications. *Compr Rev Food Sci Food Saf* **18**, no. 6: 2025–2046. https://doi.org/10.1111/1541-4337.12506

Zhu, Y. U., Chu, J., Lu, Z., et al. 2018. Physicochemical and functional properties of dietary fiber from foxtail millet (*Setaria italic*) bran. *J Cereal Sci* **79**: 456–461. https://doi.org/10.1016/j.jcs.2017.12.011

6 Millets During Pregnancy and Lactation
A Maternal Health Promoter

Neelam Chaturvedi
Division of Food Science and Nutrition, Faculty of Home Science, Banasthali Vidyapith, Tonk, Rajasthan, India

6.1 INTRODUCTION

Optimal nutrition during pregnancy and lactation is a critical factor for safeguarding the health of the mother and the next generations to come, as the heightened demands of essential nutrients during this period can potentially lead to some or other type of nutrient deficiency (Jouanne et al 2021). Furthermore, more attention should be given to maternal nutrition as pregnancy outcomes are influenced by it, along with a risk of developing pregnancy-related disorders. Addressing the pivotal role of nutrition during pregnancy, millets emerge as a nutrient-dense and sustainable food choice to be included in the maternal diet (Figure 6.1).

Millets are small-seeded ancient grains belonging to the family Poaceae and have been a part of staple diets of various civilizations across the globe. Naturally gluten-free, these cereal grains are packed with fiber, proteins, minerals, and vitamins along with bioactive compounds and provide greater nutritional benefits as compared to major cereals (Kumar et al 2024). Indians can trace back the cultivation of millets to the Indus Valley Civilization, attributed to their significant nutrient content and ability to thrive in arid and semi-arid conditions.

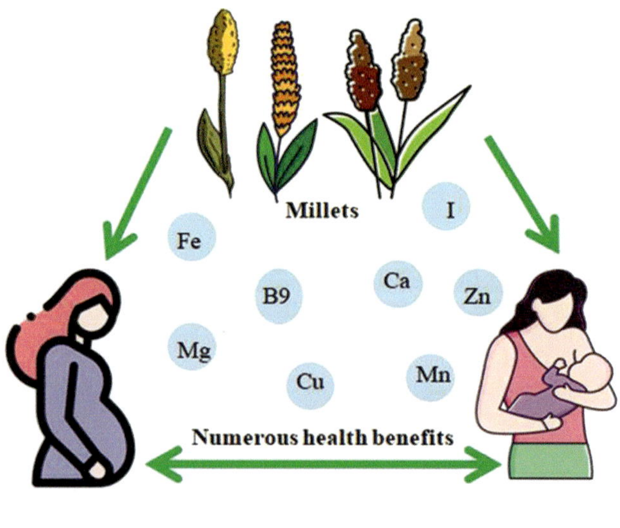

FIGURE 6.1 Millet-based nutrition for maternal health.

DOI: 10.1201/9781003686668-6

6.2 CULTURAL SIGNIFICANCE OF MILLETS: AN ANCIENT GRAIN WITH MODERN RELEVANCE

The term 'millet' is derived from the Latin word 'Milum', meaning grain. Archeological evidence suggests that millets have been growing for thousands of years and their domestication started in China, India, and Africa, around 8000 years ago (Senthamil et al 2023). The ethno-botanical importance of millets has been well documented in several ancient texts in India as well as in the texts from around the world, and owing to the presence of significant amounts of essential nutrients, millet has been part of the staple diets of several civilizations. The Vedas mention millets and elaborate upon their potential health benefits; the Harappan Civilization, which flourished around 2500 BCE, had millets as an essential part of its agriculture and diet (Haaland 2012). The Atharva Veda recognized Shayamaka (little millet) as food for birds and stranded travelers; the Rig Veda mentioned several millets such as Priyangu (foxtail millet), Anu (proso millet), and Shayamaka and acknowledged them for their ability to thrive in harsh environmental conditions (Veerabadhran et al 2023).

With the advent of the Green Revolution in India during the 1960s and the government's policies regarding food safety and security, a significant decline in millet consumption and cultivation has been observed. However, over the past few years, the awareness regarding the nutritional profile and environmental sustainability of millets has been regaining prominence, leading to a resurgence in their cultivation and consumption (Anbukkani et al 2017). In the years 2018–2019, the government of India took a significant step in spreading awareness regarding millets by recognizing them as 'Nutri-Cereals' (Ramdas et al 2023). Furthermore, the United Nations General Assembly has declared the proclaimed year 2023 as the 'International Year of Millets', to highlight the role of millets in enhancing food security and food safety, reducing nutrient deficiency and malnutrition, and addressing the global problem of climate change and sustainable agricultural practices (Kane-Potaka et al 2021).

6.3 NEED FOR MACRO- AND MICRONUTRIENTS DURING PREGNANCY AND LACTATION

Despite the presence of a large body of evidence, highlighting the role of optimal maternal nutrition during pregnancy and lactation, nearly 20–30% of all pregnant women are still affected by various nutritional deficiencies (Mousa et al 2019). Maternal diet should contain sufficient calories to satisfy the typical needs as well as those of the growing tissues, placenta, and fetus, and additional energy is required to support all the structural and hormonal changes. Hence, ensuring an adequate energy intake during pregnancy and lactation is paramount to avoid insufficient or excessive gestational weight gain, both of which are associated with complications and undesirable birth outcomes such as miscarriages, low birth weight, poor fetal growth, infant morbidity, and mortality (Hill & Hill 2024).

Following conception, protein metabolism undergoes various alterations to support fetal growth and development and maintain metabolic balance within the mother's body, and later to prepare the mother for lactation as protein is an essential structural and functional part of breast milk. Maternal protein also plays an important role in fetal programming and fetal gene expression. Protein deficiency during pregnancy can contribute to intrauterine growth restriction (IUGR) leading to poor postnatal growth rate, and during lactation, it can lead to delayed lactogenesis, reduced milk volume, and adverse impact on the growth and development of the infant (Ji et al 2017).

Millets are rich in micronutrients such as iron, calcium, zinc, magnesium, and various vitamins making them an exceptional promoter of maternal health. To support the growing tissues and fetus, blood volume in mothers increases, often leading to iron deficiency. Millets are naturally rich in iron, can help in the prevention of anemia, and aid in hemoglobin production, accommodating the elevated needs, whereas the calcium present in millets is instrumental for the growth and

TABLE 6.1
Macronutrient Content of Different Millets

Millet	Protein (g/100 g)	Carbohydrate (g/100 g)	Fats (g/100 g)	Crude Fiber (g/100 g)	Total Energy (kcal/100 g)
Pearl millet	11.4 ± 0.8	69.10 ± 1.52	4.87 ± 0.12	2.0 ± 0.55	363.0
Foxtail millet	11.34 ± 0.91	67.30 ± 5.70	3.33 ± 0.76	8.23 ± 1.66	352 ± 1.41
Finger millet	7.44 ± 0.87	71.52 ± 3.59	1.43 ± 0.12	3.60	353 ± 1.41
Banyard millet	10.76 ± 1.11	56.88 ± 6.86	3.53 ± 1.19	12.8 ± 2.4	300
Kodo millet	9.94 ± 1.6	63.82 ± 7.94	3.03 ± 1.03	8.20 ± 2.3	349.5 ± 4.95

Source: Kumar et al (2018).

mineralization of fetal growth, along with the maintenance of maternal calcium reserves (Kam et al 2016). Additionally, millets are a rich source of folate and B-group vitamins, which are crucial for fetal development as their deficiency in mothers can lead to neural tube defects in infants. The low glycemic index of millets helps in the regulation of glucose metabolism, thereby reducing the risk of gestational diabetes (Sadh et al 2024). Therefore, incorporating millet into the maternal diet can be pivotal in reducing nutritional inadequacies. Based on the scale of cultivation, consumption, and economic importance, millets are classified into major millets, including finger, sorghum, and pearl millet, and minor millets such as kodo, barnyard, proso, little, and foxtail millets. The nutrient composition of millets comprises carbohydrates, proteins, fats, and crude fiber, along with significantly high concentrations of essential fatty acids such as linolenic, linoleic, and oleic acids and essential amino acids such as methionine and cysteine (Gowda et al 2022). Macro- and micronutrient content of various millets is mentioned in Tables 6.1 and 6.2 (Kumar et al 2018).

6.4 NEED FOR BIOACTIVE COMPONENTS FOR MATERNAL HEALTH

The increased metabolic and physiological activity during pregnancy demands an adequate amount of bioactive compounds to maintain maternal homeostasis for promoting optimal growth and development of the fetus. These compounds include essential fatty acids, minerals, antioxidants, vitamins, etc. and are crucial in reducing the risk of various pregnancy-related ailments, reducing

TABLE 6.2
Micronutrient Content of Different Millets

Micronutrients (mg/100 g)	Pearl Millet	Foxtail Millet	Finger Millet	Banyard Millet	Kodo Millet
Calcium	35 ± 8.9	31 ± 11	348 ± 3.5	18.33 ± 6.0	32.33 ± 4.6
Iron	10.3 ± 7.0	3.5 ± 1.2	4.27 ± 0.6	17.47 ± 2.0	3.17 ± 1.3
Phosphorus	339	300	250	–	300
Zinc	–	60.6	60.6	57.45 ± 1.9	32.7 ± 2.2
Thiamine	0.03 ± 0.01	0.60	0.40 ± 0.1	0.33	0.15
Niacin	1.11 ± 1.3	0.55 ± 0.6	0.80 ± 0.9	0.10	0.09
Riboflavin	1.48 ± 1.9	1.65 ± 2.22	0.60 ± 0.7	4.20	2.0

Source: Kumar et al (2018).

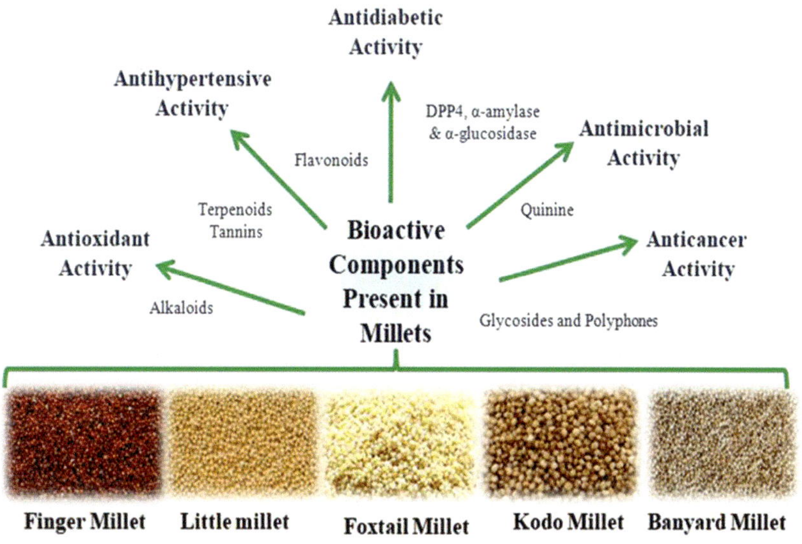

FIGURE 6.2 Bioactive components present in millets.

inflammation, and enhancing immunity (Centers for Disease Control and Prevention (CDC) 2024). Fruits and vegetables along with whole grains such as millets are a rich source of various bioactive compounds that are necessary for a healthy pregnancy. Owing to the indispensable role of these bioactives, it is crucial to integrate them into the maternal diet (Pal et al 2024).

The bioactive profile of millets includes compounds such as polyphenols, flavonoids, and antioxidants, which contribute to several health benefits. These bioactive compounds can potentially help protect the mother as well as the fetus from inflammation and oxidative stress and prevent the risk of various maternal complications such as gestational diabetes, and preeclampsia. The notable bioactive compounds present in millets are quercetin, kaempferol, ferulic acid, myricetin, and catechins (Sadh et al 2024). The presence of significant amounts of these bioactive compounds in millets can address various nutritional challenges that can occur during pregnancy and lactation (Figure 6.2).

6.5 NUTRITIONAL RECOMMENDATIONS DURING PREGNANCY AND LACTATION

Nutritional demand of pregnant and lactating women is significantly higher as compared to that of non-pregnant/non-lactating women, to accommodate all the physiological changes that occur in mothers' bodies and fetal growth. Therefore, meeting nutritional needs is crucial during pregnancy and lactation. The Indian Council of Medical Research (ICMR) has proposed Recommended Daily Allowances (RDA) for all the essential nutrients to ensure adequate intake (Gopalan et al 2024), as mentioned in Table 6.3.

Deficiency of various micronutrients among pregnant and lactating women is prevalent globally i.e., 54.6 and 52.2% of all pregnant and lactating women suffer from iron deficiency, almost 66.4% suffer from calcium deficiency, and 93.6% are affected by vitamin D deficiency. These deficiencies adversely impact maternal health and are directly linked with increased cases of anemia, gestational hypertension, maternal mortality, and obstetric issues (Anitha et al 2021).

The requirement for iron, during pregnancy and lactation, rises significantly to 29–40 mg/day, and inefficiency in meeting the demand can lead to iron deficiency anemia (IDA), leading to nutrient deficiency worldwide (Singh & Kaur 2018). The need for calcium goes up by

TABLE 6.3
Recommended Daily Allowances for Pregnant and Lactating Women

Nutrients	Non-Pregnant/ Non-Lactating Women	Pregnancy		Lactation	
		2nd Trimester	3rd Trimester	0–6 Months	7–12 Months
Protein (g/d)	45.7	+9.5	+22.0	+16.9	+13.2
CHO (g/d)	130	175	175	200	23.2
Calcium (mg/d)	1000	1000		1200	
Magnesium (mg/d)	325	385		325	
Iron (mg/d)	29	40		23	
Zinc (mg/d)	13.2	14.5		14	
Iodine (µg/d)	150	250		280	
Thiamine (mg/d)	1.7	2.0		2.1	
Riboflavin (mg/d)	2.4	2.7		3.0	2.9
Niacin (mg/d)	14	+2.5		+5	+5
Vitamin B6 (mg/d)	1.9	2.3		+0.26	+0.17
Folate (µg/d)	220	570		330	330
Vitamin B12 (µg/d)	2.5	+0.25		+1.0	
Vitamin C (mg/d)	65	+15		+50	
Vitamin A (µg/d)	840	900		950	
Vitamin D (IU/d)	600	600		600	

Source: Gopalan et al (2024).

1000–1200 mg/day and insufficient calcium intake can lead to decreased bone mineralization in the mother as well as the fetus, gestational hypertension, and preterm birth. Zinc deficiency can lead to congenital deformities caused by altered nucleic acid metabolism, IUGR, and a high risk of infections, eclampsia, and preterm delivery. Demand for zinc rises to 14 mg/day during pregnancy (Jouanne et al 2021). Various studies have linked gestational diabetes, fetal growth disorders, gestational hypertension, preeclampsia, and preterm birth with magnesium deficiency (Dalton et al 2016). Congenital heart defects and neural tube defects in infants are directly linked with maternal folate deficiency owing to its pivotal role in the synthesis of nucleic acids and amino acid metabolism (Marangoni et al 2016). The need for iodine during pregnancy is elevated up to 220–250 µg/day due to the production of hCG (human chorionic gonadotropin) hormone (Zimmermann 2012).

Adequate levels of all the essential vitamins are necessary to maintain maternal and fetal health as their deficiency can lead to serious health outcomes for mother and fetus. Vitamin D deficiency during pregnancy and lactation often leads to fatigue, back pain, and symptomatic osteomalacia and to prevent these adverse impacts, 10–15 µg vitamin D is recommended per day. Pyridoxine (vitamin B6) is an important vitamin for preventing nausea during pregnancy (Jouanne et al 2021). Lactating mothers have an increased nutrient need to accommodate and support the production of nutrient-rich milk for the infant, mineralization of infant bones, immune-protective role, and physical and cognitive development of the infant, including maternal tissue repair. Additionally, breastfeeding mothers need adequate amounts of protein, calcium, vitamin C, vitamin D, and B-group vitamins. Adequate intake of all the essential nutrients is imperative for maternal and fetal health; likewise, this nutrient need also continues during the postnatal period, highlighting the necessity of adequate nutrition throughout pregnancy and lactation.

6.6 NUTRITIONAL BENEFITS OF VARIOUS MILLETS DURING PREGNANCY AND LACTATION

Millets such as finger millet, foxtail millet, barnyard millet, etc. are the powerhouse of essential nutrients and their inclusion in the maternal diet can garner numerous health benefits for maternal as well as fetal health (Figure 6.3).

6.6.1 Foxtail Millet (Kangni)

Foxtail millet is a nutrient-dense grain and contains appreciable amounts of various essential nutrients such as dietary fiber (6–7 g/100 g) which helps in preventing digestive issues that are commonly observed during pregnancy. It has about 2.8 mg/100 g of iron content which supports hemoglobin production that helps in maintaining a healthy blood volume. Foxtail millet can be very helpful in combating muscle cramps that are often observed during pregnancy due to its high calcium content, i.e., 31 mg/100 g (Sharma & Niranjan 2017). Owing to its rich dietary fiber content, foxtail millet has a low glycemic index which is extremely beneficial in the prevention and management of gestational diabetes. Therefore, the incorporation of foxtail millet in the maternal diet in various forms such as laddu, roti, porridges, etc. can effectively support the nutritional demands as well as aid in the control and prevention of various pregnancy-related complications.

6.6.2 Finger Millet (Ragi)

Ragi is referred to as 'women-friendly' millet due to its exceptionally high calcium content, i.e., 344 mg/100 g. It is a superfood that must be incorporated into the maternal diet for the maintenance and development of maternal as well as fetal bone health. Calcium is one of the most important minerals for the production of breast milk, and its deficiency can lead to depletion of calcium reserve in the body, leading to long-term impact on maternal bone health. IDA, the most prevalent micronutrient deficiency across the world, with adverse birth outcomes, can easily be managed and reversed through the incorporation of finger millet in the maternal diet, because of its high iron content (3.9 mg/100 g). Additionally, finger millet also contains appreciable amounts of magnesium and potassium that help in reducing muscle cramping and maintaining electrolyte balance during

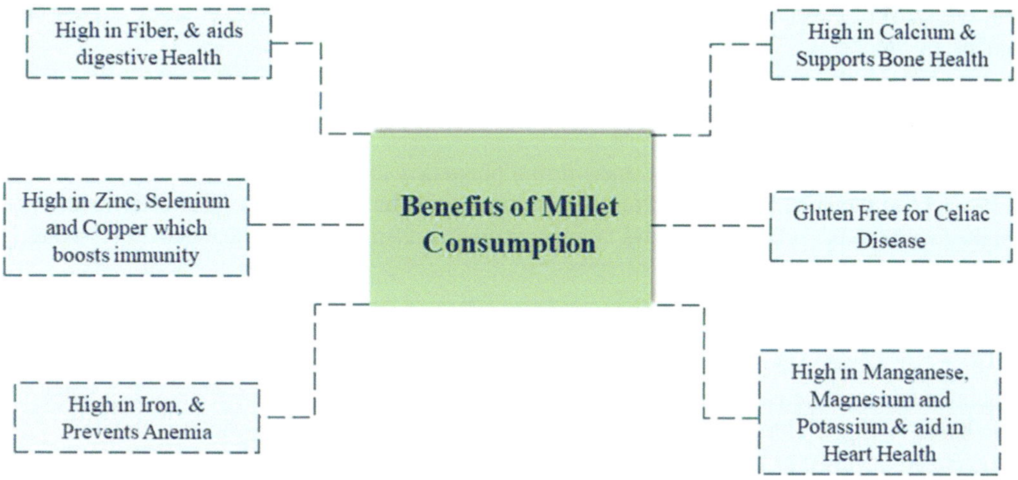

FIGURE 6.3 Health benefits of millet consumption.

pregnancy. A study conducted by Hemamalin and Babitha (2019) has elucidated the positive impact of ragi intake on iron and calcium levels of expectant and lactating mothers.

6.6.3 Pearl Millet (Bajra)

It is rich in various essential nutrients making it a highly nutritious grain that can help address various deficiencies and complications that occur during pregnancy and lactation. The presence of magnesium (114 mg/100 g) in this millet can help in the prevention of complications such as gestational hypertension. The folate content of pearl millet is about 45 μg/100 g, which is advantageous in mitigating fetal neural tube defects (Goswami et al 2020). The high protein content of pearl millet helps in fetal growth, and repair and maintenance of maternal tissues. Gestational diabetes can be effectively managed with the intake of pearl millet due to the presence of dietary fiber in it. Hence, the inclusion of pear millet in various food preparations for pregnant and lactating mothers can offer numerous advantages.

6.6.4 Barnyard Millet (Sanwa)

It is an energy-dense and highly nutritious grain that has several health benefits to offer. Owing to its low glycemic index, the barnyard millet aids in ensuring proper glucose metabolism. The bioactive content present in the barnyard millet is rich in several antioxidants, which can effectively manage the oxidative stress and inflammation, experienced during pregnancy and lactation. Furthermore, the insoluble fiber content of the millet aids in cholesterol management which can be potentially helpful in managing gestational hypertension (Bhatt et al 2020). Barnyard millet is a very versatile millet and can easily be integrated into the maternal diet through soups, rotis, khichdi, etc.

6.6.5 Sorghum (Jowar)

It is known for its high nutrient content; sorghum is an excellent source of various macro- and micronutrients such as copper, iron, calcium, and B-group vitamins such as niacin and thiamin. These are highly beneficial in maintaining maternal health. The presence of phenolic compounds and flavonoids makes the antioxidant profile of sorghum very rich, aiding in the mitigation of oxidative stress and providing additional help and support to the maternal immune system (Xiong et al 2019). The addition of sorghum in maternal diets can be done easily due to its adaptability in various types of flavors. It can be used to make value-added products such as cookies, cakes, soups, salads, porridges, etc.

6.7 HARNESSING MILLETS TO MITIGATE MATERNAL HEALTH RISKS

The altered physiological state of women during pregnancy and lactation can pose several risks to maternal health which are essential to address, for positive birth outcomes. The inclusion of millet in the maternal diet is one of the ways to manage pregnancy-related complications through diet.

6.7.1 Millets and Iron Deficiency

The global prevalence of IDA during pregnancy and lactation is very high and it is the most common maternal hematological condition. IDA occurs when the concentration of hemoglobin in the blood is 11 gm/dl or less (Garzon et al 2020). The most common symptoms experienced by women suffering from IDA are fatigue, shortness of breath, lightheadedness, pica, tachycardia, etc. Furthermore, deficiency in iron during pregnancy and lactation can hamper various physiological and cellular activities that are essential for the growth and development of the fetus. Mothers deficient in iron can experience a delay in postpartum recovery. IDA can lead to a weakened immune system making the mother susceptible to various infections, and the milk produced by iron-deficient mothers can potentially cause iron deficiency in the infant (Annamraju & Pavord 2016).

One of the key strategies to combat IDA is the inclusion of foods that are naturally rich in iron, such as barnyard and finger millet in the maternal diet. Chandel et al (2014) in their study, analyzed the iron content of various millets such as foxtail, kodo, finger, and barnyard and concluded that the iron concentration of barnyard millet was highest among all the other types, i.e., 40.2 ppm, reinstating the use of millets in combating iron deficiency.

6.7.2 Millets and Preeclampsia

Preeclampsia is a pregnancy-related complication characterized by high blood pressure and protein in urine that usually arises after the 20th week of pregnancy. It affects about 2–15% of all pregnancies and is one of the most prevalent conditions that poses a significant risk for both mother and the fetus, with an increase in the rates of maternal mortality and morbidity. Women suffering from it exhibit symptoms such as edema of the face, hands, and feet, sudden weight gain, nausea, vision problems, etc. (Chang et al 2023). Various risk factors such as endometriosis, abnormalities in the placenta, heredity, etc. can contribute to the high rates of incidence of preeclampsia during pregnancy (Briceño-Pérez et al 2009).

The dietary management of preeclampsia includes the inclusion of calcium-rich foods such as finger millet which are naturally abundant in calcium, which is directly related to the regulation of blood pressure. Additionally, the inclusion of millets with high protein and fiber content can also contribute to the prevention and management of preeclampsia (Rani et al 2021).

6.7.3 Millets and Gestational Diabetes Mellitus

The inability of the body to produce sufficient insulin during pregnancy gives rise to gestational diabetes mellitus (GDM), leading to a spike in blood glucose levels. Women with GDM often exhibit generic symptoms like an increase in thirst, polyuria, fatigue, and increased episodes of infection. This makes it imperative for pregnant women to undergo regular screening, as it may lead to preterm birth, babies with respiratory distress syndrome, and increased risk of obesity and type 2 diabetes (Hinkle et al 2016). The findings of Wang et al (2021) elucidated that 14% of the total pregnancies worldwide suffer from GDM, with slight regional variations.

Dietary management is very crucial for the prevention of GDM which includes the incorporation of food groups that have low glycemic index, making millets an ideal choice. Vetriventhan et al (2021) concluded that the fiber content of millets is 2.3–4 times higher than that of the major cereals such as rice and wheat, which is substantial in controlling sugar spikes. Several studies have established that millet such as finger millet can potentially have antidiabetic properties, owing to its low glycemic load and ability to modulate gut microbiome (Singh et al 2022). Additionally, millets also have several micronutrients and bioactive compounds that have a positive impact on the prevention of GDM.

6.7.4 Millets and Constipation

Owing to hormonal changes such as an increase in progesterone and the pressure from a growing fetus, constipation is the most common complication that occurs during pregnancy. Management of constipation includes an increase in the intake of fiber-rich foods such as millet, as fiber adds bulk to the stool and retains water, promoting regular bowel movements (Anagha 2023). The gut-regulating effect of millets also plays a significant role in relieving digestive issues; additionally, to further maximize the digestive benefits of millets, processing such as soaking and fermentation can be done. Dishes such as millet-based soups, porridges, and khichdi can be included in the maternal diet as an effective strategy to combat constipation and also millets being gluten-free are especially beneficial for women with gluten intolerance (Sadh et al 2024).

6.7.5 Millets and Morning Sickness

Early in pregnancy, women may experience symptoms such as nausea and vomiting, called morning sickness due to the high rate of occurrence in the morning, but can happen at any time of the day. The major factor responsible for morning sickness is a rapid surge in hormones, especially estrogen and hCG, that can have a direct impact on the digestive tract (Anagha 2023). Owing to the fiber content, millets have a positive impact on morning sickness. Millets are an alkaline-forming food group that help to balance acidity in the stomach that can potentially help in relieving the symptoms of morning sickness. Sudden drop in blood glucose levels can also elevate the symptoms of morning sickness; hence, the complex carbohydrates present in the millets may help in mitigating the problem by a gradual release of energy (Mishra & Singh 2024). Additionally, the presence of micronutrients such as magnesium and B-group vitamins can also contribute significantly to combating morning sickness.

6.8 MILLET-BASED FOODS FOR COMPREHENSIVE MATERNAL HEALTH AND WELLNESS

With the increasing awareness regarding the nutrient profile of the millets, their inclusion in the maternal diet is encouraged to garner various health benefits that they can offer. The essential nutrients present in the millets not only support the general needs of expectant mothers but can effectively meet the increased need for various nutrients during pregnancy and lactation. Several studies have shown the positive impact of millet-based food items on the reduction of the incidence rate of various micronutrient deficiencies and millets as an effective strategy for the management of pregnancy-related complications such as anemia, constipation, gestational hypertension, etc. (Narayan et al 2019). Inclusion of millets in the maternal diet in the form of everyday food is very easy due to the flavor profile of millets. Foods like flatbreads, porridge, breakfast flakes, and ready-to-eat snacks or cookies can all be made out of millets or a blend of millets for maximizing the benefits. Furthermore, malt made out of millet is another nutrient-rich option for expectant and lactating mothers as the malting enhances the bioavailability of micronutrients. Traditional Indian recipes made out of millets include idli, dosa, aape appam, laddus, kheer, roti, etc. Gaudadhe et al (2023) have highlighted ways through which millets can be incorporated into the daily diets of pregnant and lactating women as mentioned in Table 6.4.

TABLE 6.4
Millets and Their Potential Food Preparations

Millet	Food Products
Sorghum	Roti, ugali, popped sorghum, malt food, roasted mixed grains.
Pearl millet	Roti, ugali, fermented food products, roasted mixed grains, porridge
Finger millet	Roti, dumplings, cookies, ragi-malt, ragi-mudde, cake, idli
Little millet	Roti, cookies, cake, idli, kheer
Foxtail millet	Upma, dosa, cookies, kheer
Banyard millet	Khichdi, porridge, pancakes, laddu
Proso millet	Millet soup, upma, porridge, idli
Kodo millet	Chivda, pancakes, kheer

Source: Gaudadhe et al (2023).

6.9 LIMITATIONS AND CONSIDERATIONS

Despite the presence of a plethora of evidence suggesting the innumerable benefits of millets for lactation and pregnancy, there still is a huge gap in the consumption of millets. Additionally, comprehensive human trials are essential for evaluating digestibility, allergenic potential, and suitability of millets for diverse populations to form informed dietary guidelines. Certain challenges are associated with the usage of millet in day-to-day life that must be taken into consideration for maximum benefit, such as the following:

1. *Presence of anti-nutritional factors*: Millets have high phytic acid content which hinders the bioavailability of mineral ions like calcium, magnesium, iron, zinc, along with the presence of various types of enzyme inhibitors such as protease inhibitors, alpha-amylase inhibitors, and trypsin inhibitors which can negatively impact amino acid metabolism (Rajakumar et al 2023), hence requiring proper processing techniques.
2. *Shelf-life management*: The high nutritional content of millets and a naturally high enzymatic activity make millets prone to spoilage, making proper pre-treatment and specialized storage conditions mandatory for millets, contributing to the increase in cost (Harish et al 2024).
3. *Lack of awareness*: The general population remains largely unaware of the numerous health benefits that millet can impart, resulting in its low demand.
4. *Agricultural challenges*: Millet cultivation is often associated with poor market linkage, high labor cost, and lack of processing facilities, resulting in low yields and reducing its accessibility to consumers.

6.10 CONCLUSION

The nutrient profile of millets offers an exceptional opportunity for enhancing maternal health, garnering them the status of superfoods. Millets serve as a comprehensive solution for the complications that can arise during pregnancy and lactation such as micronutrient deficiencies, anemia, digestive issues, GDM, gestational hypertension, preeclampsia, etc. Additionally, the essential nutrients present in the millet also foster the proper growth and development of the fetus, as maternal deficiency can have an adverse impact on the fetal birth outcomes, such as preterm delivery, low birth weight, congenital malformations, etc. The ability of millets to thrive in harsh and drought-prone conditions makes them a sustainable source of holistic nutrients. Going forward, integration of millets in maternal diets should be prioritized along with educating pregnant and lactating women regarding all the benefits of millets through various means such as campaigns, workshops, etc. Bridging nutritional knowledge of millets with practical applications can significantly transform maternal health outcomes.

REFERENCES

Anagha, K. 2023. Millets: Nutritional importance, health benefits, and bioavailability: A review. *He Pharma Innovation Journal*, *12*(8), 223–227.

Anbukkani, P., Balaji, S. J., & Nithyashree, M. L. 2017. Production and consumption of minor millets in India-A structural break analysis. *Annals of Agricultural Research*, *38*(4), 1–8.

Anitha, S., Kane-Potaka, J., Tsusaka, T. W., Botha, R., Rajendran, A., Givens, D. I., Parasannanavar, D. J., Subramaniam, K., Prasad, K. D. V., Vetriventhan, M., & Bhandari, R. K. 2021. A systematic review and meta-analysis of the potential of millets for managing and reducing the risk of developing diabetes mellitus. *Frontiers in Nutrition*, *8*. https://doi.org/10.3389/fnut.2021.687428

Annamraju, H., & Pavord, S. 2016. Anaemia in pregnancy. *British Journal of Hospital Medicine*, *77*(Sup10), 584–588. https://doi.org/10.12968/hmed.2016.77.10.584

Bhatt, S., Singh, S., Singh, P., & Pandey, V. 2020. Chemical composition of Jhingora (Indian barnyard millet) varieties cultivated in Uttarakhand and their uses. *Journal of Food Science and Technology*, *57*(5), 1789–1797.

Briceño-Pérez, C., Briceño-Sanabria, L., & Gracia, P. V. 2009. Prediction and prevention of preeclampsia. *Hypertension in Pregnancy*, *28*(2), 138–155. https://doi.org/10.1080/10641950802022384

Chandel, G., Kumar Meena, R., & Dubey, M. 2014. Nutritional properties of minor millets: neglected cereals with potentials to combat malnutrition. *Current Science*, *107*(7), 1109–1111.

Chang, K., Seow, K., & Chen, K. 2023. Preeclampsia: Recent advances in predicting, preventing, and managing the maternal and fetal life-threatening condition. *International Journal of Environmental Research and Public Health*, *20*(4), 2994–2996. https://doi.org/10.3390/ijerph20042994

Dalton, L. M., Fhloinn, D. M. N., Gaydadzhieva, G. T., Mazurkiewicz, O. M., Leeson, H., & Wright, C. P. 2016. Magnesium in pregnancy. *Nutrition Reviews*, *74*(9), 549–557. https://doi.org/10.1093/nutrit/nuw018

Garzon, S., Cacciato, P. M., Certelli, C., Salvaggio, C., Magliarditi, M., & Rizzo, G. 2020. Iron deficiency Anemia in pregnancy: Novel approaches for an old problem. *Oman Medical Journal*, *35*(5), e166. https://doi.org/10.5001/omj.2020.108

Gaudadhe, N. N., Raut, A. A., Bisht, K., & Bisht, K. 2023. Assessment of production trends, nutritional benefits, constraints, policy support, processing and value addition of millets for achieving higher productivity and nutritional security. *Indian Journal of Fertilisers*, *19*(10), 1020–1031.

Gopalan, C., Rama Shastri, B.V., & Balasubramaniam, S.C. 2024. *Nutritive Value of Indian Foods*. National Institute of Nutrition, Indian Council of Medical Research.

Goswami, S., Asrani, P., Ali, T. P. A., et al. 2020. Rancidity matrix: Development of biochemical indicators for analysing the keeping quality of pearl millet flour. *Food Analytical Methods*, *13*(10), 2147–2164. https://doi.org/10.1007/s12161-020-01831-2

Gowda, N. N., Siliveru, K., Prasad, P. V., Bhatt, Y., Netravati, B. P., & Gurikar, C. 2022. Modern processing of Indian millets: A perspective on changes in nutritional properties. *Foods*, *11*(4), 499.

Haaland, R. 2012. Crops and culture: Dispersal of African millets to the Indian subcontinent and its cultural consequences. *Dhaulagiri Journal of Sociology and Anthropology*, *5*, 1–30. https://doi.org/10.3126/dsaj.v5i0.6354

Harish, M. S., Bhuker, A., & Chauhan, B. S. 2024. Millet production, challenges, and opportunities in the Asia-pacific region: A comprehensive review. *Frontiers in Sustainable Food Systems*, *8*. https://doi.org/10.3389/fsufs.2024.1386469

Hemamalin, K., & Babitha, B. 2019. A study on effect of millet intake on iron levels of pregnant and lactating women in the Tadepalli mandal Guntur district. *International Journal of Food and Nutritional Sciences*, *8*(1), 862–871.

Hill, D. J., & Hill, T. G. 2024. Maternal diet during pregnancy and adaptive changes in the maternal and fetal pancreas have implications for future metabolic health. *Frontiers in Endocrinology*, *15*. https://doi.org/10.3389/fendo.2024.1456629

Hinkle, S. N., Louis, G. M. B., Rawal, S., Zhu, Y., Albert, P. S., & Zhang, C. 2016. A longitudinal study of depression and gestational diabetes in pregnancy and the postpartum period. *Diabetologia*, *59*(12), 2594–2602. https://doi.org/10.1007/s00125-016-4086-1

Ji, Y., Wu, Z., Dai, Z., Wang, X., Li, J., Wang, B., & Wu, G. 2017. Fetal and neonatal programming of postnatal growth and feed efficiency in swine. *Journal of Animal Science and Biotechnology/Journal of Animal Science and Biotechnology*, *8*(1). https://doi.org/10.1186/s40104-017-0173-5

Jouanne, M., Oddoux, S., Noël, A., & Voisin-Chiret, A. S. 2021. Nutrient requirements during pregnancy and lactation. *Nutrients*, *13*(2), 692. https://doi.org/10.3390/nu13020692

Kam, J., Puranik, S., Yadav, R., Manwaring, H. R., Pierre, S., Srivastava, R. K., & Yadav, R. S. 2016. Dietary interventions for Type 2 diabetes: How millet comes to help. *Frontiers in Plant Science*, *7*. https://doi.org/10.3389/fpls.2016.01454

Kane-Potaka, J., Anitha, S., Tsusaka, T. W., Botha, R., Budumuru, M., Upadhyay, S., Kumar, P., Mallesh, K., Hunasgi, R., Jalagam, A. K., & Nedumaran, S. 2021. Assessing millets and sorghum consumption behavior in Urban India: A Large-Scale Survey. *Frontiers in Sustainable Food Systems*, *5*, 680776–680777. https://doi.org/10.3389/fsufs.2021.680777

Kumar, A., Tomer, V., Kaur, A., Kumar, V., & Gupta, K. 2018. Millets: A solution to agrarian and nutritional challenges. *Agriculture & Food Security*, *7*(1), 31. https://doi.org/10.1186/s40066-018-0183-3

Kumar, V., Yadav, M., Awala, S. K., Valombola, J. S., Saxena, M. S., Ahmad, F., & Saxena, S. C. 2024. Millets: A nutritional powerhouse for ensuring food security. *Planta*, *260*(4), 101–104. https://doi.org/10.1007/s00425-024-04533-9

Marangoni, F., Cetin, I., Verduci, E., Canzone, G., Giovannini, M., Scollo, P., Corsello, G., & Poli, A. 2016. Maternal diet and nutrient requirements in pregnancy and breastfeeding. an Italian consensus document. *Nutrients*, *8*(10), 629–630. https://doi.org/10.3390/nu8100629

Mishra, S., & Singh, R. 2023. Potential health-benefits of millets "Nutri-Cereals" – A review. *Journal of Primary Care & General Practice*, *6*(5), 1–10.

Mousa, A., Naqash, A., & Lim, S. 2019. Macronutrient and micronutrient intake during pregnancy: An overview of recent evidence. *Nutrients*, *11*(2), 443–444. https://doi.org/10.3390/nu11020443

Narayan, J., John, D., & Ramadas, N. 2019. Malnutrition in India: status and government initiatives. *Journal of Public Health Policy*, *40*, 126–141.

Pal, S., Agnihotri, U., Singh, R., Shukla, A., & Dev, R. 2024. Plant derived bioactive compounds during pregnancy: A comprehensive review. *International Journal of All Research Education and Scientific Methods*, *12*(11), 3237–3244.

Rajakumar, R., Ammal, U. B., Sankar, R., Selvaraj, S., Jayalakshmi, C., Umamageswari, M., & Pai, V. G. 2023. Anti-Nutritional Factors in Millets and Their Reduction Strategies. In *Sensitizing the Millet Farming, Consumption and Nutritional Security – Challenges and Opportunities.*

Ramdas, S., Joseph, J., Panathady, A. M., Devi, S., T., Swaminathan, N., & Pouchepparadjou, A. 2023. Status of Millets in India: Trends and Prospects. In A. Pouchepparadjou, V. Krishnan, N. Swaminathan, R. Sendhil, L. Umamaheswari, T. Sivasakthi Devi, S. Parthasarathi, V. Vengadessan, & M. Umamageswari (Eds.), *Sensitizing the Millet Farming, Consumption and Nutritional Security- Challenges and Opportunities* (pp. 15–25).

Rani, G. S., Swaminathan, A., & Vijayaraghavan, R. 2021. Effectiveness of physical activity and finger millet-based food supplement on biochemical parameters and bone mineral density among premenopausal women. *Evidence-Based Complementary and Alternative Medicine*, *2021*, 1–7. https://doi.org/10.1155/2021/4757991

Sadh, P. K., Kamboj, A., Kumar, S., Chawla, P., Kumar, R., Saharan, B. S., Kumar, D., Duhan, S., Nehra, M., Goyal, C., Brar, B., Joshi, S., & Duhan, J. S. 2024. Perspectives of millets for nutritional properties, health benefits and food of the future: A review. *Discover Food*, *4*(1). https://doi.org/10.1007/s44187-024-00266-6

Senthamil, E., Tamilmounika, R., & Kowsalya, V. 2023. Cultural heritage of Millets. *Farm Chronicle – An Agriculture Newsletter*, *2*, 77–81.

Sharma, N., & Niranjan, K. 2017. Foxtail millet: Properties, processing, health benefits, and uses. *Food Reviews International*, *34*(4), 329–363. https://doi.org/10.1080/87559129.2017.1290103

Singh, S., & Kaur, K. 2018. Maternal outcome in cases of severe anaemia in labour. *International Journal of Reproduction Contraception Obstetrics and Gynecology*, *7*(3), 1201. https://doi.org/10.18203/2320-1770.ijrcog20180918

Singh, V., Gupta, V., Bhardwaj, R., & Tripathi, K. 2022. Anti-diabetic prospects of dietary bio-actives of millets and the significance of the gut microbiota: A case of finger millet. *Frontiers in Nutrition*, *9*, 997358.

Veerabadhran, V., Palakuru, H. R., Pratap, G. P., Rajeshwari, B., Prasad, G. P., Srikanth, N., & Acharya, R. 2023. A critical review of the history and practices of millets in India. *Journal of Drug Research in Ayurvedic Sciences*, *8*(Suppl 1), S18–S25. https://doi.org/10.4103/jdras.jdras_113_23

Vetriventhan, M., Upadhyaya, H. D., Azevedo, V. C., Allan, V., & Anitha, S. 2021. Variability and trait-specific accessions for grain yield and nutritional traits in germplasm of little millet (*Panicum sumatrense* Roth. Ex. Roem. & Schult.). *Crop Science*, *61*(4), 2658–2679. https://doi.org/10.1002/csc2.20527

Wang, H., Li, N., Chivese, T., Werfalli, M., Sun, H., Yuen, L., & Yang, X. 2021. IDF Diabetes Atlas: Estimation of global and regional gestational diabetes mellitus prevalence for 2021 by International Association of Diabetes in Pregnancy Study Group's criteria. *Diabetes Research and Clinical Practice*, *183*, 109050. https://doi.org/10.1016/j.diabres.2021.109050

Xiong, Y., Zhang, P., Warner, R. D., & Fang, Z. 2019. Sorghum grain: From genotype, nutrition, and phenolic profile to its health benefits and food applications. *Journal of Food Science and Technology*, *56*(7), 3501–3512.

Zimmermann, M. B. 2012. The effects of iodine deficiency in pregnancy and infancy. *Paediatric and Perinatal Epidemiology*, *26*(s1), 108–117. https://doi.org/10.1111/j.1365-3016.2012.01275.x

7 Millets
An Immunity-Boosting Treasure

Bhavna, Shivangi Singh Chauhan, and Sangeeta C. Sindhu
Department of Foods & Nutrition, CCS Haryana Agricultural University, Hisar, India

7.1 INTRODUCTION

The COVID-19 pandemic took the whole world by storm. Other than being devastating, it also taught us some important lessons. Suddenly hygiene and immunity-boosting natural foods became as important as taking vaccine shots in time. The sudden focus on immunity-booster foods brought Ayurveda into limelight and people became more conscious of food on their plates. Rightly has someone said, "Eat what comes from plants; not what we make in plants". The pandemic aroused significant interest in immunity boosting through natural foods. One of the significant dietary shifts during this period was toward millets (Gonella et al 2022).

The growing interest in millets is actually a connection being explored to our ancient grains that present to us nature's nutritional power. Millets stand out as a true "superfood" that has been cherished for centuries across various cultures. Millets find mention in ancient medicine scriptures of India (Ayurveda) as well as that of China (Jarosz et al 2024). During the COVID-19 pandemic, millets gained popularity due to their known potential to boost immunity. Packed with essential nutrients and offering a range of health benefits, millets rapidly gained recognition not just as a versatile, gluten-free alternative but also as an immunity-boosting powerhouse. Rich in antioxidants, vitamins, and minerals, millets support the body's natural defense system, helping to enhance immune function, combat inflammation, and improve overall health. Post Covid, we have reached an era where immunity has become more crucial than ever. Thus, interweaving millets into our daily diet could be a simple yet effective way to fortify our body's defenses through nourishment. Whether consumed as a wholesome grain, flour, or in other creative forms, millets offer a treasure trove of benefits that make its comeback, a valuable addition to the modern diet.

This chapter navigates through the understanding of the concept of immunity, interrelationship of nutrients and immunity and the scientific evidence in favor of millets as an immunity-boosting treasure.

7.2 IMMUNITY – THE BASIC CONCEPT AND REGULATION

Immunity refers to "the body's ability to resist or defend itself against harmful organisms, such as pathogens (bacteria, viruses, fungi, and parasites), as well as foreign substances and abnormal cells (e.g., cancer cells)". This defense system involves complex interactions between different components of the immune system, including cells, proteins, and tissues, which work together to recognize and eliminate threats. Typically, immunity can be innate (non-specific immunity) or acquired (specific immunity).

7.2.1 Innate Immunity

Innate immunity is the "body's first line of defense against pathogens" and is present from birth. It provides a general response to pathogens, regardless of their specific type. It is a long-term immunity

DOI: 10.1201/9781003686668-7

in which our body produces the antibodies on its own. Our body has mainly four types of natural defense to prevent the entry of pathogens. These include the following:

- *Physical barriers*: Skin, mucous secretions, tears, earwax, and stomach acid act as natural physical barriers to prevent pathogens from entering the body.
- *Phagocytes*: White blood cells like macrophages and neutrophils circulate through the body searching for any foreign substance. They engulf and destroy these foreign substances, defending the body against pathogens. Major examples of phagocytes include macrophages, mast cells, neutrophils, eosinophils, basophils, dendritic cells, and natural killer cells.
- *Inflammation*: Inflammation forms a key defense mechanism against both infectious and non-infectious threats. Whenever tissues get damaged, the body releases chemicals that change vascular flow and cause leakage of fluid from blood vessels into the tissues. This results in swelling, redness, and increased regional temperature to isolate and destroy pathogens. Inflammation, however, can be harmful if it occurs in healthy tissues or goes on for too long.
- *Complement proteins*: Complement proteins are soluble proteins that are produced by liver and are circulated in an inactive state. These proteins play an important role in initiating the inflammatory response by changing vascular flow and permeability, clearing immune complexes, increasing the number of leukocytes, modulating immunoglobulin production, opsonizing microbial pathogens by binding to them and marking them for destruction by phagocytes.

7.2.2 Acquired Immunity

Acquired immunity develops over time and is more specific to particular pathogens. It can recognize and fight specific invaders more effectively after an initial exposure. The acquired immunity may be active or passive. It is called as active when the body produces its own immune response to a specific pathogen, either through exposure to the pathogen or vaccination. This may happen naturally by infection or artificially by vaccination. In the case of vaccination, the immune system is exposed to a harmless version of a given pathogen (e.g., a killed or weakened virus) and generates immunity without causing illness. On the other hand, when immunity is transferred from another source, such as through the placenta (from mother to fetus) or via antibody-containing blood products (e.g., immunoglobulin shots), it is known as passive immunity. Passive immunity provides temporary protection, as the body does not produce its own immune response (Janeway et al 2005).

The acquired immunity is either antibody-mediated or cell-mediated (Figure 7.1).

- *Antibody-mediated immunity*: Reactions carried out by antibodies are called "humoral immune reactions". Antibody-mediated immunity relates to B cells or the B lymphocytes which develop in the fetal liver. Post birth, B cells are known to develop in the bone marrow from hematopoietic stem cells. The process is called hematopoiesis. When a B cell encounters an antigen, it is stimulated to proliferate into a plasma cell. This leads to expansion of the number of plasma cells, which are capable of secreting antibody to the given antigen (Gombart et al 2020). The contact of B cells with antigen and their interactions with T cells, macrophages, or complement regulate their replication and differentiation into plasma cells. After the initial encounter with antigen, B cells also differentiate into memory B cells after activation. These memory of B cells remember the antigen and can facilitate a rapid activation to create plasma cells and antibodies if the antigen is encountered again.
- *Cell-mediated immunity*: Cell-mediated immunity is conferred through T cells. There are two types of T cells: cytotoxic T cells (CD8+ T cells or killer T cells), which are directly

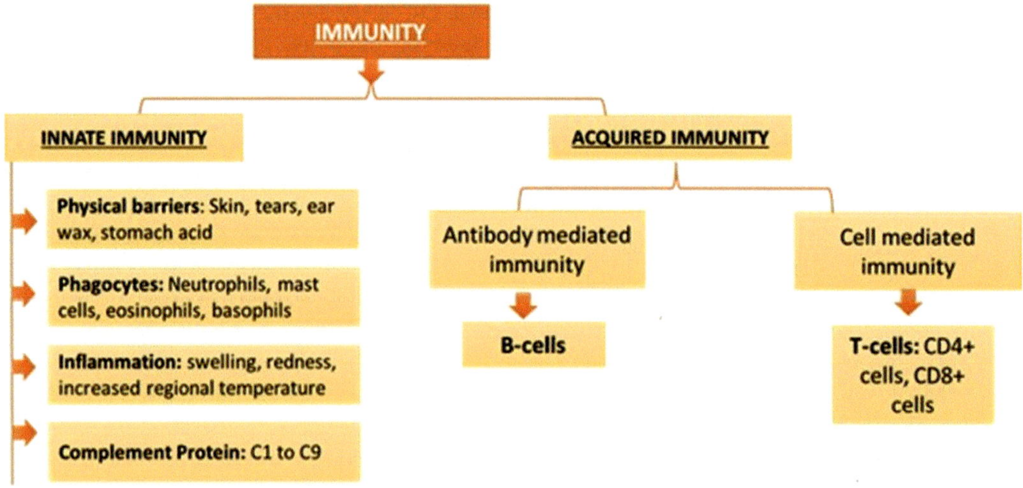

FIGURE 7.1 The basic regulation of immunity.

involved in killing infected cells/tumor cells (Jasenosky et al 2015), and T_4 helper cells (CD4+ cells), which send signals to other cells to coordinate an attack. The cytotoxic CD8 T cells release two types of preformed cytotoxic protein: the granzymes and perforin. Granzymes induce apoptosis in target cells while perforin creates holes in the membrane of target cells. The granzymes enter the target cell through these punched holes. The CD4 T cells on the other hand differentiate into CD4 Th_1 and CD4 Th_2 effector cells. Th_1 cells are mainly involved in the eradication of virus-infected cells and intracellular pathogens within peripheral tissues. Interferon IFNγ is their signature cytokine and they also produce tumor necrosis factor TNF-α. Th_2 cells, on the other hand, are defined by the transcription factor GATA-3. Other cytokines secreted by Th_2 cells include IL-4, IL-5, and IL-10 (Howard et al 2022).

7.3 ROLE OF NUTRITION IN IMMUNITY

Food and disease share a strong relationship. Food is a complex matrix capable of supplying the nutrients along with other dietary compounds that are essential to life and have beneficial synergic effects on health. Food not only nourishes our body but also supports optimal immunological response. Balanced nutrition provides not only the building blocks for immune cell synthesis but also provides energy for their proliferation and maturation. It supports an individual's immunity by providing adequate nutrients in sufficient concentrations to the immune cells. The nutrients along with the non-nutrient components of food support the body's ability to fight infections, regulate inflammation, and maintain immune cell health. The immune system requires a variety of nutrients to function optimally. Innate immunity is the first wall of defense that falls in a malnourished individual. In fact, low immunity and undernutrition form a vicious cycle, boosting each other. Both upper respiratory and enteric infections are part of this vicious cycle. The importance and role of nutrition in immunity is very much evident from the famous phrase "Let food be thy medicine and medicine be thy food".

7.3.1 Nutrients

There are a large number of micro- and macronutrients, such as minerals and vitamins, as well as some amino acids, cholesterol, and fatty acids that are known to have an impact on immune activity.

These are involved in cell proliferation and diverse macrophages' activities. Major nutrients that play a role in immune health are as follows:

- *Protein and amino acids*: Protein is essential to produce antibodies, enzymes, and immune cells. Dietary deficiency of protein or amino acids impairs the immune function of animals and humans and increases their susceptibility to infectious disease. Amino acids are required for the synthesis of cytokines and antibodies. They are involved in regulation of key metabolic pathways of the immune response. Amino acids such as L-arginine and L-tryptophan are essential for macrophage-mediated immune activity. The tryptophan metabolism leads to the synthesis of the cofactor NAD+, which is involved in redox reactions and electron transfer. Major tryptophan metabolites are bioactive. These metabolites play important roles in barrier integrity and immunosuppression in tumors. The inflamed organs and tumors use kynurenine pathway for tryptophan metabolism that involves Indoleamine 2,3-dioxygenase 1 (IDO1). IDO 1 deprives invading bacteria as well as tumor cells of the essential amino acid tryptophan (Seo and Kwon 2023). The kynurenine pathway serves as a basic negative feedback mechanism to resolve inflammation. It also acts as a compensatory mechanism to manage increased energy demand.

  Arginine contributes to the production of nitric oxide (NO) in macrophage cells. NO is a signaling molecule that gives an anti-inflammatory effect under normal physiological conditions but induces inflammation due to overproduction in abnormal situations. NO not only determines the cytotoxicity of macrophages in the fight against antigens such as pathogenic bacteria and parasites; it is also a vasodilator, a neurotransmitter, a regulator of nutrient metabolism, and a killer of bacteria, fungi, parasites, and viruses, including coronaviruses, such as SARS-CoV and SARS-CoV-2 (the virus causing COVID-19). Under the action of NO synthase (iNOS), our body converts arginine into NO (Wu et al 2021; Munteanu and Schwartz 2022).

  Moreover, arginine and methionine together lead to the synthesis of polyamines. Polyamines are important for cell growth and development. They are involved in transcription, translation, signaling, and post-translational modifications. Due to their ability to maintain cell membrane stability and keep DNA homeostasis, they stimulate cell proliferation (Sagar et al 2021; Munteanu and Schwartz 2022). Furthermore, degradation of methionine leads to the synthesis of glutathione, which acts as an antioxidant and helps in the prevention of oxidative stress, activation of T cells, regulation of NK and T cell cytotoxicity.

  Glutamine is a non-essential amino acid that has roles in the functioning of a number of immune cells including neutrophils, macrophages, and lymphocytes. It serves as a precursor for nucleotide synthesis in rapidly dividing immune cells during an immune response. The rate of glutamine consumption by immune cells is observed to be greater than that for glucose during infection (Childs et al 2019). In catabolic conditions such as infection or inflammation, glutamine is released into the circulation. The significant glutamine depletion observed in the plasma and tissues during critical illness has provided a rationale for its use in clinical nutrition supplementation (Cruzat et al 2018).
- *Fat-soluble vitamins*: Vitamin-rich foods are known as protective foods due to their well-known roles in enhancing immunity against diseases. Vitamin A, also known as the anti-infective vitamin, is required for normal differentiation of epithelial tissues and production of mucous which is essential for maintaining the integrity of epithelial tissues (e.g., skin, lungs, and gut), which serve as physical barriers against infections. Furthermore, vitamin A enhances antibody responses, thus improving the body's ability to recognize and neutralize pathogens (Rasheed and Rayner 2021). Retinoids directly stimulate the expression of interferon-stimulated genes (ISGs), including RIG-I (retinoic acid-inducible gene I) and IRF-1 (IFN regulatory factor 1). Interferons (IFNs) are produced by macrophages in response to

infection or foreign body stimuli. Furthermore, vitamin A stimulates the expansion and differentiation of Th_1 and Th_2. It promotes the Th_2 anti-inflammatory response by repression of IL-12 and IFNγ which are synthesized by Th_1 lymphocytes (Carazo et al 2021).

Vitamin D enhances the pathogen-fighting effects of monocytes and macrophages. Adequate levels of vitamin D have been linked to a lower risk of infections such as the flu and respiratory illnesses (Gombart et al 2020). Immune cells, including dendritic cells, macrophages, and T and B cells, express a high number of vitamin D receptors (VDRs) and 1α-hydroxylase (vitamin D-activating enzyme). Ligation of VDR by $1,25(OH)_2D_3$ elicits the production of antimicrobial proteins, influences cytokine production by immune cells, and exerts inhibitory effects on NF-κB (Childs et al 2019; El-Sharkawy and Malki 2020).

Vitamin E is a natural antioxidant that is known to protect the polyunsaturated fatty acids (PUFAs) in the membrane from oxidation, regulates the production of reactive oxygen species (ROS) and reactive nitrogen species (RNS), and modulates signal transduction (Lee and Han 2018). The protective role is clearly validated by the fact that vitamin E is present in high concentrations in immune cells. Vitamin E in nature occurs as eight analogues, of which alpha-tocopherol (αT) reaches high plasma levels and is the only form of vitamin E recognized to meet human requirements (Lewis et al 2019; Meydani and Blumberg 2020).

Vitamin K comprises a group of substances with chlorophyll quinone bioactivity. In nature, it exists in the form of K_1 and K_2. Better known for its role in blood coagulation, it plays an important role in immunity, inflammation, and metabolism also. When vitamin K levels are high, MGP (matrix gamma-carboxyglutamic acid protein) levels are high, and IL-6 levels are low and vice versa. MGP is a potent calcification inhibitor in the lung tissue and plays an important role in asthma and other lung inflammatory diseases such as COVID-19 (Jespersen et al 2023). Interleukin-6 (IL-6) can act as both a pro-inflammatory cytokine and an anti-inflammatory myokine.

Vitamin K also participates in the biological activation of a range of VK-dependent proteins (VKDPs). VKDPs such as the dependent protein growth arrest-specific gene 6 (Gas6) and protein S. Gas-6 regulates neuro-inflammation and reduces hippocampal neuronal cell death (Xie et al 2024).

- *Water-soluble vitamins*: Vitamins B_1 (thiamine), B_2 (riboflavin), B_3 (niacin), B_5 (pantothenic acid), B_6 (pyridoxine), B_7 (biotin), B_9 (folate), and B_{12} (cobalamin), commonly known as B complex vitamins, are essential micronutrients for all cellular life. B vitamins are key intermediates in the form of essential cofactors of various metabolic pathways. Most B-vitamins have antioxidant and anti-inflammatory roles. Vitamin B1 or thiamine exerts an antioxidative role through protective action on sulfhydryl groups from the surface of neutrophils. As a result, the synthesis of cytokines from macrophages is blocked (Peterson et al 2020). Similarly, riboflavin's role as a regulator of oxidative stress is evident from the presence of several FAD-dependent enzymes, such as glutathione reductase (Zangelmi et al 2023).

  Folate is another important B-vitamin that plays an important role in the synthesis and repair of DNA and is crucial for the proliferation of immune cells (T and B cells and macrophages). It also helps in the formation of red and white blood cells, supporting the immune system in responding to infections. Folate deficiency leads to impaired immune function, thus reducing production of immune cells and weakening immune responses (Suardi et al 2021).

  Vitamin C enhances the production and functioning of white blood cells, particularly neutrophils and lymphocytes, which are critical for fighting infections. Additionally, it acts as an antioxidant, protecting immune cells from oxidative stress during infection. It functions as an electron donor to reduce molecular oxygen (Gombart et al 2020). Vitamin C inhibits the action of the pro-inflammatory cytokines and initiation of the NF-κB reaction (Bozonet et al 2015) and supports caspase-dependent apoptosis as well as cell cycle arrest mediated by human carcinogenesis related to genes p53/p21 (Zhou et al 2020). Further, vitamin C inhibits necrosis by inhibiting platelet activation through the CXCL12/CXCR4 pathway (Gui et al 2023).

- *Minerals*: Minerals play an important role in the optimal functioning of both the innate defense system and the adaptive immune response. Zinc is an essential element for maintaining the structure and function of immune cells. Zinc deficiency results in impaired function of neutrophils and macrophages. It is essential for the proliferation and differentiation of T cells, Th17 and Th9 cells, and cytokines (Weyh et al 2022). The pro-inflammatory factor NF-κB can be inhibited by zinc (Brieger et al 2013). Zinc is involved in long-term retardation of oxidative processes by inducing the expression of metallothionein. Metallothionein is a cysteine-rich protein involved in metal detoxification and acts as cytoprotective agents. Zinc also increases the activation of antioxidant proteins and enzymes, such as glutathione and catalase (Gombart et al 2020).

  Iron is required for the production of red blood cells and for the activation and proliferation of T and B lymphocytes (Punt et al 2009). Macrophages require iron for phagocytosis, antigen presentation, and cytokine production (Nairz et al 2010). Neutrophils rely on iron for their oxidative burst, which is used to kill pathogens. Similarly, Selenium is incorporated into proteins as selenocysteine. Selenoproteins such as glutathione peroxidases (GPx) and thioredoxin reductases (TrxR) help maintain the balance of reactive oxygen species (ROS) by neutralizing it. This supports the integrity and function of immune cells, such as T lymphocytes and macrophages (Shahidin et al 2025).

7.3.2 Bioactive Non-Nutrients

There are bioactive phytochemicals which although do not directly contribute toward nutrition but result in significant physiological effects, such as enhancing immune function, reducing inflammation, and providing antioxidant protection. These compounds work synergistically to promote overall health and immunity. They impact metabolic pathways, have an antioxidant and anti-inflammatory action, and are also known to reduce intestinal absorption of glucose and fat.

Major bioactive non-nutrients include polyphenols, phytosterols, saponins, and phytates.

- *Polyphenols*: Polyphenols are aromatic compounds that plants produce in response to stress or injury. These secondary metabolites are made up of one or more hydroxyl groups attached to a benzene ring. Based on their chemical structure, they can be divided as follows: phenolic acids (hydroxybenzoic and hydroxycinnamic acids), flavonoids (flavanols, flavones, isoflavones, flavanones, and anthocyanins), lignans, and curcuminoids. Polyphenols exert antioxidant activity by capturing free radicals. Also, these phenolic compounds lower the production of superoxide anions and hydrogen peroxide (H_2O_2), thereby preserving the activity of glutathione reductase and glutathione peroxidase. Certain polyphenols like hesperidin, naringenin and resveratrol increase the expression of NF-E2-related factor 2 (NRF2), a key regulator of antioxidant enzyme expression. This results in a favorable redox state and reduced oxidative stress (Ribeiro de Melo et al 2019; Xia et al 2024).

  Scientific evidence indicates that dietary polyphenols can influence dendritic cells and have an immunomodulatory effect on macrophages. These phytochemicals support increased proliferation of B cells and T cells while suppressing Type 1 T helper (Th_1), Th_2, Th17, and Th9 cells. They reduce inflammation by suppressing the pro-inflammatory cytokines, inhibit tumor necrosis factor-alpha (TNF-α), and cause induction of apoptosis (Shakoor et al 2021).

- *Phytosterols*: Phytosterols are plant-derived sterols structurally similar and functionally analogous to cholesterol. Sitosterol and campesterol followed by stigmasterol are the most abundant phytosterols in food. Although phytosterols have mostly been in focus for cholesterol-lowering activity, some evidence also suggests additional biological actions such as immunomodulatory properties. Phytosterols can alleviate the inflammatory response and nitric acid production (Nattagh-Eshtivani et al 2022). They also inhibit the release of TNF-α, cyclooxygenase 2 (COX-2), and phosphorylated extracellular signal-regulated protein kinase (p-ERK). COX-2 is an enzyme that is expressed in response to inflammatory stimuli and produces pro-inflammatory prostaglandins. Similarly, p-ERK is a signaling protein and a key regulator of pro-inflammatory responses in microglia in Alzheimer's disease.
- *Saponins*: Saponins are bioactive glycosides derived from the secondary metabolism of plants. Saponins are known for activities including inhibition of platelet aggregation, anticoagulant, and anti-inflammatory (Nattagh-Eshtivani et al 2022). Saponins can reduce the production of pro-inflammatory cytokines like tumor necrosis factor-α (TNF-α) and interleukin-1β (IL-1β) and inhibit the NF-κB signaling pathway as well as reduce the activity of cyclooxygenase-2 (COX-2) and prostaglandin E2 (PGE2) (Passos et al 2022).
- *Phytic acid*: Phytic acid, also known as phytate or inositol hexa phosphate (IP6), is the main form of phosphorus storage in seeds. Being negatively charged, it strongly binds to metal cations of calcium, iron, potassium, magnesium, manganese, and zinc, forming insoluble complexes. Its ability to chelate with iron and remove it from circulation has been related to its use as an antioxidant. Reduced iron-mediated oxidative reactions, especially the formation of free radicals, avoid cellular injury and DNA damage (De Vos et al 2022).

In addition, it also promotes cell repair and regeneration by activating intracellular signaling pathways (Chen and Xu 2023). Markiewicz et al (2022) reported that phytic acid reduced the pro-inflammatory response of human cancer colonocytes to gut bacteria, while being neutral for the bacteria-treated healthy colonocytes. Likewise, Armah (2019) observed that "overweight or obese individuals with high PA intake were associated with a lower risk of inflammation-related chronic diseases". The protective effects might be exerted by activating the antioxidant protein sestrin2 and inhibiting the p-38 MAPK signaling pathway (Liu et al 2020; Chen & Xu 2023).

7.3.3 Fiber and Gut Microbiome in Immunity

For a pathogen to cause an infection in the gastro-intestinal (GI) tract, it has to overcome three main hurdles: the intestinal microbiota, the intestinal epithelial layer, and the mucosal immune system. The intricate interplay between the gut microbiota and intestinal epithelium leads to constant immune signaling. Almost 70–80% of immune cells are present in the gut. Food plays an important role in the complex interactions of the immune system and the gut microbiome (Wiertsema et al 2021). Any alterations to gut microbiota, usually induced by diet, stress, or drug treatment, result in inflammation, reduce resistance to pathogen colonization, and therefore increase infection susceptibility of the individual.

The symbiotic relationship between the host and gut microorganisms comprises its role in immune regulation, metabolic homeostasis, and even neurological functions. Dysbiosis often results in the development of inflammatory conditions leading to numerous chronic diseases, including obesity, type 2 diabetes, and cardiovascular disorders. The gut microbiome form metabolites such as short-chain fatty acids (SCFA), tryptophan metabolites, and bile acid derivatives from dietary components. These microbial metabolites possess immune protective abilities.

> SCFAs enhance the production of antimicrobial peptides and mucus by specialized intestinal epithelial cells; stimulate the maturation and expansion of regulatory T cells in colon, which dampens the local inflammatory responses and support proliferation of innate lymphoid cells (ILC3), which release

IL22. Interleukin-22 (IL-22) is a protein that plays role in the induction of antimicrobial molecules by epithelial cells.

(Luu et al 2019; Wiertsema et al 2021)

Dietary components, specifically dietary fibers, prebiotics, and probiotics, are known to affect the interaction between the host and pathogen, both directly and indirectly through the microbiome. "Prebiotics are non-digestible food ingredients that beneficially affect the host by selectively stimulating the growth and/or activity of one or a limited number of bacteria in the Colon" (Gibson et al 2017). Dietary fibers are considered prebiotics only if they are selectively utilized by host organisms, providing a health benefit, e.g., galacto-oligosaccharides, fructo-oligosaccharides, human milk oligosaccharides, and inulin. However, dietary fibers such as beta-glucans, arabinoxylans, pectins, and resistant starches, although not typical prebiotics, but still have prebiotic properties. These soluble fibers exhibit gel-forming properties by absorbing water resulting in increased food viscosity. The gut microflora (*Bacteroides* and *Bifidobacterium*) metabolize these soluble fibers to produce SCFAs during colonic fermentation. These dietary fibers along with prebiotics act as substrate for fermentation and thereby promote the growth of beneficial bacteria in the gut, thus inhibiting the growth of pathogens through niche exclusion and SCFA production. Direct interactions of prebiotics and dietary fiber with epithelial and immune cells also contribute to preventing infection. "Dietary fibres such as beta-glucans and arabinoxylans have been shown to activate the CLR dectin-1, an important receptor involved in the induction of trained immunity, which increases immune responses against secondary infections" (Wiertsema et al 2021). Human milk oligosaccharides, arabinoxylan, and pectin also interact with TLRs (Toll-like receptors), resulting in induction of tolerogenic dendritic cells via intestinal epithelial cells and protection of the GI tract from exaggerated TLR signaling. Exaggerated TLR signaling can lead to chronic inflammation and autoimmune diseases.

7.4 IMMUNITY-BOOSTING NUTRIENT TREASURE OF MILLETS

Millets, which are a group of small-seeded grasses, have long been recognized for their nutritional benefits. The pandemic of COVID-19 further amplified their importance due to their positive impact on immunity, digestive health, and overall well-being. The majority of infections like bronchitis, pneumonia, pulmonary inflammation, fever, and fibrosis are mediated by pro-inflammatory cytokines, which are preventable to some extent by nutrients and bioactive non-nutrient phytochemicals.

Millets are an abundant source of bioactive compounds along with essential micronutrients like magnesium, potassium, iron, and B-vitamins (especially folate), which play a vital role in supporting the immune system. It was the impressive nutrient profile of millets that has fetched them the name "nutricereals". The nutritional content of millets may vary depending upon variety and geographical locations. Millets in general contain about 65–75% carbohydrates, 7–15% proteins, 2–5% fat, and 8–15% fiber (Jacob et al 2024). Not only do millets have a higher content of essential amino acids compared to conventional cereals, they also have better protein digestibility due to prolamins. Various *in vitro* and animal research studies provide significant evidence of health-improving properties of millet-based bioactive peptides (Sachdev et al 2023).

The non-nutrient components of millets, chiefly polyphenols, flavonoids, phenolic acids, saponins, tannins, and other phytochemicals, contribute toward reducing oxidative damage within the body (Jacob et al 2024). Bioactive phytochemicals such as lignans, flavonoids, phenolics, beta-glucan, inulin, and pigments account for the majority of health benefits associated with the consumption of millets. In addition to these, millets provide soluble and insoluble fiber, which aid digestion and help in enhancing immune responses by promoting the growth of beneficial gut bacteria. Millets comprise a 15–20% dietary fiber component along with non-starchy polysaccharides,

TABLE 7.1
Nutritional Profile of Millets in Relation to Immunity Boosting Components

Millets	Protein (g/100 g)	Dietary Fiber (g/100 g)	Iron (mg/100/g)	Thiamine B_1 (mg/100 g)	Riboflavin B_2 (mg/100 g)
Pearl millet	10.96	11.49	6.42	0.25	0.20
Sorghum	9.97	10.22	3.95	0.35	0.14
Ragi	7.16	11.18	4.62	0.37	0.17
Little millet	8.92	6.39	1.26	0.26	0.05
Kodo	8.92	6.39	2.34	0.29	0.20
Foxtail[a]	12.30	8[b]	1.1[b]	0.59	0.11
Barnyard[a]	6.20	10.1[b]	15[b]	0.33	0.10
Proso[a]	12.50	2.5[b]	3.8[b]	0.41	0.28

Source: Longvah et al., 2017.
[a] Gopalan et al., 2023.
[b] Jacob et al., 2024.

arabinoxylan, and β-glucan (Mutshinyani et al 2020). Table 7.1 presents a glimpse of the nutritional profile of various millets which helps in boosting immunity.

7.5 SCIENTIFIC EVIDENCE ON MILLETS AND IMMUNOMODULATION

Millets support health and immunity in a number of ways.

7.5.1 Controlling Inflammation

Inflammation is a normal immune response of the innate immune system that makes physiological conditions unfavorable for the survival of pathogens or foreign-invading bodies. However, inappropriate activation of inflammation or the inability to turn off inflammation can cause unwanted tissue damage, leading to the development of chronic diseases. A major clinical use of the immune stimulants is to treat cancer and to ease the immune-deficient status, like AIDS. Srinivasan et al (2020) evaluated the immune-stimulating effect of phenolic acid-bound arabinoxylan (PA-AXs) isolated from barnyard (PA-AX-B) and foxtail (PA-AX-F) millets. In RAW 264.7 cells, both PA-AX-B and PA-AX-F exhibited significant immune stimulation as established by increased release of NO, ROS, and cytokines (TNF-α, IL-1β, and IL-6) in a dose-dependent manner. Another study by He et al (2022) also established that "millet bran peptides could significantly reduce the levels of inflammatory factors, including tumor necrosis factor-α (TNF-α), interleukin-1β (IL-1β) and prostaglandin E2 (PGE2), in the LPS-induced RAW 264.7 cell. This property can have hepatoprotective and cardioprotective significance". Alzahrani et al (2022) tested the anti-inflammatory effects of whole pearl millet grain powder and its ethanol extract. Obese rats fed a high-fat diet were used as experimental models. Authors observed that "serum levels of interleukine-6 (IL-6), interleukine-10 (IL-10), C-reactive protein (CRP), tumor necrosis factor (TNF-α), and adiponectin progressively decreased in a dose dependent manner". The antioxidant and immunomodulatory activities of a water-soluble polysaccharide from foxtail millet (FM-D1) were evaluated in vitro by Zhang et al (2025).

> FM-D1 exhibited moderate2,2-diphenyl-1-picrylhydrazyl (DPPH) and 2,2′-Azinobis-(3-ethylbenzthiazoline-6-sulphonate) (ABTS) radical scavenging capacity and total antioxidant capacity (TAOC). FM-D1 stimulated macrophage proliferation and inhibited the production of nitric oxide (NO) and inflammatory factors (TNF-α, IL-1β, and IL-6) in lipopolysaccharide (LPS)-stimulated RAW 246. 7 cells.

7.5.2 Apoptosis

The programmed cell death or apoptosis is a characteristic cellular process which plays an important part in the development of normal and cancer cells. Usually, the main cause of cancer is dysregulation of apoptosis due to alternations in the DNA. A normal cell will generally repair the alternation or would die, while cancer cells survive with the transformations and continue to proliferate in an uncontrolled manner, resulting in tumor formation. Components from millets have been shown to induce apoptosis in cancer cells thereby controlling further proliferation.

Han and Kim (2023) examined the antitumor effect of proso millet grains.

> The 80% ethanol (EtOH) extract of Proso millet grains exerted potency to toxicity against human breast cancer MDA-MB-231 cells whereas normal mammary epithelial MCF-10A cells exhibited a significantly lesser extent of sensitivity. Along with the cytotoxicity, TUNEL-positive apoptotic nucleosomal DNA fragmentation and several apoptotic responses including BAK/BAX activation, mitochondria membrane potential loss, mitochondrial cytochrome c release into the cytosol, and degradation of polymerase (PARP) were detected.

The bound polyphenols of foxtail millet (*Setaria italica*) inner shell were observed to induce breast cancer cell death and elevate the autophagy level simultaneously (Zhang et al 2023).

> The addition of an autophagy inhibitor blocked polyphenol induced breast cancer cell death, indicating that excessive autophagy induced cell death. Furthermore, oil redO and BODIPY staining also confirmed that lipids, which are important inducers of autophagy, accumulated in breast cancer cells treated with foxtail polyphenol. Glycerophospholipids were the main accumulated lipids. Elevated PCYT1A expression was responsible for glycerophospholipid accumulation. Polyphenol extract contained ferulic acid and *p*-coumaric acid, which induced PCYT1A expression and breast cancer cell death.

It shows that polyphenol extract from foxtail millet promoted lipid accumulation which induced the autophagic death.

Hajri et al (2024) investigated the

> anticancer effects of polyphenol-rich (apigenin, caffeic acid, and luteolin) fractions, extracted from pearl millet (*Pennisetum glaucum*), using three different cellular models of breast cancer, namely triple negative HCC1806, ER-positive HCC1428, and HER2-positive AU565 cells. Encapsulated polyphenolic extract induced apoptotic cell death in breast cancer cells, whereas it was ineffective against non-tumorigenic MCF10F cells. Encapsulated polyphenolic extract was also found to be cytotoxic against drug-resistant doxorubicin-induced senescent breast cancer cells that were accompanied by increased levels of apoptotic and necrotic markers, cell cycle inhibitor p21 and proinflammatory cytokine IL8. In the non-proliferating AU565 cells, the cytotoxic autophagy, was also induced, as judged by elevated levels of beclin-1 and LC3b.

Similarly, Mahanta et al (2024) evaluated

> anti-carcinogenic potential of *Levilactobacillus brevis* (MTTC 4460) fermented finger millet. The fermented millet formulation exhibited anti-proliferative and anti-migratory effects on MDA-MB-231 and HCT116 cancer cell lines. Western blot analysis revealed that the formulation elicited apoptotic responses mediated by the Bcl-2 family of proteins in cancer cell lines while demonstrating no discernible impact on normal cells.

7.5.3 Oxidative Burst

Phagocytes engulf and destroy invading organisms. Neutrophils produce a concentrated burst of ROS that causes oxidative stress in pathogens. This causes damage to critical cellular components like DNA, proteins, and lipids within the pathogen resulting in cell death. The respiratory burst is part of the normal immune response just like inflammation. However, prolonged and continuous exposure to ROS causes damage to healthy tissues that can lead to chronic disease. The rich phytochemical content of millets makes them potential natural antioxidants which have been proved in several scientific studies.

"The oxidation resistance and anti-inflammatory effect of three millet prolamins peptides (MPP) were evaluated in human keratinocyte HaCaT cells and RAW264.7 murine macrophages" (Ji et al 2020). Authors reported that

> MPP effectively reduced the production of reactive oxygen species(ROS) as well as malondialdehyde (MDA) but increased the level of glutathione (GSH) in H_2O_2-induced HaCaT cells, showing anti-oxidant bioactivity in cells. In addition, MPP were able to significantly alleviate inflammation by inhibiting the yield of nitric oxide (NO) and pro-inflammatory cytokines (TNF-α, interleukin IL-6 and IL-1β) in (lipopolysaccharide) LPS-stimulated RAW264.7 murine macrophages.

Theodoro et al (2021) investigated the effects of germinated millet flour on oxidative stress. Wistar rats fed with a high-fat, high-fructose diet were used as an experimental model. "The germinated millet increased ($p<0.05$) IL-10, PPARα protein, total antioxidant capacity of the liver and the activity of SOD and catalase". In another study, Srinivasan et al (2021) investigated the immunomodulating effect of phenolic acid-bound arabinoxylans (PCA-AXs) extracted from little (PCA-AX-L) and kodo (PCA-AX-K) millet seeds in RAW 264.7 cells. The phenolic acid content was higher in PCA-AX-K than in PCA-AX-L. It was observed that the PCA-AX-L–treated cells showed higher release of NO, ROS, and cytokines than PCA-AX-K–treated cells. The mRNA expressions of TNF-α, iNOS, and COX-2 were upregulated by PCA-AX-L and downregulated by PCA-AX-K in a dose-dependent manner. Furthermore, the ERK and NF-κB were found to be activated by PCA-AX-L and inhibited by PCA-AX-K. The higher phenolic content in PCA-AX-K could modulate the immune response by downregulating ERK and NF-κB signaling pathways, and thus, it could act as an immunomodulator.

7.5.4 Macrophage Proliferation

Proliferation means an increase in the number or amount of something. The immune system is constantly producing cells, chemical messengers, and proteins to carry out its functions. The production of macrophages is ramped up when it encounters a foreign invader. Therefore, evaluation of effectiveness of macrophage activation can assess the immune-stimulatory activity. The stimulation of macrophages eliminates the pathogen from the host either directly (phagocytosis) or indirectly via the release of various inflammatory mediators. This process of macrophage proliferation requires energy, building blocks, and various cofactors to produce the substances needed to mount an effective immune response. NO is a critical mediator of many biological functions and can be considered a critical marker of macrophage activation.

Cao et al (2021) observed that

> deproteinated non-starch polysaccharide (ECPs-II) from finger millet, remarkably stimulated RAW 264.7 cells by inducing nitric oxide (NO) production, upregulating inducible nitric oxide synthase (iNOS) and various pro-inflammatory cytokines including interleukin (IL)-1β, IL-6, IL-10, and tumor necrosis factor alpha (TNF-α). Furthermore, the RAW 264.7 cells were activated after ECPs-II treatment via NF-κB and mitogen-activated protein kinase signaling (MAPK) pathways induced by a cluster of differentiation 40 (CD40) expression. NF-κB is a transcription factor important for activation and function of B lymphocytes.

7.5.5 Promoting Gut Microbiota

Being rich in carbohydrates and fiber, millets support a diverse and healthy gut microbiome and contribute toward reducing the risk of dysbiosis. Gut microorganisms can utilize carbohydrates and produce microbial metabolites. These metabolites act as signaling molecules between the gut microbiota and the host. This has implications for the prevention and management of various gut-related diseases, including inflammatory bowel diseases (IBD), constipation, and colorectal cancer. The positive impact of millets on the gut microbiome has been validated by a number of scientists.

Ren et al (2022) demonstrated that the "four weeks of 48% foxtail millet supplementation significantly increased the relative abundance of *Bifidobacterium* and concentration of butyrate in fecal samples of rats with streptozotocin induced diabetes". Authors suggested that the hypoglycemic effects of foxtail supplementation might be partially mediated by gut microbiota. Similarly, Sori et al (2023) demonstrated that

> kodo and kutki millets could positively modulate the gut microbial diversity which was directly related to the production of the metabolites. However, both millets stimulated the growth of different bacteria. More specifically, *Bifidobacterium* and *Prevotella* were abundant in Kodo millet, whereas Kutki millet stimulates the growth of *Lactobacillus*. Variations in metabolites such as SCFAs concentration, amino acids and other metabolites between different millet groups could also be attributed to the cumulative effects of microbial metabolism and cross-feeding of microbes.

Soni et al (2024) studied

> the *in vitro* prebiotic activity of pearl millet (*Pennisetum glaucum* L.), finger millet (*Eleusine coracana* L.), sorghum (*Sorghum bicolor* L.), and foxtail millet (*Setaria italica* L.). The prebiotic activity was performed by using them as a sole carbon source in DeMan–Rogosa–Sharpe agar media with probiotic strains *Lactobacillus plantarum* [Microbial Type Culture Collection (MTCC) 1407], *Lactobacillus paracasei* (Microbial Culture Collection 4490), *Lactobacillus rhamnosus* (MTCC 1408), and *Saccharomyces boulardii*. The growth of all microorganisms was confluent on their respective Petri plates under anaerobic conditions as observed on positive control plates.

Similarly, Mondal et al (2022) and Mondal et al (2023) demonstrated high prebiotic activity of pearl millet oligosaccharide and polysaccharide, respectively. A number of authors have reported using millets as a source of prebiotics in developed food products and beverages (Arya and Shakya 2021; Peerkhan et al 2024; Farzana et al 2024).

Wang et al (2022) demonstrated that

> millet-derived selenylated soluble dietary fiber promoted intestinal health in mice with DSS-induced colitis. In female mice, Se-SDF markedly alleviated body weight loss, decreased colon length, reduced histological damage scores, and enhanced IL-10 expression to maintain the barrier function of intestinal mucosa compared to male mice. The 16 SrRNA sequence analysis further indicated that pretreatment with Se-SDF restored the gut microbiota composition in female mice by increasing the relative abundance of Lactobacillus and the Firmicutes/Bacteroidetes ratio.

In another study,

> polyphenol-rich extracts (PREs) from Finger millet (FM) and Kodo millet (KM) were assessed for modulating effects on selected human gut bacteria. Fecal batch fermentation of FM-PRE and KM-PRE enhanced the abundance of selected beneficial bacteria, such as *Bifidobacterium* spp. *Lactobacillus* spp. and the production of SCFAs. Moreover, the millet polyphenols protected the intestinal cells against DSS-induced intestinal barrier dysfunction by reducing inflammatory cytokines, TEER by ~40%, FITC-dextran fluorescence and up-regulating the expression of tight junction genes, thereby improving gut functions.
>
> **(Maurya et al 2024)**

7.6 CONCLUSION

Millets are a promising dietary option for promoting immunity because of its nutritional treasure of bioactive nutrients, high fiber content, and prebiotic effect. The prebiotic effect supports the diversity and composition of the gut microbiome and thereby contributes toward immunologic properties. The consumption of millets as part of a diverse and balanced diet holds great potential for promoting and preserving immunity and gut health, and preventing chronic diseases like IBD, obesity, diabetes, and even cancer.

In conclusion, millets represent not only an ancient and nutritionally rich food source but also a modern functional food with the potential to support natural immunity, making them an important component of sustainable, health-promoting diets for the future.

REFERENCES

Alzahrani, N. S., Alshammari, G. M., El-Ansary, A., Yagoub, A. E. A., Amina, M., Saleh, A., & Yahya, M. A. 2022. Anti-hyperlipidemia, hypoglycemic, and hepatoprotective impacts of pearl millet (*Pennisetum glaucum* L.) grains and their ethanol extract on rats fed a high-fat diet. *Nutrients, 14*(9), 1791.

Armah, S. M. 2019. Association between phytate intake and c-reactive protein concentration among people with overweight or obesity: Across-sectional study using NHANES 2009/2010. *International Journal of Environmental Research and Public Health, 16*(9), 1549.

Arya, S. S., & Shakya, N. K. 2021. High fiber, low glycaemic index (GI) prebiotic multigrain functional beverage from barnyard, foxtail and kodo millet. *LWT, 135*, 109991.

Bozonet, S., Carr, A., Pullar, J., & Vissers, M. 2015. Enhanced human neutrophil vitamin C status, chemotaxis and oxidant generation following dietary supplementation with vitamin C-rich Sun Gold kiwifruit. *Nutrients, 7*, 2574–88.

Brieger, A., Rink, L., & Haase, H. 2013. Differential regulation of TLR-dependent MyD88 and TRIF signaling pathways by free zinc ions. *Journal of Immunology, 191*, 1808–17.

Cao, R. A., Palanisamy, S., Ma, N., Talapphet, N., Zhang, J., Wang, C., & You, S. 2021. Extraction, structural characterization, and immunostimulatory activity of soluble non-starch polysaccharides of finger millet. *Process Biochemistry, 111*, 40–50.

Carazo, A., Macáková, K., Matoušová, K., Krčmová, L. K., Protti, M., & Mladěnka, P. 2021. Vitamin A update: Forms, sources, kinetics, detection, function, deficiency, therapeutic use and toxicity. *Nutrients, 13*(5), 1703.

Chen, W., & Xu, D. 2023. Phytic acid and its interactions in food components, health benefits, and applications: A comprehensive review. *Trends in Food Science & Technology, 141*, 104201.

Childs, C. E., Calder, P. C., & Miles, E. A. 2019. Diet and immune function. *Nutrients, 11*(8), 1933. https://doi.org/10.3390/nu11081933

Cruzat, V., Macedo Rogero, M., Noel Keane, K., Curi, R., & Newsholme, P. 2018. Glutamine: Metabolism and immune function, supplementation and clinical translation. *Nutrients, 10*(11), 1564.

De Vos, W. M., Tilg, H., Van Hul, M., & Cani, P. D. 2022. Gut microbiome and health: Mechanistic insights. *Gut, 71*(5), 1020–1032.

El-Sharkawy, A., & Malki, A. 2020. Vitamin D signaling in inflammation and cancer: Molecular mechanisms and therapeutic implications. *Molecules, 25*(14), 3219. https://doi.org/10.3390/molecules25143219

Farzana, T., Abedin, M. J., Abdullah, A. T. M., Reaz, A. H., Bhuiyan, M. N. I., Afrin, S., & Satter, M. A. 2024. Enhancing prebiotic, antioxidant, and nutritional qualities of noodles: A collaborative strategy with foxtail millet and green banana flour. *PLoS One, 19*(8), e0307909.

Gibson, G. R., Hutkins, R., Sanders, M. E., Prescott, S. L., Reimer, R. A., Salminen, S. J., & Reid, G. 2017. Expert consensus document: The International Scientific Association for Probiotics and Prebiotics (ISAPP) consensus statement on the definition and scope of prebiotics. *Nature Reviews Gastroenterology & Hepatology, 14*(8), 491–502.

Gombart, A. F., Pierre, A., & Maggini, S. 2020. A review of micronutrients and the immune system-working in harmony to reduce the risk of infection. *Nutrients, 12*(1), 236.

Gonella, K., Nayak, S. P., Garg, M., & Kotebagilu, N. P. 2022. Impact of the COVID-19 pandemic on immune boosting food consumption and overall dietary pattern among selected Indian adults: An observational study. *Clin Epidemiol Glob Health* 15, 101056. doi: 10.1016/j.cegh.2022.101056.

Gopalan, C., Ramasastry, B. V., Balasubramanian, S. C., Narasinga Rao B.S., Deosthala, Y.G. & Pant, K.C. 2023. *Nutritive Value of Indian Foods*. National Institute of Nutrition, Indian Council of Medical Research, Hyderabad.

Gui, M., Huang, J., Sheng, H., Chen, Y., Yang, Z., Ma, L., Wang, D., Xu, L., Sun, W., Liu, J., Xu, Y., Chen, E., Zhao, B., & Mao, E. 2023. High-dose vitamin C alleviates pancreatic necrosis by inhibiting platelet activation through the CXCL12/CXCR4 pathway in Severe Acute Pancreatitis. *Journal of Inflammation Research*, 2865–2877. https://doi.org/10.2147/JIR.S415974

Hajri, L., Lewińska, A., Rzeszutek, I., Oklejewicz, B., Wojnarowska-Nowak, R., Krogul-Sobczak, A., & Wnuk, M. 2024. Anticancer activity of encapsulated pearl millet polyphenol-rich extract against proliferating and non-proliferating breast cancer cells *in vitro*. *Cancers*, *16*(9), 1750.

Han, C. R., & Kim, Y. H. 2023. Apoptotic effect of proso millet grains on human breast cancer MDA-MB-231 cells is exerted by activation of BAK and BAX, and mitochondrial damage-mediated caspase cascade activation. *Journal of Life Science*, *33*(1), 15–24. https://doi.org/10.5352/JLS.2023.33.1.15

He, R., Liu, M., Zou, Z., Wang, M., Wang, Z., Ju, X., & Hao, G. 2022. Anti-inflammatory activity of peptides derived from millet bran in vitro and in vivo. *Food & Function*, *13*(4), 1881–1889.

Howard, F. H., Kwan, A., Winder, N., Mughal, A., Collado-Rojas, C., & Muthana, M.. 2022. Understanding immune responses to viruses—Do underlying Th1/Th2 cell biases predict outcome? *Viruses 14*(7):1493. https://doi.org/10.3390/v14071493

Jacob, J., Krishnan, V., Antony, C., Bhavyasri, M., Aruna, C., Mishra, K., & Visarada, K. B. 2024. The nutrition and therapeutic potential of millets: An updated narrative review. *Frontiers in Nutrition*, *11*, 1346869.

Janeway, C. A., Travers, P., Walport, M., & Shlomchik, M. J. 2005. A detailed source covering both the adaptive and innate immune systems. In *Immunobiology* (6th ed.). Garland Science.

Jarosz, L., Smith, A. L., Brown, M., & Wang, Y. 2024. Millets in ancient medicine: An exploration of ayurvedic and Chinese texts. *Journal of Ancient Medical Studies*, *42*(3), 213–225.

Jasenosky, L., Scriba, T., Hanekom, W., & Goldfeld, A. E. 2015. T cells and adaptive immunity to *Mycobacterium tuberculosis* in humans. *Immunological Reviews*, *264*, 74–87.

Jespersen, T., Kampmann, F. B., Dantoft, T. M., Jørgensen, N. R., Kårhus, L. L., Madsen, F., & Thysen, S. M. 2023. The association of vitamin K status with lung function and disease in a general population. *ERJ Open Research*, *9*(5).

Ji, Z., Mao, J., Chen, S., & Mao, J. 2020. Anti oxidant and anti-inflammatory activity of peptides from foxtail millet (*Setaria italica*) prolamins in HaCaT cells and RAW264. 7 murine macrophages. *Food Bioscience*, *36*, 100636.

Lee, G. Y., & Han, S. N. 2018. The role of vitamin E inimmunity. *Nutrients*, *10*(11), 1614.

Lewis, E. D., Meydani, S. N., & Wu, D. 2019. Regulatory role of vitamin E in the immune system and inflammation. *IUBMB Life*, *71*(4), 487–494.

Liu, J., Li, Y., Mei, C., Ning, X., Pang, J., Gu, L., & Wu, L. 2020. Phytic acid exerts protective effects in cerebral ischemia-reperfusion injury by activating the anti-oxidative protein sestrin 2. *Bioscience, Biotechnology, and Biochemistry*, *84*(7), 1401–1408.

Longvah, T., A<u>n</u>anta<u>n</u>, I., Bhaskarachary, K., & Venkaiah, K. 2017. Indian Food Composition Tables. *National Institute of Nutrition*, Indian Council of Medical Research, Hyderabad, pp. 2–58.

Luu, M., Pautz, S., Kohl, V., Singh, R., Romero, R., Lucas, S., & Visekruna, A. 2019. The short-chain fatty acid pentanoate suppresses autoimmunity by modulating the metabolic-epigenetic crosstalk in lymphocytes. *Nature Communications*, *10*(1), 760.

Mahanta, S. K., Nayak, P. P., Muduli, K., Elangovan, S., Paramasivan, S. S., Mallick, P. K., & Panda, S. K. 2024. Optimisation of *Levilactobacillus brevis*-fermented finger millet (*Eleusine coracana*) and evaluation of its effects on cancer cells (HCT116 and MDA-MB-231). *Methods*, *229*, 30–40.

Markiewicz, L. H., Ogrodowczyk, A. M., Wiczkowski, W., & Wróblewska, B. 2022. Phytate hydrolysate differently modulates the immune response of human healthy and cancer colonocytes to intestinal bacteria. *Nutrients*, *14*(20), 4234.

Maurya, R., Shandilya, C., Raina, N., Rawat, A., Devi, K., Kumar Bhadada, S., & Kiran Kondepudi, K. 2024. Effect of millet polyphenol-rich extracts on human fecal bacteria and dextran sulfate sodium-induced human intestinal epithelial cell derangements. *Food Biotechnology*, *38*(1), 42–63.

Meydani, S. N., & Blumberg, J. B. 2020. Vitamin E and the Immune Response. In *Nutrient Modulation of the Immune Response* (pp. 223–238). CRC Press.

Mondal, S., Agrawal, S., Balasubramanian, A., Maji, S., Shit, S., Biswas, P., Ghosh, S., Islam, S. S., & Dey, S. 2023. Structural analysis of a water insoluble polysaccharide from pearl millet and evaluating its prebiotic activity. *International Journal of Biological Macromolecules*, *253*, 126469.

Mondal, S., Balasubramanian, A., Biswas, P., Agrawal, S., Ghosh, S., & Dey, S. 2022. Characterization of pearl millet oligosaccharides and evaluation of their prebiotic potential. *Bioactive Carbohydrates and Dietary Fibre*, *28*, 100324.

Munteanu, M., & Schwartz, D. 2022. Nitric oxide production and its implications in human health. *Journal of Medical Research*, *35*(4), 301–315.

Mutshinyani, M., Mashau, M. E., & Jideani, A. I. O. 2020. Bioactive compounds, antioxidant activity and consumer acceptability of porridges of finger millet (*Eleusine coracana*) flours: Effects of spontaneous fermentation. *International Journal of Food Properties*, *23*(1), 1692–1710.

Nairz, M., Theurl, I., & Weiss, G. 2010. Iron and innate immunity: From mechanisms to clinical translation. *Frontiers in Pharmacology*, *1*(148).

Nattagh-Eshtivani, E., Barghchi, H., Pahlavani, N., Barati, M., Amiri, Y., Fadel, A., & Ghavami, A. 2022. Biological and pharmacological effects and nutritional impact of phytosterols: A comprehensive review. *Phytotherapy Research*, *36*(1), 299–322.

Passos, F. R. S., Araújo-Filho, H. G., Monteiro, B. S., Shanmugam, S., deSouzaAraújo, A. A., da Silva Almeida, J. R. G., & Quintans, J. D. S. S. 2022. Anti-inflammatory and modulatory effects of steroidal saponins and sapogenins on cytokines : A review of pre-clinical research. *Phytomedicine*, *96*, 153842.

Peerkhan, N., Pandey, M., & Bhandari, Y. 2024. Formulation of prebiotic, low glycemic index millet soups using foxtail, barnyard and kodo millet. *Discover Food*, *4*(1), 62.

Peterson, C., Rodionov, D., Osterman, A., & Peterson, S. N. 2020. B vitamins and their role in immune regulation and cancer. *Nutrients* 12, 3380. 10.3390/nu12113380

Punt, J. A., DenHaan, J. M. M., & Weersing, K. 2009. *Immunology* (6th ed.). Elsevier.

Rasheed, A., & Rayner, K. J. 2021. Macrophage responses to environmental stimuli during homeostasis and disease. *Endocrine Reviews*, *42*(4), 407–435.

Ren, X., Wang, L., Chen, Z., Zhang, M., Hou, D., Xue, Y., & Shen, Q. 2022. Foxtail millet supplementation improves glucose metabolism and gut microbiota in rats with high-fat diet/streptozotocin-induced diabetes. *Food Science and Human Wellness*, *11*(1), 119–128.

Ribeiro de Melo, P. V., Andrade, P. A., Hermsdorff, H. H. M., DosSantos, C. A., Cotta, R. M. M., Estanislau, J. D. A. S. G., Campos, A. A. D. O., & Rosa, C. D. O. B.. 2019. Dietary non-nutrients in the prevention of non-communicable diseases: Potentially related mechanisms. *Nutrition 66*, 22–28.

Sachdev, N., Goomer, S., Singh, L. R., Pathak, V. M., Aggarwal, D., & Chowhan, R. K. 2023. Current status of millet seed proteins and its applications: A comprehensive review. *Applied Food Research*, *3*(1), 100288.

Sagar, M., Kapoor, A., & Gupta, R. 2021. The role of arginine and methionine in polyamine synthesis and cell growth. *Journal of Cellular Biochemistry*, *122*(10), 1514–1524. https://doi.org/10.1002/jcb.29545

Seo, S. K., & Kwon, B. 2023. Immune regulation through tryptophan metabolism. *Experimental & Molecular Medicine*, *55*(7), 1371–1379.

Shahidin, Wang, Y., Wu, Y., Chen, T., Wu, X., Yuan, W., Zhu, Q., Wang, X., & Zi, C., 2025. Selenium and selenoproteins: Mechanisms, health functions, and emerging applications. *Molecules*, *30*(3), 437. https://www.mdpi.com/1420-3049/30/3/437

Shakoor, H., Feehan, J., Apostolopoulos, V., Platat, C., Al Dhaheri, A. S., Ali, H. I., & Stojanovska, L. 2021. Immunomodulatory effects of dietary polyphenols. *Nutrients*, *13*(3), 728.

Soni, H., Bhagwat, P., Singh, G., Tandon, S., Yadav, S., Parihar, A. S., Lale, S. K., Prasad, S. B., Thakur, A., Kumar, V., Charde, V., Jagtap, C. Y., Arya, J. C., Narasimhaji, C. V., Srikanth, N., Acharya, R., & Acharya, R. 2024. In vitro prebiotic activity of millets with selected probiotic microorganisms. *Journal of Drug Research in Ayurvedic Sciences*, *9*(6), 384–394.

Sori, N., Poyil, N. C., & Khan, M. 2023. In vitro fermentation of kodo and kutki millets by human gut microbiota: Gut microbiota and metabolomic analysis. *Food Bioscience*, *56*, 103343.

Srinivasan, A., Aruldhas, J., Perumal, S. S., & Ekambaram, S. P. 2021. Phenolic acid bound arabinoxylans extracted from Little and Kodo millets modulate immune system mediators and pathways in RAW 264. 7 cells. *Journal of Food Biochemistry*, *45*(1), e13563. https://doi.org/10.1111/jfbc.13563

Srinivasan, A., Ekambaram, S. P., Perumal, S. S., Aruldhas, J., & Erusappan, T. 2020. Chemical characterization and immunostimulatory activity of phenolic acid bound arabinoxylans derived from foxtail and barnyard millets. *Journal of Food Biochemistry*, *44*(2), e13116. https://doi.org/10.1111/jfbc.13116

Suardi, C., Cazzaniga, E., Graci, S., Dongo, D., & Palestini, P. 2021. Link between viral infections, immune system, inflammation and diet. *International Journal of Environmental Research and Public Health*, *18*(5), 2455. https://doi.org/10.3390/ijerph18052455

Theodoro, J. M. V., Martinez, O. D. M., Grancieri, M., Toledo, R. C. L., Martins, A. M. D., Dias, D. M., & Martino, H. S. D. 2021. Germinated millet flour (*Pennisetum glaucum* (L.) R. Br.) reduces inflammation, oxidative stress, and liver steatosis in rats fed with high-fat high-fructose diet. *Journal of Cereal Science*, *99*, 103207.

Wang, H., Fu, Y., Zhao, Q., Hou, D., Yang, X., Bai, S., & Shen, Q. 2022. Effect of different processing methods on the millet polyphenols and their anti-diabetic potential. *Frontiers in Nutrition*, *9*, 780499.

Weyh, C., Krüger, K., Peeling, P., & Castell, L. 2022. The role of minerals in the optimal functioning of the immune system. *Nutrients*, *14*(3), 644. https://doi.org/10.3390/nu14030644

Wiertsema, S. P., van Bergenhenegouwen, J., Garssen, J., & Knippels, L. M. 2021. The interplay between the gut microbiome and the immune system in the context of infectious diseases throughout life and the role of nutrition in optimizing treatment strategies. *Nutrients*, *13*(3), 886. https://doi.org/10.3390/nu13030886

Wu, G., Meininger, C. J., McNeal, C. J., Bazer, F. W., & Rhoads, J. M. 2021. Role of L-Arginine in Nitric Oxide Synthesis and Health in Humans. In: Wu, G. (ed) *Amino Acids in Nutrition and Health. Advances in Experimental Medicine and Biology*, vol 1332. Springer, Cham. https://doi.org/10.1007/978-3-030-74180-8_10

Xia, J., Wan, Y., Wu, J. J., Yang, Y., Xu, J. F., Zhang, L., & Peng, C. 2024. Therapeutic potential of dietary flavonoid hyperoside against non-communicable diseases: Targeting underlying properties of diseases. *Critical Reviews in Food Science and Nutrition*, *64*(5), 1340–1370. https://doi.org/10.1080/10408398.2022.2115457

Xie, Y., Li, S., Wu, D., Wang, Y., Chen, J., Duan, L., & Li, Y. 2024. Vitamin K: Infection, inflammation, and auto-immunity. *Journal of Inflammation Research*, 1147–1160. https://doi.org/10.2147/JIR.S445806

Zangelmi, E., Ruffolo, F., Dinhof, T., Gerdol, M., Malatesta, M., Chin, J. P., & Peracchi, A. 2023. Deciphering the role of recurrent FAD-dependent enzymes in bacterial phosphonate catabolism. *iScience*, *26*(11). https://doi.org/10.1016/j.isci.2023.108108

Zhang, H., Peng, C., Zhang, W., Liu, H., Liu, X., Sun, C., & Cao, X. 2025. Structural characterization of foxtail millet (*Setaria italica*) polysaccharides and evaluation of its antioxidant and immuno-stimulatory activities. *Antioxidants*, *14*(1), 113. https://doi.org/10.3390/antiox14010113

Zhang, L. C., Liu, Y. N., La, X. Q., Li, S. T., Wen, L. N., Liu, T., Li, H., Li, A., Wu, H., Wu, C., & Li, Z. Y. 2023. The bound poly phenols off oxtail millet (*Setaria italica*) inner shell inhibit breast cancer by promoting lipid accumulation-induced autophagic death. *Food and Chemical Toxicology*, *177*, 113855. https://doi.org/10.1016/j.fct.2023.113855

Zhou, J., Chen, C., Chen, X., Fei, Y., Jiang, L., & Wang, G. 2020. Vitamin C promotes apoptosis and cell cycle arrest in oral squamous cell carcinoma. *Frontiers in Oncology*, *10*, 976. https://doi.org/10.3389/fonc.2020.00976

8 Millets' Role in Weight Management

Swati Shukla
Department of Food and Nutrition, College of Community Sciences,
G.B. Pant University of Agriculture & Technology,
Pantnagar, Uttarakhand, India

8.1 OVERVIEW OF WEIGHT MANAGEMENT AND DIETARY NEEDS

8.1.1 Definition and Components of Weight Management

Obesity is one of the most prevalent public health issues affecting all the strata of the community in developed as well as developing nations equally. If remain unchecked, it can be the leading cause of various chronic inflammatory disorders like hypertension, cardiovascular diseases (CVDs), and diabetes mellitus. For instance, 1 kg reduction of weight in overweight and prediabetes individual has been related with 16% reduced risk of developing diabetes mellitus. Among other factors, lifestyle is one of the key aspects in prevention and management of higher weight. Adopting a healthy lifestyle, including regular physical activity, mindful eating, and stress management, is crucial to prevent and effectively manage obesity and its associated complications (Asritha 2021).

Weight management is a holistic approach of maintaining a healthy weight with the assistance of physical activity, a balanced diet, and behavioral factors like social, psychological, and environmental, which, in turn, impact an individual's behavioral patterns (Kim 2021; Sarte and Quinto 2024).

8.1.2 Importance of Diet in Achieving and Maintaining a Healthy Weight

Healthy eating is one of the key behavioral modifications required for a healthy weight. It infers not only to the quantity of food consumed but also the quality of food on your plate. As per ICMR-NIN (2018), a healthy plate must include a variety of fresh fruits and vegetables, legumes, pulses, healthy fats, and whole grains to not only get a balance of macronutrients but also an efficient supply of vitamins and minerals. As whole grains constitute a major portion of a calories, the nutrient value matters. The better the quality of grain is, the better the nutrient density of the plate (Asritha, 2021).

8.1.3 Millets as a Functional Food in Weight Control

8.1.3.1 Nutritional Profile of Millets

In recent years, millet consumption has been an uprising trend. Millets are small-seeded grains cultivated for centuries as staples across the world. Once seen as 'poor man's food', millets are now valued for their nutrition, food security, and sustainability. These are rich in protein, complex carbohydrates, dietary fiber, vitamins, minerals, and antioxidants.

These are gluten-free and low in glycemic index (GI), promoting satiety, regulating appetite, blood sugar levels, and healthy weight management. Millets exhibit anti-inflammatory and antioxidant properties owing to their high antioxidant content. This, in turn, helps promote better prevention and destruction of oxidative stress-causing free radicals. These properties make millets a

DOI: 10.1201/9781003686668-8

TABLE 8.1
Nutrient Profile of Some Common Millets and Cereal Grains (Per 100 g)

Millets and Cereal Grains	Protein (g)	Fat (g)	Dietary Fiber (g)	Carbohydrates (g)	Ca (mg)	Fe (mg)	Mg (mg)	Cu (mg)	Zn (mg)	Thiamine (mg)	Riboflavin (mg)	Niacin (mg)
Finger millet	7.16	1.92	11.18	66.82	364	4.62	146	0.67	2.53	0.37	0.17	1.34
Pearl millet	10.96	5.4	11.49	61.7	27.35	6.42	124	0.54	2.76	0.25	0.20	0.86
Sorghum	9.97	1.73	10.22	67.68	27.6	3.95	133	0.45	1.96	0.35	0.14	2.10
Little millet	10.13	3.89	7.72	65.55	16.06	1.26	91.4	0.34	1.82	0.26	0.05	1.29
Kodo millet	8.92	2.55	6.39	66.19	15.27	2.34	122	0.26	1.65	0.29	0.20	1.49
Cereals												
Wheat	10.59	1.47	11.23	64.72	39.36	3.97	125	0.49	2.85	0.46	0.15	2.68
Rice	7.94	0.52	2.81	78.24	7.49	0.65	19	0.23	1.2	0.05	0.05	1.6

Source: Longvah et al (2017).

powerful grain, a 'nutri-cereal', beneficial against several health conditions, boosting overall health and well-being (Maurya et al 2023).

8.1.3.2 Comparison of Millets with Other Grains in Weight Management

The nutritional value of millets is comparable to some of the major cereal grains like wheat, rice, and oats, as they are plentiful in nutrients like carbohydrates, protein, dietary fiber, and micronutrients like vitamins and minerals, as shown in Table 8.1. Millets are an abundant source of essential nutrients and phytonutrients.

Millets are also rich in health-enhancing phytonutrients like phytocyanins, polyphenols, phytosterols, and lignin. A study conducted by Kalam Azad et al (2019) reported around 50 different phenolic compounds and their derivatives, like flavones, ferulic acid, and flavonols, that act as potent antioxidants and detoxifying agents.

In addition, polyphenols can obstruct the lipogenic pathway and obesity linked enzymes like pancreatic lipase, which mitigates fat synthesis and storage. These compounds can also elevate thermogenesis, which increases energy expenditure and, subsequently, more calorie burning (Mamun et al 2024; Gowda et al 2022).

8.1.4 Rise in Popularity of Millets for Weight Loss Diets

8.1.4.1 Trends in Millet Consumption

Millets have always been a staple food in traditional diet habits, but somewhere lost in the modernization of lifestyle and eating habits. Researchers have analyzed the consumption pattern of millets during the independence era and current times to compare between the years 1977–78 and 2011–12. In rural areas, sorghum was consumed in relatively higher quantities, followed by pearl millet, finger millet, and small millets. Between 1977–78 and 2011–12, the largest decline in consumption was observed for small millets (97.62%), followed by sorghum (88.41%), finger millet (83.33%), and pearl millet (68.67%) in rural households. In urban households, per capita consumption of sorghum decreased by 82.44%, pearl millet by 64.86%, and finger millet by 59.44% over the same period.

TABLE 8.2
Health Benefits of Millets

	Nutrients	Health Benefits
Millets	High fiber and complex carbohydrates Gluten-free High micronutrients Phytonutrients	Low glycemic index – encourages slow release of blood glucose. Helps in diabetes. Improved digestive health and gut health Anti-cholesterol effect – helps reduce cholesterol levels Anti-hypertensive – helps regulate blood pressure Anthropometric effect – positive impact on BMI and reduced fat mass Helpful in celiac disease Supports healthy metabolism Combats oxidative stress and prevents disease risk Supports overall well-being

Sources: Sabuz et al (2023), Ambati and Sucharitha (2019), Kaur et al (2024).

Overall, the drop in millet consumption was more evident in rural areas compared to urban areas (Sukumaran et al 2022).

However, recent reports suggest that millet consumption is experiencing a resurgence in India and across the globe owing to factors like growing health consciousness, increased awareness around the health benefits of millets, gluten-free trend, product diversification, and, even, government initiatives. Production and consumption of millets is witnessing an elevated rise. In fact, an opportunity for revival of this grain at a global platform has been presented by the United Nations, which declared year 2023 as the International Year of Millet.

In terms of statistics and data, the Indian Development Review reported an increase in the production of millets in India. The projected millet yield has increased two folds since 1966, with yield of 1208 kg/ha in the time 2021–22. Meanwhile, experimenters prognosticate that transnational request is anticipated to witness a composite periodic growth rate (CAGR) of 4.5 between 2021 and 2026 (Dhaniya et al 2024).

8.1.4.2 Health Benefits Beyond Weight Management

Owing to their versatility, failure resistance, and high nutritive value, millets are considered an eventuality to address global food security as well as environmental challenges. Hence, new and advanced research are emerging more frequently around preventive and therapeutic properties of millets. In fact, these nutri-cereals are mentioned in old textbooks of India and China for their medicinal value.

For this reason, the health benefits of millets are not limited only to weight management, as shown in Table 8.2.

8.2 NUTRITIONAL COMPONENTS OF MILLETS FOR WEIGHT MANAGEMENT

8.2.1 Macronutrient Composition

8.2.1.1 Carbohydrates and Fiber

8.2.1.1.1 Slow-Digesting Carbs and Their Role in Satiety

Carbohydrates are the principal source of energy in the body. However, its function and health benefits can be numerous depending on the quality as well. When it comes to millets, carbohydrates constitute the majority of their composition, accounting for about 60–70% of their composition. In millets, starch makes up about half to nearly four-fifths of the seed's weight, in the form of amylopectin and amylose. The amylose-to-amylopectin ratio determines starch digestibility, classified as rapidly, slowly, or resistant starch (RS) based on how long it takes to break down. The amylose and RS in millets slow their digestion, contributing to better blood sugar control and improved gut health.

The key factor attributing to this characteristic is its lower surface area. Because of its limited surface area, when compared to amylopectin, amylose chain is less readily available to digestive enzymes, making its digestion and release into bloodstream a slow process. Therefore, millets containing amylose takes longer time to digest, remain in the gut tract for long and provide prolonged satiety. Consequently, this leads to reduced food intake and better calorie control (Anderson and Woodend 2003).

8.2.1.1.2 High Fiber Content for Appetite Control and Digestion

Millets are a notable source of dietary fiber, with content varying between approximately 2 and 14%, depending on the specific millet variety. The high fiber content contributes to increased gastric volume and reduced gastric emptying rate, which together result in prolonged distension of the stomach. This mechanical effect enhances the sensation of satiety and helps regulate appetite over a longer duration. Improved satiety facilitates better control over calorie intake and lowers the hunger index, thereby suppressing unnecessary cravings that may otherwise lead to episodes of uncontrolled binge eating and subsequent weight gain.

Additionally, the delayed delivery of nutrients to the small intestine slows the rate of carbohydrate absorption, which likely explains the blunted postprandial glycemic response observed with millet consumption. These physiological effects of dietary fiber in millets contribute to better glycemic control and effective weight management (Anitha et al 2024).

8.2.1.2 Protein Content

8.2.1.2.1 Protein's Role in Increasing Metabolism and Reducing Hunger

Millets are a valuable source of dietary protein, contributing approximately 7–12% of their weight, and are notable for their relatively higher content of essential amino acids – particularly lysine, methionine, and cysteine – compared to conventional cereals. They also contain prolamin, a key storage protein, which provides important amino acids such as phenylalanine, proline, and glutamic acid (Zhang et al 2024).

In the context of metabolism, protein has the highest thermic effect of food (TEF) among the macronutrients, meaning that approximately 20–30% of its calorie content is expended during digestion, absorption, and metabolism. This elevated energy cost, combined with protein's role in preserving and supporting muscle mass as well as enhancing resting energy expenditure, contributes to an increased metabolic rate (Drummen et al 2018).

Moreover, protein plays a crucial role in regulating appetite and satiety. It is well-established that protein-rich foods are more satiating than isocaloric amounts of carbohydrates or fats. During digestion, the breakdown of dietary protein releases amino acids, which act as signals to stimulate the secretion of gastrointestinal satiety hormones, including cholecystokinin (CCK) and glucagon-like peptide-1 (GLP-1). These hormones slow gastric emptying and promote the sensation of fullness, thereby aiding in appetite control and reducing subsequent energy intake.

Another mechanism attributed to protein role in weight management is through its impact on liver gluconeogenesis. High-protein and low-carbohydrate diets can stimulate hepatic gluconeogenesis to maintain plasma glucose levels and enhance glucose homeostasis, which, in turn, has a positive influence on satiety, as otherwise decreased levels of glucose can be appetite-stimulating (Pesta and Samuel 2014).

Thus, the unique protein composition of millets not only contributes to their nutritional value but also supports metabolic health and weight management through both thermogenic and satiety-promoting mechanisms.

8.2.1.2.2 Amino Acid Profile and Muscle Retention

When weight is lost, there is also equally the risk of weight loss associated with loss of lean body mass, which if remain unchecked, can be harmful, increasing the risk of low muscle mass and impaired muscle function. Studies have reported that people with higher weight have higher muscles mass, but the quality is poor, and that if weight is lost with a dietary strategy, in addition to high protein intake, the loss of lean muscle mass can be minimized with relatively lower impact on strength. This can be attributed to high protein in diet which can help preserve lean body and muscle mass (Cava et al 2017).

The amino acid profile of millets is rich in some essential amino acids like isoleucine, leucine, methionine, valine, phenylalanine, though typically low in lysine. In non-essential amino acids category, millets have significant number of amino acids as well, such as alanine, aspartic acid, glutamic acid, and serine (Amadou et al 2013).

Suryawan et al (2011) have discussed the role of leucine, which, in particular, is a branched-chain amino acid and known to stimulate muscle protein synthesis through stimulation of the mTORC1 (mammalian target of rapamycin complex 1) pathway, which involves phosphorylation of protein kinase, initiating the mRNA translation for muscle synthesis. In addition, preserving muscle mass during weight loss and its sustenance for long is crucial as fat-free or lean tissue preserves resting energy expenditure and supports metabolic health.

To attain the complete supply of all essential amino acids, millets can be paired with other complementary protein sources like beans, legumes, nuts, dairy or lean meat sources. This is also helpful in improving the overall protein quality of the diet. Additionally, adequate protein intake during hypocaloric diets attenuate the loss of fat-free mass and enhances satiety paired with high TEF, which supports long-term weight management (Romano et al 2024).

8.2.1.3 Healthy Fats

8.2.1.3.1 Role of Fats in Satiety and Overall Health

Dietary fat is one of the macronutrients that is less talked about and is always considered a villain when it comes to weight gain and obesity. However, with advancements in science, it is now established that not all fats are bad. Saturated fats, also known as unhealthy or 'bad' fats have the tendency to cause inflammation, to deposit in arteries and around vital organs causing increase in weight. However, unsaturated fatty acids like PUFA (polyunsaturated fatty acids) and MUFA (monounsaturated fatty acids) have been associated with healthy weight and metabolism.

Dietary fats play a significant role in weight management through various mechanisms. This nutrient is known to modulate satiety, supporting hormonal and cellular functions. Dietary fats with a chain length of more than 12 carbons, as in the case of MUFA and PUFA, are known to stimulate the secretion of satiety hormones like CCK and PYY (peptide YY). This, in turn, helps in preventing overeating and excess calorie intake (Samra 2010).

Besides aiding appetite regulation, fats also help in nutrient digestion and act as carriers for fat-soluble vitamins (A, D, E, and K), which are required by the body for various metabolic processes. Obesity-associated dyslipidemia is a common consequence of higher visceral fat, disturbing the lipid metabolism, release of free fatty acids from enlarged adipose tissues and consequently, release of pro-inflammatory cytokines causing inflammation. Studies have shown that replacing saturated fats with unsaturated fatty acids and, particularly, MUFA, the levels of HDL (High-Density Lipoprotein) increases while LDL (Low-Density Lipoprotein), total cholesterol (TC), and triglycerides tend to reduce (Sacks and Katan 2002).

In addition, chronic low-grade inflammation is one of the root causes of weight gain and obesity, which affects and impairs insulin sensitivity. This further creates a vicious cycle of higher production of free radicals, impaired insulin sensitivity, and weight gain. Healthy fats are also known to exhibit anti-inflammatory properties, which help to reduce systemic inflammation by downregulating some of the prominent pro-inflammatory cytokines in adipose tissue, such as MCP-1 (monocyte chemoattractant protein-1), TNF-α (tumor necrosis factor-alpha), and IL-6 (interleukin-6). Healthy fats like EPA and DHA also help in modifying the composition of the cell membrane that prevents the translocation of pro-inflammatory cytokines like TNF-α and IL-6 (Teng et al 2014).

Therefore, moderate intake of healthy fats can be beneficial for healthy weight management, extending sustainable weight loss and even cardiometabolic health.

8.2.1.3.2 Types of Fats Found in Different Millet Varieties

Millets contain moderate amounts of fats, typically ranging between 2 and 8%. As for the type, millets majorly contain unsaturated fatty acids, prominently alpha linoleic acid and oleic acid, which are beneficial for improving lipid levels, inflammation, and metabolic health (Jacob et al 2024).

8.2.2 Micronutrient Benefits for Weight Management

8.2.2.1 Vitamins

Dietary interventions have been considered as an effective strategy in reducing body weight and body mass index (BMI), where major attention has been given to the role of macronutrients. However, considering the role of metabolic parameters in the management of obesity, micronutrients like vitamins and minerals are equally crucial.

8.2.2.1.1 B Vitamins in Energy Metabolism

Millets are rich sources of Vitamin B complex, notably thiamine (B1), riboflavin (B2), niacin (B3), and folate (B9). These vitamins act as a coenzyme assisting in various metabolic pathways for assimilation of nutrients like carbohydrate, protein, and fat and converting them into usable energy. For instance, thiamine catalyzes many biochemical reactions involved in the metabolism of glucose as a cofactor for pyruvate dehydrogenase and alpha-ketoglutarate, which participate in the citric acid cycle for TAP/energy production (Lee 2023).

B vitamins also exhibit anti-inflammatory and antioxidant properties, diminishing the vicious cycle of oxidative stress and inflammation. Researchers have found that intestinal stress can impair folic acid absorption, causing its deficiency and forming a vicious cycle. It has also been seen that deficiency of B vitamins, particularly of folic acid and vitamin B_6, can raise the levels of homocysteine, which is known to hinder fat oxidation. Thus, adequate B vitamin intake ensures efficient energy metabolism, supporting physical activity and fat oxidation during weight loss interventions (Fu et al 2023).

8.2.2.1.2 Vitamin E and Antioxidant Effects

Vitamin E, though present in small amounts in millets, acts as a fat-soluble antioxidant, protecting cell membranes from cellular oxidative damage by neutralizing reactive oxygen species (ROS). As it is a well-established fact, oxidative stress is often elevated in obesity and weight loss efforts; therefore, vitamin E helps reduce inflammatory markers, improve insulin sensitivity, and support healthy lipid levels restoration during weight loss (Wong et al 2017).

8.2.2.2 Minerals

8.2.2.2.1 Magnesium, Zinc, and Their Roles in Metabolism

Magnesium is an abundant mineral present in millets, which acts as a cofactor in over 300 enzymatic reactions. It is engaged in ATP (Adenosine Triphosphate) production, nutrient utilization, insulin transmission, and glucose regulation. Magnesium is also known to stimulate the secretion of CCK, a satiety hormone, hence regulates appetite, controls calorie intake, and weight management. Magnesium also helps in improving sleep quality, which directly affects metabolism and indirectly, weight management.

As we know, oxidative stress is a major pathophysiology behind metabolic dysfunction that triggers cellular damage with oxidation of biomolecules. Zinc acts as a cofactor for many enzymes that play a protective role against oxidative damage. It also stimulates production of metallothioneins, a protein effective in lowering the concentration of harmful hydroxyl radicals and ROS (Marreiro et al 2017).

Zinc also impacts insulin signaling and glucose metabolism as this mineral plays a crucial role in insulin synthesis, its storage, and secretion within the pancreas. It also assists fatty acid metabolism by stimulating adipogenesis, influencing gene expression, and acting as a cofactor for enzymes involved in lipid metabolism (Kreft and Štrukelj 2021; Olechnowicz et al 2018).

8.2.2.2.2 Iron for Sustained Energy and Combating Fatigue

Iron deficiency is associated with obesity because of increased body fat and inflammation that impairs the body's capacity to absorb the mineral (Alshwaiyat et al 2021). Millets are a good source of non-heme iron, particularly pearl millet and barnyard millet at 16.9 and 15.2 g per 100 g (IIMR (Indian Institute of Millets Research), 2025).

Iron is critical for hemoglobin production and oxygen transport, directly influencing endurance, activity performance, and energy levels. Sometimes, with calorie-deficit diet during a weight management regimen, the intake of micronutrients such as vitamins and minerals may fall short of recommended levels. Ensuring adequate iron intake during weight loss prevents fatigue and supports higher activity levels, promoting sustained weight reduction (Beard and Tobin 2000).

8.3 SATIETY AND APPETITE CONTROL WITH MILLETS

8.3.1 Role of Dietary Fiber in Enhancing Fullness

8.3.1.1 Types of Fiber in Millets and Their Digestive Effects

Millets provide about 15–20% dietary fiber – nearly double that of rice and similar to whole wheat – with both soluble (β-glucans, arabinoxylans, pectins) and insoluble (cellulose, hemicellulose) fiber concentrated in the seed coat and bran (Jacob et al. 2024).

Millets have shorter amylose chains, which are densely packed; therefore, their hydrolysis is a slow process. In addition, due to effective levels of dietary fiber and RS combined with their low GI, millets have a positive impact on digestive health and especially satiety (Anitha et al 2024).

The suggested mechanisms indicate that high fiber in millets increases gastric volume and extends the gastric emptying time, resulting in a longer stay in the gastrointestinal tract. This causes a feeling of fullness or satiety. Fiber also supports slowed digestion and release of glucose into the bloodstream, increasing insulin sensitivity and better controlled glycemic response. This gradual and sustained rise in blood glucose can help regulate appetite and reduce hunger (Bornet et al 2007).

As fiber stays longer, it also triggers insulinotropic hormone like GLP-1, an endogenous satiation signal which helps stimulate insulin secretion, slows gastric emptying, and thus helps with better satiety (Wu et al 2023).

Millets contain natural enzymes such as phytase and polyphenol oxidase, which help break down nutrients like carbohydrates and proteins into simpler forms. This supports digestion, enhances nutrient availability, and helps reduce gastric discomfort.

Moreover, with a unique combination of both soluble and insoluble fibers, millets have a positive impact on gut microbiome while providing efficient support in the digestion process.

Insoluble fibers, as the name implies, do not dissolve and instead add bulk to the stool, aiding in regular bowel movements and reducing the risk of constipation. In contrast, soluble fibers dissolve to form a viscous gel and function as prebiotics. These prebiotics serve as a food source for gut microbiota, supporting the growth and activity of beneficial bacteria (Maurya et al 2023).

8.3.1.2 Impact on Gut Health and Metabolism

Besides their role in digestive health and satiety, dietary fibers and RS in millets have a very specific role in the gut microbiome. The fiber in millets acts as a prebiotic, resulting in enhanced growth and functioning of good gut bacteria. Research has demonstrated that intake of millets has been linked with the percentage abundance of beneficial bacteria like Lactobacilli and Bifidobacteria. It facilitates colonic fermentation by the gut microbes, leading to the production of crucial metabolites called short-chain fatty acids (SCFAs) like acetate, butyrate, and propionate. These SCFAs play a key role in a wide array of health areas, like maintaining the integrity of the gut barrier and preventing the translocation of toxins into the bloodstream. These metabolites also help inhibit the growth of pathogenic bacteria, protect against inflammation, and regulate the gut–brain axis and various hormones (Maurya et al 2023).

The nature of gut microbiota and SCFAs also plays a critical role in the host metabolism. Studies have shown that gut dysbiosis can be a pathophysiology behind many of the most common metabolic conditions. SCFAs help support against weight gain and higher adiposity by increasing energy expenditure and fat oxidation. They can also improve insulin sensitivity and boost the secretion of GLP-1, which in turn leads to better calorie control and ultimately better glycemic control. SCFAs also support glucose homeostasis. SCFAs like acetate and butyrate activate receptors such as GPR43 and GPR41, which help release hormones like insulin, GLP-1, and PYY, and help improve fat metabolism and lower blood sugar levels. In the liver, SCFAs block the pathway of glycolysis and gluconeogenesis while triggering glycogen synthesis.

Imbalance in SCFAs is also associated with metabolic dysfunction–associated steatotic liver disease, as alteration in healthy gut microbiome and associated SCFAs can affect glucose homeostasis, lipid metabolism, inflammation, and liver health (Facchin et al 2024).

8.3.2 Low Glycemic Index and Blood Sugar Regulation

8.3.2.1 Effect of Millets on Blood Glucose and Insulin Response

In today's trend of busy schedules, better control of glycemic response is not solely attributed to metabolic fluctuations but is deeply rooted within the lifestyle and kind of diet one consumes.

Millet is one such underutilized crop that offers wide benefits, including glucose homeostasis and blood sugar regulation, owing to its low GI. Food's ability to modulate the blood glucose levels is called the GI. The higher the GI, the more quickly the blood sugar rises, whereas a low GI implies a slow and gradual rise in blood glucose levels. Unlike cereals like wheat and rice, millets have higher dietary fiber, non-starch polysaccharide, and RS content, which helps in the slower digestion of starchy foods by intestinal enzymes and thus, delayed glucose absorption and mild glycemic response (Ahamed et al 2024).

Millets are also a rich source of protein, which helps in stimulating insulin sensitivity and secretion, resulting in better glycemic response. This macronutrient slows down the rate of gastric emptying and, thereby, reduces the absorption of simple molecules like glucose (Anitha et al 2021b).

Hence, it is evident that regular consumption of millets can help improve insulin sensitivity by preventing regular blood glucose spikes and strengthening body cells, becoming more responsive to insulin and utilizing glucose more efficiently.

8.3.2.2 Benefits of Stable Blood Sugar for Appetite Control

American Diabetes Association (2022) has emphasized the significance of stable blood sugar and appetite. Elevated blood sugar levels can irregularly amplify hunger and food cravings. Although one might assume that excess blood sugar can help suppress appetite, the underlying mechanism is more complex. With irregular blood glucose spikes, the insulin sensitivity reduces and becomes more unresponsive to the amount of glucose in the bloodstream.

In the absence of adequate insulin, glucose fails to enter the brain across the blood–brain barrier efficiently, leaving the brain in a perceived state of energy deficit despite systemic higher blood sugar levels. Now, the brain depends on a continuous supply of glucose for its functioning and metabolic needs and in the condition of perceived deficit, it activates neural and hormonal pathways that stimulate hunger and encourage more food intake.

This creates a negative feedback loop: with higher food consumption further exacerbating blood glucose levels and spikes, particularly when insulin action or availability is insufficient to maintain glucose homeostasis. Therefore, it becomes imperative to maintain blood sugar levels within, healthy range to break this vicious cycle.

8.3.3 Millet-Based Meals for Sustained Energy

8.3.3.1 Slow-Digesting Carbs for Longer Energy Release

Starch is the major component of millets ranging from 50 to 79% of total seed weight. Based on its digestibility pattern, starch is categorized into three types – rapidly digestible starch (RDS) which digests within 20 minutes, slow digestible starch (SDS) which digests between 20 and 120 minutes; and RS which takes over 120 minutes for digestion.

Millets have a high proportion of RS that takes maximum time to get hydrolyzed and, thus, results in more controlled and slow release of glucose into bloodstream. In fact, various processing techniques like cooking and cooling, germination and fermentation facilitate restructuring of starch molecules and influences starch hydrolysis and glucose release. For instance, protein makes a barrier between starch molecules and digestive enzymes, hence, slowing down its digestion (Gowda et al 2025).

8.3.3.2 Millet Porridge, Salads, and Grain Bowls for Extended Satiety

The slow digestible and RS in millets not only provide steady and sustained supply of energy but also contribute to extended satiety, making them beneficial for weight management.

Millet is one such grain that has been a staple since ancient times all across the world. Therefore, dishes made with millet such as porridge, salads, and grain bowls can be an efficient way to harness the benefits. A warm bowl of millet porridge, cooked with vegetables, offers a nutritious power breakfast that releases glucose slowly into bloodstream and keeps one full for longer without any craving or hunger pangs for long time.

Similarly, a millet salad or grain bowl, when paired with protein, seasonal vegetables, and healthy fats, can be a wholesome meal in itself, keeping one full and metabolically active. Such combination of protein, high fiber, and fats can aid in sustained energy release to make the person more active whereas, such nutrients pair can also stimulate appetite hormones like GLP-1 and PYY. This is crucial to induce satiety, better portion control, and reduced tendency of overeating. Additionally, the chewy texture of millets in such preparations encourages slower eating and better portion control, which can further aid in managing body weight and sustaining energy (Hawton et al 2018).

8.4 METABOLIC BENEFITS OF MILLETS FOR WEIGHT LOSS

8.4.1 Impact on Basal Metabolic Rate (BMR)

Basal metabolic rate (BMR) is the rate of energy expenditure by humans to perform basic life sustaining functions, like blood circulation, breathing, heartbeat, and food digestion, at rest. It accounts for approximately 60–75% of total energy expenditure and has a positive relationship with weight. An individual with lower BMR expends less energy as compared to one with higher BMR. In addition to lower BMR, if the calorie intake from exogenous sources exceeds more than body's requirement, higher weight becomes inevitable. However, the dietary approaches with right set of nutrients like high fiber and high protein can help accelerating the body's slowed BMR (Nagashree et al 2015).

8.4.1.1 Protein's Thermic Effect on Metabolism

TEF, also known as diet-induced thermogenesis (DIT), is the energy utilized in response to food. Food consumption results in a brief increase in energy expenditure resulting from various steps involved in food processing like digestion, absorption, transportation to different organs and systems, assimilation, and storage. The TEF is represented as the percentage rise in energy expenditure over the BMR.

When it comes to protein, it has the highest DIT of 15–30% followed by that of carbohydrate (5–10%) and fat (0–3%). Recently studies have suggested that the TEF increases by approx. 29 kJ/4184 kJ of ingested food for each 10% increase in energy coming from protein.

The high DIT coming from protein can play an important role in energy balance and consequently on weight management. For reducing weight effectively, it is important to improve the energy expenditure to balance high calorie intake where protein can play a critical role. For instance, a study as published in American Journal of Clinical Nutrition demonstrated that subjects who had diet comprising of 29% protein had 891 kJ/day higher metabolic rate as compared to another arm of subjects consuming the same isocaloric diet with 11% protein (Mikkelsen et al 2000).

Another mechanism through DIT of protein can help in weight management is through DIT associated satiety. The likely mechanism contributing to this observation is the rise in oxygen requirement to utilize protein, which can boost satiety (Pesta and Samuel 2014).

8.4.1.2 Role of Micronutrients in Supporting Metabolic Function

As the name suggests, micronutrients (essential trace minerals and vitamins) are required in small amounts, however, plays a critical role in body's metabolism and maintenance of its healthy functioning.

Vitamins are compounds, organic in nature, and classified into water soluble or fat soluble. They function as vital regulators in the body, playing crucial roles in energy metabolism by serving as coenzymes, acting as antioxidants, and regulating gene expression. Vitamins are also essential for the metabolism of key nutrients such as carbohydrates, fats, and proteins, as well as supporting wound healing, maintaining organ health, and facilitating DNA and RNA synthesis.

Similarly, minerals are vital nutrients and represent about 5–6% of total body weight. These micronutrients are responsible for wide array of functions like providing structural components to skeletal systems like bone and teeth, regulation of neurotransmission and muscle contraction, maintenance of osmotic pressure, regulating acid-base equilibrium in the body and serving as essential component of various enzymes and hormones (National Research Council 1989, chap. 13).

Overall, these micronutrients play a crucial role in many biochemical functions serving as follows:

- *Cofactors* – These involve moderating enzymes activity or are an integral part of enzyme prosthetic group.
- *Coenzyme in metabolism* – These nutrients play an active role in some complex biochemical pathways that are essential for transitional metabolism, facilitating the utilization of major nutrients to produce energy, proteins, and nucleic acids.
- *Regulates genetic pathways* – Some trace minerals act as transcriptional regulator which binds with DNA and regulates the transcription of receptors for steroids and other hormones.
- *Antioxidant property* – Chronic oxidative stress and inflammation hinders and slows down metabolic processes. Various vitamins like A, C, and E and minerals like selenium, and zinc perform protective functions against free radicals and support healthy metabolism (Shenkin 2006).

8.4.2 Antioxidants in Millets and Their Role in Metabolic Health

8.4.2.1 Polyphenols and Flavonoids in Metabolic Health

Just like micronutrients, there are several compounds derived from plants or phytonutrients, which exhibit antioxidant potential. Polyphenols represent the largest group of phytochemicals and are found abundantly in millets as phenolic acids and flavonoids. Although polyphenols are not classified

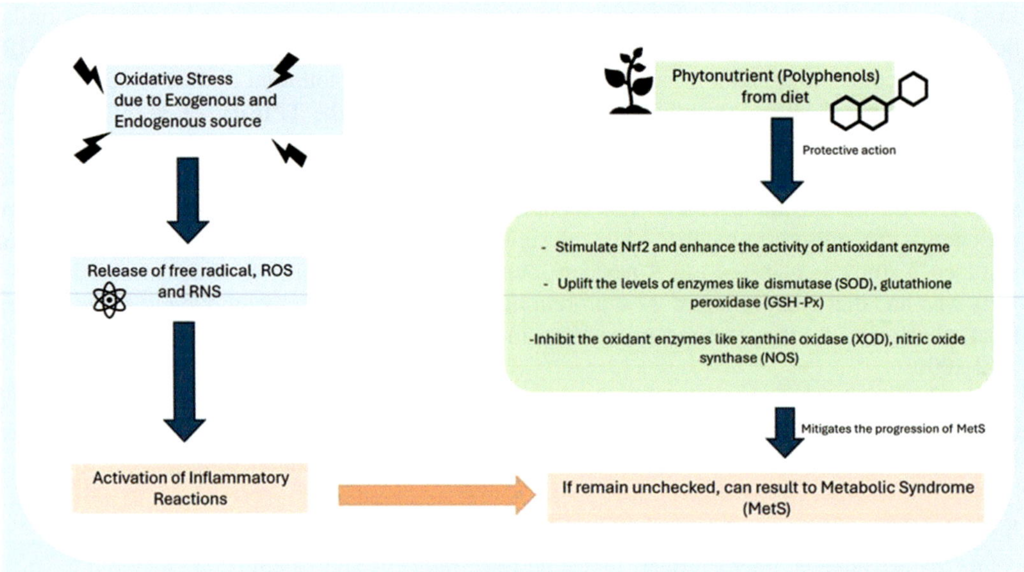

FIGURE 8.1 Protective action of polyphenols against inflammation in metabolic syndrome (MetS)

as essential nutrients, several studies have demonstrated that consuming adequate amounts of these compounds can positively impact the body's metabolic health.

Metabolic syndrome (MetS) is a commonly used clinical terminology and refers to the complex coexisting diagnosis including obesity, hypertension, dyslipidemia, and elevated blood sugar levels. It is a key contributor to the development of diabetes mellitus and CVDs. Advanced redox biology emphasizes that the central mechanism in the pathophysiology of MetS is uncontrolled systemic oxidative stress driven by free radicals and redox imbalance. In addition, if chronic oxidative stress remains unchecked, it can affect various organs and systems with the onset of disorders like diabetes, atherosclerosis, Alzheimer's disease, DNA damage, metabolic imbalance, and hormonal disturbances.

As illustrated in Figure 8.1, evidence proposes that polyphenols, at relevant doses, may help prevent or delay metabolic syndrome (MetS) by the following:

1. *Affecting the antioxidant signaling pathways* – Polyphenols are well-established to stimulate the Nrf2 (master transcription factor for antioxidant and cytoprotective genes) pathway and upregulation of antioxidant genes. In this way, it helps increase the expression of primary and phase II detoxifying enzymes, which contribute to antioxidant defense. Polyphenols also modulate MAPK signaling which is associated with Nrf2 activation and enhanced expression of antioxidant enzymes. These phytochemicals also stabilizes and helps release of Nrf2 by regulating keapl (Kelch-like ECH-associated protein 1). In normal healthy condition, keapl is Nrf2 suppressor, however, during oxidative stress, keapl is to be regulated so that Nrf2 can be activated for antioxidant defense.
2. *Induction of antioxidant enzymes* – ROS can be regulated with the help of antioxidant enzyme system like superoxide dismutase (SOD), catalase (CAT), and glutathione peroxidase (GSH-Px). Polyphenols have been seen to uplift the levels of these enzymes upon administration.
3. *Inhibition of oxidant enzymes* – Along with activation of antioxidant enzymes, it is equally important to suppress the activity of oxidant enzymes such as xanthine oxidase (XOD), lipoxygenase (LOX), nicotinamide adenine dinucleotide phosphate oxidase (NOX), nitric

oxide synthase (NOS), and cyclooxygenase (COX). These enzymes not only participate in redox reactions but also enhance the levels of cellular reactive oxygen and nitrogen species.

With these properties, polyphenols contribute to improvement in MetS and associated conditions as established by various clinical studies.

- *Hyperglycemia* – Studies have shown that administration of polyphenols like anthocyanins and flavanones has positive impact on fasting insulin, insulin sensitivity index, thus, improved insulin secretion from pancreatic cells with reduced glycated hemoglobin (HbA1C) and blood glucose levels.
- *Obesity* – Clinical studies have demonstrated that intake of polyphenols like flavonoids and gallic acid results in positive improvement in fat deposition and excess inflammation. Various anthropometric measurements like waist–hip circumference, body weight, BMI, and abdominal fat were significantly reduced while antioxidant markers like superoxide dismutase (SOD) and glutathione (GSH) were found to be increased.
- *Hypertension* – Increased blood pressure is a predominant risk factor contributing to CVDs. Polyphenols have demonstrated a positive change in blood pressure coupled with increased concentration of S-nitrosoglutathione at about 0.23 nmol/L, signifying the impactful role of oxidative stress and this process.
- *Dyslipidemia* – Elevated lipid levels is another one of the pathophysiological factors for cardiovascular damage. Studies revealed that supplementation with dietary polyphenols like as present in berries (flavan-3-ols, flavonols, and flavanones) and green tea (epigallocatechin gallate (EGCG)) helps in favorable changes were revealed in TC, LDLC, and HDLC levels with overall lipid profile and, thus, prevents dyslipidemia (Liu et al 2019).

8.4.3 Millets Thermogenic Properties and Fat Metabolism

8.4.3.1 Effect of Millets on Lipid Profiles and Fat Storage

CVD is one of the foremost causes of morbidity and mortality globally, contributing to approximately 30% of global deaths, with blood lipid levels playing a significant role. Elevated TC, low-density lipoprotein cholesterol (LDL-C), and triglycerides contribute to the development and progression of CVD, increasing mortality risk.

Millets are good source of phytonutrients like polyphenols and flavanols, which are known to counteract the damage caused by free radicals and ROS, resulting in controlled inflammation and regulated lipid profile. Similarly, being a high fiber and low GI grain, millets tend to reduce blood glucose levels, which is otherwise available for triacylglycerol synthesis (Alzahrani et al, 2022).

A systematic review and meta-analysis published in *Frontiers in Nutrition* in 2021 assessed the benefits of millets of elevated blood lipid levels or hyperlipidemia and cardiovascular risk. The analysis collated 19 clinical studies published between 2011 and 2021 including both the genders and encompassing various parameters under lipid profiles – including TC, triglycerides, HDL-C, LDL-C, and VLDL-C for duration between 21 days to 4 months. The authors reported significant reduction in TC by 8% from 189.5 ± 27.7 to 174.8 ± 28.9 mg/dl ($p < 0.01$). Similarly, triglycerides level was found to decrease by 9.5% from 154.3 ± 24.5 to 139.8 ± 23.5 mg/dl ($p < 0.01$). The levels of LDL-C were also reduced by 10%, whereas VLDL-C dipped by 9% ($p < 0.01$). Markedly, in four studies, millet consumption normalized TC and triglyceride levels (<200 and <150 mg/dl, respectively). The review also found a 6.0% increase in HDL-C (the 'good' cholesterol), which has beneficial health impact cardiovascular health (Anitha et al 2021a).

Another clinical study conducted by Hou et al (2018) demonstrated that replacing 50 g of staple food with foxtail millet for 12 weeks helped with significant reduction ($p < 0.05$) in body fat% (from 31.03 ± 1.38 to 30.16 ± 1.40), fat mass (from 21.63 ± 0.96 to 20.92 ± 0.98), and even, the BMI.

8.5 PRACTICAL INCLUSION OF MILLETS IN A WEIGHT MANAGEMENT DIET

8.5.1 Millet-Based Meal Ideas for Weight Loss

8.5.1.1 Breakfast: Millet Porridge, Smoothie Bowls, and Pancake

Beginning the day with a millet-based breakfast can help regulate hunger cravings providing satiety and support steady energy levels. Millets such as finger millet (ragi), foxtail millet, or pearl millet can be prepared as a warm porridge with vegetables, providing a low-glycemic, high-fiber meal that promotes satiety and prevents in between meals, mid-morning hunger pangs. Research shows that whole grains with high fiber and RS improve satiety by modulating gut hormones like GLP-1 and PYY, reducing overall calorie intake (Zhou et al 2008).

On the other hand, to extract benefits of RS, cooked and cooled millets can be blended into smoothie bowls with fruits, nuts like almonds, walnuts, and seeds like chia seeds and flax seeds. This enhances the content of fiber, healthy fats, and micronutrients while minimizing added sugars. Another option can be millet-based pancakes made with whole-grain millet flour and combined with protein-rich toppings such as yogurt or nut butter, with seasonal fruits on the side, can also deliver balanced macro and micronutrients to support weight loss goals.

8.5.1.2 Lunch and Dinner: Millet Salads, Grain Bowls, and Stir-Fries

For other two major meals – lunch and dinner, millets can make for an excellent substitute to refined and processed grains, attributed to their lower GI and higher fiber content, which support controlled glycemic response and extended satiety. Millet salads, combining cooked millets with seasonal vegetables, lean proteins, and healthy fats, create nutrient-dense, satisfying meals. Similarly, grain bowls featuring cooked millets as the base can be customized with plant-based proteins like legumes or beans and green, leafy, and seasonal vegetables. It can provide various health benefits, like improving gut health and regulating healthy metabolism. Millet-based stir-fries, where cooked millets replace rice or noodles, add texture and a slow-digesting starch source, which research connects with better weight management and improved carbohydrate and lipid (Bojarczuk et al 2022).

8.5.1.3 Snacks: Millet Energy Bars, Crackers, and Fermented Dishes

While the major meals are of high concern as maximum percent of calorie intake is determined during these meals, snacking can play an equally important role in influencing daily total calorie intake along with overall nutritional quality. Including millet-based snacks can help regulate hunger between meals without excess calories. For instance, millet energy bars, made with puffed millets, nuts, and natural sweeteners, offer a convenient and easy-to-carry alternative which is high in fiber, protein, and healthy fat and helps prevent uncontrolled blood sugar spikes. Whole-grain millet crackers, paired with hummus or hung curd dip, provide a crunchy, filling option with minimal refined carbohydrates. Choosing these negligibly processed, low-calorie, and nutrient-dense snacks over refined and high-sugar options supports with evidence-based strategies for sustainable weight loss.

8.5.2 Meal Timing and Portion Control with Millets

8.5.2.1 Optimal Times to Consume Millet-Based Meals

Millets are one of such versatile grains that can be included with major meal like breakfast, lunch, and dinner in the form of salads, porridge, stir fry, breads, or as snacks like puffed or roasted millets, millet crackers, and bars. As millets are rich in micronutrients, protein, and fiber, its consumption throughout the day will ensure constant, optimal supply of these essential nutrients with many health benefits. For example, studies have shown that intake of high-protein breakfast is associated with better satiety, reduced levels of ghrelin, and higher satiety hormone PYY and even better muscle mass (Leidy et al 2013; Khaing et al 2025).

It also helps with better and more controlled glucose response while prevent erratic spikes. Dalgaard et al (2024) demonstrated that high-protein breakfast is associated with higher satiety and better calorie control until lunch time, known as 'second meal effect' and was also beneficial for better concentration. Similarly, protein-rich meal at night helps with improved muscle protein synthesis with better muscle mass and muscle strength (Snijders et al 2015).

A high dietary fiber diet is associated with more regularized bowel movement, better gut health with promotion of beneficial gut bacteria and healthy metabolites. Also, daily intake of optimal dietary fiber helps support lowering the blood cholesterol and postprandial blood glucose levels with improved satiety, better calorie control, and consequently, weight management (Akbar and Shreenath 2023).

8.5.2.2 Portion Control Strategies for Weight Management

It has been proven that consuming higher portions of beverages and food rich in sugar is linked with increased calorie intake and, consequently, weight gain. And with the current lifestyle with minimal physical activity, more prominent desk jobs, and easy access to high-calorie foods, portion control becomes more important than ever.

However, the question may arise that is eating less good for health. The earlier recommendations given by nutrition organization emphasized on the benefits of eating less. However, such an approach may be challenging to adopt and sustain for long. Focusing instead on portion control and the nutritional quality of foods can promote a healthier and more sustainable diet. By replacing high-energy-dense foods with vegetables, fruits, and other nutrient-rich, low-energy-dense options, individuals can enjoy greater food volume without increasing calorie intake.

Therefore, it is highly crucial to be more aware of various ways not only just to reduce the quantity on plate but also to improve the quality of food being consumed, making it nutrient-rich.

1. *Amorphous foods* – With no proper shape or defined boundaries such as macaroni and cheese or halwa, it may become difficult to assess the portion size and may result in significant calorie intake. Therefore, it is crucial to consider pre-measured servings or smaller serving plates.
2. *Unit packaging* – For foods which comes basis defined serving units like sandwiches or packet of chips, larger pack will lead to increased energy intake. Strategies like choosing smaller serve pack with mindful moderate intake can boost self-control while restricting excess energy intake. Beverage intake is another aspect which generally gets ignored when combined with food. A research was conducted to see if there is any change in calorie intake when food and beverage combined and found that the food intake was not affected, although the energy intake changed basis serving size of beverage. With the larger portion of regular soda being served, women increased their calorie intake by 10% and men by 26%. Therefore, the concept of moderation and self-control is equally applicable for beverage as well.
3. *Restaurant portions* – In restaurants, oversized portions often go unnoticed by consumers, leading to higher energy intake and contributing to obesity risk. Strategies such as offering smaller portion options, consumer awareness around difference in calorie needs vs. nutrient needs, proper menu tagging, can help with controlled portions without compromising with satisfaction.
4. *Persistence* – Evidence show that constant exposure to large portions leads to a sustained increase in daily energy intake over time, and without suitable biological compensation,

the excess calories tend to accumulate, increasing the risk of obesity. Long-term strategies like consistently offering smaller, standardized portions are essential to as sustained effects.

Therefore, an understanding of apt portion sizes should take into account that how energy value affects the food. Also, for efficient weight management, individuals should be aware that they can enjoy filling, sufficient portions by choosing larger amounts of low-energy-dense foods while keeping portions of high-energy-dense foods limited (Rolls 2014).

8.5.3 Pairing Millets with Complementary Foods

8.5.3.1 High-Protein and High-Fiber Combinations for Satiety

Coupling millets with high-protein and high-fiber foods is an efficient dietary strategy to boost satiety, regulate appetite, and support weight management. Millets themselves are rich in dietary fiber and RS, which decelerate gastric emptying and influence the secretion of satiety hormones like GLP-1 and PYY, known to promote fullness and reduce energy intake. The fiber content can further be elevated with addition of seasonal vegetables. However, the protein content in millets is moderate (7–12%), and although it contains all nine essential amino acids, but levels of some like lysine is very less as compared to other protein sources. Therefore, combining millets with complementary proteins, such as legumes, beans, nuts, dairy, eggs, or lean meats, can help improve the overall amino acid quality of the meal and further support satiety and lean body mass preservation.

For example:

- *Millet-lentil vegetable khichdi*: The fiber and RS from millets and vegetables combined with the plant-based protein of lentils can create a slow-digesting, filling meal.
- *Pearl millet roti with vegetables and soybean curry*: This combines whole-grain fiber with high-quality plant-based protein with minimal fat and cholesterol, while rich in fiber and protein.

Such combinations also attribute to low GI of meal which helps support controlled glycemic response as compared to refined carbohydrates or millets consumed alone. Such meal combinations are wholesome, balanced that helps support better metabolic health while keeping one full for a longer time.

8.6 ANTI-NUTRIENTS IN MILLETS AND THEIR IMPACT ON WEIGHT MANAGEMENT

Though millets are abundant in essential nutrients like vitamins, minerals, fiber, and phytonutrients, these small seed grains also contain some anti-nutrient factors which need to be addressed to extract benefits. These include phytates, saponins, tannins, and trypsin inhibitors. Consuming these can negatively impact nutrient availability and digestion, gastric discomfort, and many health consequences (Singh et al 2025).

8.6.1 Understanding Anti-Nutrients and Their Functions

8.6.1.1 Phytic Acid, Tannins, and Their Effects on Digestion

Phytic acid – Phytic acid (phytate) is myo-inositol 1,2,3,4,5,6-hexakis (dihydrogen phosphate), the main storage form of phosphorus in seeds, accounting for approximately 1–5% of their weight. As a secondary metabolite, it serves as a nutrient reserve, accumulated in the seed during ripening (Samtiya et al 2021).

Even though millets contain phytates levels lesser as compared to some conventional grains like wheat flour, barley, corn, and brown rice, it is crucial to reduce its content to improve nutrients' digestion and accessibility. Phytic acid, in this form, is not a readily bioavailable type of phosphorus to monogastric animals (like poultry and humans) as the digestive tract lacks phytase enzyme, which is crucial for the release of phosphorus from the phytate molecule (Sheethal et al 2022).

Tannins – Tannins are a group of antioxidants and secondary metabolites which are generally present in cereals, bark, fruits, and vegetables. In millets, these astringent and bitter tasting compounds are majorly present in finger, foxtail, barley, sorghum, kodo millet, etc.

Although these mainly serve as protective agent for plants, when consumed, they can have negative effect on digestion as well. These can bind and form complexes with nutrients like minerals, protein, and carbohydrate. Tannins can inhibit the activity of proteolytic enzymes and form complexes with protein – affecting the nutrient digestion. If remain undigested, it can affect gut microbiota and cause digestive discomforts like constipation, inflammation, and acidity. Excess intake of tannins can interact disrupt gastrointestinal mucosa by interacting with ROS and causing oxidative stress (Singh and Kaushik 2025).

To conclude, even though the anti-nutrients like phytates and tannins can reduce the nutrient availability, these compounds also demonstrate benefits like slowed carbohydrate-digestion, modulating gut microbiota, and improved satiety. When these millets are processed and consumed suitably, the balance of nutrients and bioactive compounds can assist in effective weight management.

8.6.1.2 Potential Impacts on Mineral Absorption and Nutrient Availability

As the name suggests, the anti-nutrients have the capacity to impact the digestibility of nutrients like protein, carbohydrate, and many minerals, impairing their bioavailability and ultimately utilization by the human body.

For example, phytate or phytic acid, being a negatively charged ion, reacts and forms a bond with positively charged bivalent and trivalent mineral ions like Mg^{2+}, Ca^{2+}, Zn^{2+}, $Fe^{2+/3+}$, Mn^{2+}, and Cu^{2+}, reducing their bioavailability. Similarly, it also forms complex with carbohydrates and proteins preventing its easy availability and utilization in human body.

Tannins also are polyphenolic compounds and, thus, have great affinity for protein and minerals like magnesium, zinc, iron, and calcium, impacting their bioavailability (Singh and Kaushik 2025; Singh et al 2025).

8.6.2 Processing Techniques to Reduce Anti-Nutrients

There are various processing methods, both – traditional and modern, which can help in reducing the concentration of anti-nutrients while improving the overall nutrition quotient.

8.6.2.1 Sprouting, Soaking, and Fermenting for Optimal Nutrition

Traditional techniques like sprouting, fermentation, and soaking can be time consuming but are relatively easy and efficient in reducing the concentration of anti-nutrients.

Soaking is one of the easiest ways to lower the concentration of anti-nutrients and is the first step before fermentation or cooking. Studies have reported that soaking in water for anywhere between 12 and 18 hours, followed by discarding of water helps in efficient removal of anti-nutrients like tannins and phytates.

Another traditional method like germination or sprouting is an active phase of metabolism. This technique helps in improving the nutrient quality by modifying the chemical composition and reduces the anti-nutrients factors. For example, a study by Masud et al (2007) demonstrated that germination is one of the best methods in reducing phytate content by up to 40% owing to the activity of endogenous phytase enzyme which hydrolyze the phytic acid and thus reduces its content.

Fermentation is an age-old method of food processing. Few studies have demonstrated the beneficial effect of fermentation on elevated levels of antioxidants and nutrients while reducing the level of anti-nutrients like phytates and polyphenols. For example, Mohapatra et al. (2019) demonstrated that fermentation can lower the total phenol content by 28% and the tannin content by 30–39% in sorghum.

The process of fermentation helps in improving the aromas, flavors, and textures, and thus enriching human nutrition. It also results in bio-enhancement of nutrients like fatty acids, vitamins, amino acids, and protein due to activity of enzymes like amylase and protease, which are present inside the grain. The metabolic activity of microbes during fermentation also enhances the concentration of bioactive compounds (Samtiya et al, 2021).

8.6.2.2 Cooking Methods to Maximize Nutrient Retention

In addition to traditional processing methods, various thermal treatments such as cooking, roasting, and autoclaving have been shown to effectively reduce the levels of anti-nutritional compounds. For instance, cooking can lower the concentrations of tannins, phytates, and trypsin inhibitors by approximately 42, 75, and 95.8%, respectively. Similarly, blanching has been reported to decrease tannin content progressively with increasing temperature and duration of treatment. Autoclaving, another thermal processing technique, is considered particularly efficient; for example, pressure cooking has been shown to reduce phytates and tannins by about 20–25% and tannins alone by approximately 17%. These reductions in anti-nutrients are accompanied by improvements in the nutritional quality and digestibility of macronutrients such as proteins, enhancing their bioavailability and overall dietary value (Samtiya et al 2021; Rajakumar et al 2023).

8.6.3 Benefits of Moderate Anti-Nutrient Intake

Although anti-nutritional factors can pose challenges by reducing nutrient bioavailability, some of these compounds may also confer health benefits. Therefore, it is important to be informed about both the potential positive and negative effects of these constituents. Furthermore, their effects are often concentration-dependent and should be evaluated accordingly. With appropriate processing and awareness, the health-promoting properties of these compounds can be explored (Popova and Mihaylova 2019).

8.6.3.1 Role of Anti-Nutrients in Glycemic Control

Some of the anti-nutrients exhibit natural inhibitory activity against α-amylase and α-glucosidase, which play a key role in carbohydrate metabolism. These inhibitors get release into digestive tract upon digestion and bind to the carbohydrate-digesting enzymes forming complex. This results in restricted breakdown/hydrolysis of starch molecules and hindered digestion. This ultimately slows down glucose release in bloodstream and facilitates better glycemic control. Additional anti-nutrient protease inhibitor performs as competitive inhibitor as it behaves like substrates and attach at the active site of enzyme with low dissociation constant. Tannins also demonstrate anti-inhibitory effect against enzyme α-amylase, causing limited digestion of nutrients like carbohydrates (Salim et al 2023).

8.6.3.2 Possible Appetite-Reducing Effects of Certain Anti-Nutrients

As discussed above in detail, some anti-nutrients inhibit the function of carbohydrate-digesting enzymes, it results in more controlled and slowed digestion and release of simple glucose molecules in bloodstream resulting in better glycemic control.

This sustained release can have an influence on the typical postprandial levels of plasma glucose and probably satiety. Similarly, another anti-nutrient trypsin inhibitor increases the production of satiety hormones like CCK, which suppress appetite and thus regulate calorie control and in turn, better weight management (Duraiswamy et al 2023).

8.7 SCIENTIFIC EVIDENCE ON MILLETS AND WEIGHT MANAGEMENT

8.7.1 Studies on Millets' Effects on Body Weight and Composition

8.7.1.1 Clinical Trials on Millet Diets and Body Weight Reduction

Obesity prevalence is a global health issue affecting wellbeing and quality of life. Maintaining a healthy body weight is the foundation of preventing and managing chronic conditions such as type 2 diabetes, CVD, and metabolic syndrome. Millets, owing to their rich fiber, protein, and bioactive compound content, have been studied to assess its impact on weight management.

Evidence from clinical trials, though varied in findings, suggests a potential role of millets in weight management. In a study by Sobhana et al. (2020), multigrain flatbreads made with millets and other grains consumed for 90 days in 100 type 2 diabetic patients did not result in significant weight loss. Similarly, Singh et al. (2020) observed a non-significant reduction in body weight among 60 type 2 diabetic subjects over 12 weeks on a millet-based functional diet. In contrast, Surekha et al. (2013) reported a 2% weight reduction in 11 healthy subjects consuming a barnyard millet-based formulation over 28 days, and Ren et al (2018) demonstrated a statistically significant weight decrease in adults with impaired glucose tolerance consuming foxtail millet bread over 12 weeks (from 69.1 ± 11.6 to 68.2 ± 11.2 kg; $p = 0.004$). The most notable findings come from Geetha et al. (2019), where 60 overweight subjects consuming a millet-based mix for 120 days experienced a substantial and significant weight reduction (from 68.57 ± 10.97 to 63.23 ± 10.60 kg) (Table 8.3).

Millets have the potential to contribute to satiety, regulate glucose metabolism, and provide sustained energy, which makes them a valuable alternative to refined grains in weight control strategies.

TABLE 8.3
Impact of Millet Consumption on Weight Loss

Study	Intervention	Subjects and Duration	Outcomes
Sobhana et al (2020)	*Intervention* – multigrain flatbreads made with millets (combination of wheat, soy flour, pearl millet, sorghum, foxtail, oats, maize) *Control* – Usual diet	100 Type 2 diabetic subjects *Duration* – 90 days	No significant weight loss
Surekha et al. (2013)	Food formulation with barnyard millet in combination with carrot, black gram, and spice mix	11 Healthy subjects *Duration* – 28 days	Weight reduction of 2%
Geetha et al. (2019)	Millet-based food mix (finger millet, little millet, defatted soya flour, whole green gram, fenugreek seeds, cluster bean, drumstick leaves and curry leaves)	60 Subjects with BMI > 22.9 *Duration* – 120 days	Significant weight loss from 65.34 ± 10.97 to 63.23 ± 10.60 kg
Singh et al (2020)	Millet-based functional food rich intervention diet (millets 60%, soya bean 20%, brown rice 10%, peanuts 8%, and flex seeds 2%)	60 Type 2 diabetic subjects *Duration* – 12 weeks	Non-significant weight loss from 71.54 ± 12.20 to 68.13 ± 11.74
Ren et al (2018)	Foxtail millet steamed bread	70 Adult subjects with impaired glucose tolerance *Duration* – 12 weeks	Significant decrease of body weight (p = 0.004) from 69.1 ± 11.6 to 68.2 ± 11.2 kg

TABLE 8.4
Impact of Millet Consumption on Body Mass Index (BMI)

Study	Intervention	Subjects and Duration	Outcomes
Anushia et al (2019)	Diet counseling and tips to replace wheat and rice with millets for lunch and dinner	88 Subjects with type 2 diabetes and BMI above 23 kg/m^2 *Duration* – 3 months	Significant reduction in BMI from 30.8 ± 3.7 to 29.8 ± 3.4
Hou et al (2018)	Replaced the staple food with approx. 50 g of foxtail millet	45 Subjects with mild hypertension *Duration* – 12 weeks	Significant reduction in BMI
Geetha et al. (2019)	Millet-based food mix (finger millet, little millet, defatted soya flour, whole green gram, fenugreek seeds, cluster bean, drumstick leaves, and curry leaves)	60 Subjects with BMI > 22.9 *Duration* – 120 days	Significant reduction in BMI from 27.84 ± 4.14 to 26.95 ± 4.06
Anitha et al (2021a)	Systematic review and meta-analysis – 50–200 g of millets per day	900 Subjects *Duration* – Ranging from 21 days to 3 months	Reduction in BMI by 7% from 28.5 ± 2.4 to 26.7 ± 1.8 kg/m^2
Vissapragada (2021)	Millet-based diet for breakfast and dinner	4 Weeks	Significant reduction in BMI from 28.8 to 26.6 kg/m^2

8.7.1.2 Observational Studies on Millet Consumption Patterns and BMI

BMI is an extensively used scale of body fat and a critical indicator of overweight and obesity, which are prominent risk factors for various chronic disorders. Recent clinical evidence suggests that replacing refined grains with millets in the daily diet can significantly improve BMI by promoting satiety, enhancing metabolic health, and regulating energy intake.

As shown in Table 8.4, a study by Anushia et al (2019), dietary counseling encouraging replacement of wheat and rice with millets at lunch and dinner for three months in 88 individuals with type 2 diabetes led to a significant BMI decrease of 29.8 ± 3.4 from 30.8 ± 3.7. Similarly, Hou et al (2018) reported a significant BMI reduction in 45 mildly hypertensive adults who replaced their staple food with ~50 g of foxtail millet daily over 12 weeks.

In a longer intervention, Geetha et al. (2019) provided a millet-based mix (containing finger millet, little millet, legumes, and greens) for 120 days to 60 overweight individuals, resulting in BMI reduction from 27.84 ± 4.14 to 26.95 ± 4.06 kg/m^2. Supporting these findings, Anitha et al (2021a) conducted a systematic review and meta-analysis of studies (n = 900) with millet intakes ranging from 50 to 200 g/day over 21 days to 3 months, showing a mean BMI reduction of 7%, from 28.5 ± 2.4 to 26.7 ± 1.8 kg/m^2.

Additionally, a short-term study by Vissapragada (2021) demonstrated that a millet-based breakfast and dinner over just four weeks reduced BMI from 28.8 to 26.6 kg/m^2.

Jointly, these findings highlight the potential of millets as a dietary intervention for improving BMI and managing overweight and obesity. Their high fiber content, low GI, and nutrient density make them an effective alternative to refined cereals for promoting healthier body composition.

8.7.2 Comparative Studies: Millets vs. Other Grains in Weight Loss

8.7.2.1 Weight Management Benefits of Millets Over Rice, Wheat, and Refined Grains

Millets have been progressively studied and researched for their role in weight management. Lately, the research has become more intense to assess the comparative benefits of millets with conventional and staple grains like wheat, rice, and refined cereals. The unique nutritional composition of millets – high dietary fiber, low GI, RS, and rich polyphenols with vitamins and minerals – contributes to improved satiety, reduced postprandial glucose and insulin spikes, controlled calorie intake, and combating inflammation. These aspects make the nutri-cereals beneficial for weight loss and obesity prevention.

Several comparative studies have demonstrated the superiority of millets over rice, wheat, and refined grains in supporting weight management:

- *Caloric and nutrient density*: Millets, unlike conventional and staple cereals, have less calorie and comparatively, higher nutrient content like higher protein, vitamins and minerals, dietary fiber, and RS per gram. This allows individuals to nourish their body with right set of nutrients without excess calorie consumption. This approach can be helpful in better and sustainable weight management (Ambati and Sucharitha 2019).
- *Lower GI and satiety*: Millets generally have lower GI. Descriptive statistics show that the mean GI of millets (52.7 ± 10.3) is approximately 36% lower compared to common staples like milled rice (71.7 ± 14.4) and refined wheat (74.2 ± 14.9) (Anitha et al 2021b). The low GI property of millets is attributed to higher dietary fiber, RS, and protein as compared with staples like wheat and rice. Consequently, this helps with reduced hunger, increased satiety, and better weight control.
- *Improved body weight and BMI*: A systematic review and meta-analysis of randomized controlled trials (RCTs) by Anitha et al (2021a) demonstrated that millet-based diets led to a 7% reduction in body weight along with significant reduction in BMI compared to rice or refined wheat-based diets. This is because of higher fiber intake and lower energy density of millet-based meals.
- *Improved lipid profile*: In the same study, it is demonstrated that replacing wheat/rice with millets have positive impact on lipid profile – higher HDL and reduced LDL-C, VLDL-C, TC, and even, triacylglycerol. This, in turn, is important for obese individuals at risk of metabolic syndrome. For example, randomized trials with foxtail and barnyard millet have shown significant weight loss and improved lipid markers over wheat- and rice-based controls (Ugare et al 2014).

8.7.3 Health Benefits Beyond Weight Loss

8.7.3.1 Impact on Gut Health, Cardiovascular Health, and Inflammation

Due to the nature of nutritional components present in millets, the health aspects of these nutritious grains are not just limited to weight loss and improved lipid profile, but it also helps in other crucial health aspects needed for overall wellbeing.

For instance, role of millets in gut health is an area of expanding interest. Gut health is the fundamental base for overall health. It absorbs nutrients that act as energy fuel for whole body, and it contains gut microbiota that contributes to overall health with the help of metabolites. In fact, dysbiosis or imbalanced microbiota is associated with chronic disease. Millets, owing to its rich nutritional profile with high dietary fiber, RS ad polyphenols, supports gut health.

Studies have demonstrated that millet intake is associated with increased abundance of beneficial gut bacterial taxa like Bifidobacteria and Lactobacilli, which are known for their probiotic properties, promoting growth of good bacteria and prevent pathogenic bacteria. This is associated with soluble fiber and RS content in millets. These actives are being digested by gut bacteria leading to the production of metabolites like SCFAs (acetate, butyrate, and propionate). Among these, butyrate plays a crucial role in keeping the gut health intact by providing energy to colon cells, promoting gut barrier integrity, and reducing inflammation. The polyphenols in millets as well exhibit anti-inflammatory and antioxidant activities – protecting gut health against free radicals and oxidative stress. The insoluble fibers in millets also support gut motility providing bulk to stools and preventing the risk of constipation (Singh et al 2023).

Similarly, CVD is one of the principal causes of mortality and morbidity and contributes to 30% of total death worldwide. Millets, owing to its rich profile with essential nutrients like dietary fiber, phytonutrients, and unsaturated fats, have been proven beneficial against CVDs. A meta-analysis conducted by Anitha et al (2021a) assessed and demonstrated that millets consumption in amount ranging from 50 to 200 g for duration of 21 days to 2 years have positive impact on lipid profile. It helps elevating levels of 'good cholesterol' – HDL-C and reduces the levels of 'bad cholesterol' – LDL-C, VLDL-C, triacylglycerol, and TC. The inclusion and intake of millets replacing wheat and rice have also showed positive impact on blood pressure parameters viz. systolic and diastolic values.

In addition, it is proven fact that chronic, unchecked inflammation is the root cause for many metabolic disturbances and disorders. Whole grains like millets are good source of unsaturated fatty acids, polyphenols, and other phytonutrients, which are known for their antioxidant and anti-inflammatory properties. The polyphenols present in millets have shown to restrain the activity of pro-inflammatory cytokines like IL-1β, IL-6, IL-8, and boost the expression of anti-inflammatory cytokines like IL-10, by blocking the nuclear factor-kappaB (NF-κB)-p65 nuclear translocation (Shi et al 2017).

8.7.3.2 Benefits in Managing Diabetes and Metabolic Syndrome

Diabetes mellitus is one of the most prevalent lifestyle disorders globally. It is projected that by 2045, world will have 700 million of diabetics against 463 million as in 2019, referring to 51% surge (Anitha et al 2021b).

Because of good protein, dietary fiber, RS, and bioactive content, millets are known to play a significant role in regulating glycemic response. For instance, protein in millet has shown positive impact with reduce glucose levels and increased adiponectin. It also inhibits the activity of f dipeptidyl peptidase-IV (DPP-IV), which helps in sustainable release of GLP-1. These mechanisms stimulate pancreatic beta cells and trigger insulin release with improved insulin sensitization. Similarly, dietary fiber in millets has shown restrictive action over digestive enzymes like α-glucosidase and α-amylase, which results in slowed digestion of starch and gradual release of glucose in bloodstream. As a result, the glycemic response tends to improve.

Even the bioactive compounds in millets exhibit hypoglycemic effect via various mechanisms – these inhibits key digestive enzymes like α-amylase and glucosidase, responsible for post-meal blood glucose spike. Individual with higher BMI exhibits high inflammation and oxidative stress which, in turn, disrupt insulin signaling pathways and further promote inflammation. Therefore, oxidative stress plays a key role in onset and progress of diabetes. The phenolic compounds present in millets demonstrate antioxidant effect, mitigating the oxidative stress and associated damage.

There are various molecular mechanisms as well, through which millets play protective and preventive role against elevated blood sugar levels:

1. Millet intake activates the phosphoinositide 3-kinase/protein kinase B pathway, which is responsible for downregulation of glucose synthesis via gluconeogenesis. It also boosts the pathway leading to glucose uptake by GLUT4 translocation.
2. It also triggers the activity of glycolytic enzymes like phosphofructokinase-1, which promote glucose breakdown, its efficient utilization for energy production and ultimately, better glucose tolerance.
3. Millets may improve glucose homeostasis by increasing leptin levels, which regulate appetite, energy expenditure, insulin sensitivity, and glucose metabolism. Leptin modulates neuropeptide Y, anandamide receptors, α-MSH, and CCK, enhancing satiety and reducing food intake, thereby supporting glycemic control.
4. Healthy gut microbiome plays a key role in glucose homeostasis, and millet consumption has been associated with modulation of gut bacteria to balance glucose metabolism. As a prebiotic, millets provide the food and promotes the growth of good bacteria and

associated SCFAs, which subsequently helps with healthy glucose management. For instance, *Bifidobacterium* enhances muscle glycogen synthesis and reduces hepatic gluconeogenesis, thereby improving glucose regulation (Kumar et al 2025).

8.8 PRACTICAL GUIDELINES FOR INTEGRATING MILLETS INTO WEIGHT MANAGEMENT PLANS

8.8.1 Choosing the Right Types of Millets

8.8.1.1 Comparison of Millet Types for Specific Weight Management Goals

Diverse millet types offer exclusive nutritional profiles which are unique and can be aligned with specific weight management objectives. For instance, finger millet (ragi) and pearl millet are rich in dietary fiber; thus, it can be beneficial for promoting satiety and controlled calorie intake. Millets like foxtail millet, proso millet, and pearl millet contains higher protein and thus more suitable for individuals focusing on preserving lean body mass. Foxtail millet has comparatively lesser carbohydrate so can be preferred by people who look for weight management and simultaneously better glycemic response. Similarly, pearl millet provides higher iron levels, thus can be consumed by individuals who struggle with lower energy levels and frequent episodes of fatigue. Finger millet is one of the highest sources of calcium, thus an excellent choice for maintaining bone health (Dayakar Rao et al 2017).

8.8.1.2 Recommended Millets for Different Dietary Needs (e.g., Low-Carb, High-Fiber)

Individuals can choose from wide variety of millets basis their dietary needs. For example, if an individual plans to go on low-carbohydrate diets, he may choose from Pearl millet and finger millet with carbohydrate content of 61 and 60 g, respectively, as compared to other millets. People who want to focus on high fiber intake for satiety, gut health, and regulated glycemic response, can opt for millet varieties like pearl millet, finger millet, and sorghum, which has high fiber concentration in terms of both soluble and insoluble fiber. In fact, people with gluten intolerance can choose any millet, as they are naturally gluten-free, making them an excellent substitute to wheat-based grains (Dayakar Rao et al 2017).

8.8.2 Planning a Balanced Diet with Millets

8.8.2.1 Ideal Daily Intake of Millets in Weight Management Diets

Although there is no one-size-fits-all recommendation, there are certain standard guidelines that can help in determining ideal daily intake of food groups including millets. In line with 'Health Plate concept' advocated by Indian Council of Medical Research – about one-third of the plate should consist of whole grains and cereals. Among that one-third, at least half of the recommended cereals can be covered by whole grains and millets and can be consumed to the extent of 30–40% of total recommended cereals in raw weight, totaling of up to 45% calories coming from cereals and millets (ICMR 2024).

However, it is important to exercise caution regarding the portion control, as even healthy grains can contribute to excess calorie intake if over-consumed. Opting unprocessed or minimally processed millets while maintaining balanced diet and restricting added fats or sugars in preparation further supports weight management.

8.8.2.2 Balancing Millets with Other Food Groups

Millets are great source of several essential nutrients like protein, dietary fiber, and micronutrients, but it is crucial to have a balanced diet with inclusion of other food groups like seasonal fresh fruits and vegetables, legumes, beans, healthy fats, etc. This helps in extracting benefits from each food while meeting the daily nutrient requirement. According to the Healthy Plate Concept, the remaining two-thirds of the plate must be filled with vegetables, fruits, and protein-rich foods, nuts, and seeds, ensuring a diverse and balanced meal.

Millets, as the grain component, should be consumed in combination with legumes, pulses, dairy, eggs, fish, or lean meats to improve the protein quality, supplying all the essential amino acids. Half the plate should be covered with seasonal, fresh, and colorful vegetables and fruits, which add fiber, vitamins, minerals, and phytonutrients to the meal.

Adding a small portion of healthy fats, such as seeds, nuts, or a drizzle of plant-based oil, helps boosting the absorption of nutrients especially fat soluble one like Vitamin A, D, and also improves meal palatability and satisfaction.

Such a diverse and balanced plate, with healthy substitution of refined grains with millets, aligns with ICMR's guidelines for weight management and prevention of chronic diseases.

8.8.3 Lifestyle and Behavioral Considerations in Weight Management

8.8.3.1 Importance of Consistency and Variety in Millet-Based Diets

Weight management is a holistic approach where diet or exercise alone may not be beneficial. It must be a comprehensive effort where even behavioral modifications need to be addressed. Following a strict regimen might give results in short term, but it is the long-term habits which plays a crucial role to be on track and maintain the desired weight management goals. Consistency is one such behavioral aspect that helps achieve targeted weight loss goal not only in short term but also to maintain the lost weight in a more sustainable manner in long-term. Including a variety of millet-based meals – porridges, salads, rotis, grain bowls, and snacks – can prevent dietary monotony and improve compliance. Consistently replacing refined grains with whole millets improves metabolic markers over time (Gorin et al 2004).

8.8.3.2 Strategies for Mindful Eating and Meal Satisfaction

Mindful eating is another classical example of behavioral strategy based on cognitive and sensory consciousness that stimulates healthier relationships with food and thus, supports weight management. Kristeller and Wolever (2010) highlight that the food intake is not only limited to the food quality and quantity but also controlling response to emotional states, conscious food selection, and focusing on qualities like taste, texture, aesthetics, and aroma, developing satiety cue and developing self-acceptance. These can help controlling energy intake and better meal satisfaction.

When inclined to more of nutrient dense foods besides just calorie count while selecting healthy foods like millets over refined cereals, such mindfulness eliminates the chances of overeating while maximizing satiety and health benefits. Millets possess chewy texture and complex flavors, which when consumed consciously, encourage slower eating, and greater sensory enjoyment. Research shows that eating slowly and mindfully enhances the activation of satiety-related hormones (e.g., CCK and PYY), reduces subsequent calorie intake, and lowers the hedonic drive to eat beyond physiological needs (Andrade et al 2008).

In addition, aesthetic appearance of food with well-seasoned and colorful millet-based meals improves the pleasure resulting from eating. This, in turn, fosters satisfaction and helps prevent unnecessary snacking later. For example, combining millets with variety of fresh and colorful vegetables, legumes, and beans, and moderate amounts of healthy fats with seasonings, spices, and herbs not alone boosts the nutritional quality but even upgrades the sensory depth.

Also, mindful awareness of the eating experience such as appreciation for the food and identifying and acknowledging the feeling of satiety can also lower down the emotional or stress-induced eating behaviors which are often associated with weight gain.

8.9 FUTURE PERSPECTIVES AND RESEARCH DIRECTIONS IN MILLETS AND WEIGHT MANAGEMENT

8.9.1 Millet Innovations for Weight Management

8.9.1.1 Millet-Based Products and Their Role in Modern Diets

With rising awareness of the relationship between diet, metabolic health, and chronic disease, demand for nutrient-rich, high-fiber, and low-GI foods is rising. Millets offer a promising alternative to refined grains, providing fiber, slowly digestible and RS, and bioactive compounds like polyphenols, that improve postprandial glycemic control, enhance satiety, and help reduce energy intake – key for weight management. Studies show that incorporating millets into common foods, replacing the staples like wheat and rice, in the form of breads, snacks, millet-based cereals, porridges, soups, and beverages lowers blood glucose and insulin responses while promoting fullness, particularly benefiting those with overweight or glucose intolerance.

Innovations such as ready-to-eat millet flakes, gluten-free pastas, high-protein bars, and in fact, low GI millet-based food varieties can help meet urban consumers' demand for convenient, healthy, and culturally acceptable options amidst their busy lifestyle.

8.9.1.2 Potential of Millets as Functional Foods in Weight Management

As a well-established fact, it is now proven that millets are rich in bioactive compounds such as phenolics, flavonoids, protein, micronutrients, and dietary fiber, which have functional properties beyond basic nutrition. Wide array of research suggests that these compounds exert anti-inflammatory, antioxidant, and lipid-lowering effects, while providing satiety and regulating metabolic health, can counteract obesity-related metabolic fluctuations. These nutrients can further be enhanced with thermal or non-thermal treatments like fermentation, germination, or cooking, to improve the nutrient amount and availability and further improving its functional potential.

8.9.2 Emerging Areas of Research

8.9.2.1 New Findings on Millet Bioactive and Their Effects on Obesity

Beyond the major and well-known macro and micronutrients in millets, these also contain wide array of bioactives like dietary fiber, phenols, flavonoids like ferulic acid, caffeic acid, catechin, coumarin, ergosterol, vanillic acid, and quercetin (Sadh et al 2024). These bioactives exhibit health-promoting properties like antioxidant, anti-inflammatory, and modulate pathways involved in fat metabolism, appetite regulation, glycemic control, and gut microbiota composition. This, in turn, supports body weight regulation. Therefore, understanding these mechanisms could pave the way for designing targeted millet-based interventions for obesity prevention and management

8.9.2.2 Long-Term Health Outcomes and Millet Consumption

There are numerous studies and clinical trials done on short-term basis with promising effects of millets on body weight, glycemic control, and lipid profiles, there is a need for long-term, large-scale cohort studies to establish sustained benefits and their relationship with optimal consumption patterns. Another area of exploration can be prospective research to clarify the dose–response relationships, the impact of different millet types, and interactions with genetic and lifestyle factors in diverse populations.

8.10 CONCLUSION

The nutri-cereals millets promote healthy weight management owing to their rich nutrition profile – high dietary fiber, protein, RS, micronutrients, and unsaturated fats. This profile plays a crucial role via different mechanisms in weight management: promoting satiety, reducing glycemic and insulin responses, improving lipid metabolism, supporting gut health, and counteracting free radicals and inflammation. These coarse grains are affordable, versatile, and suitable for gluten-free diets. However, anti-nutrients and cultural acceptability should be addressed through appropriate processing techniques and awareness campaigns to maximize their benefits. Millets are not only beneficial for individual health but also for environmental health. They require less water and fewer inputs compared to rice or wheat, with a lower carbon footprint, better climate resilience, and biodiversity, making them environmentally sustainable. Promoting millet consumption aligns with global calls for sustainable, resilient food systems and offers a pathway to addressing both obesity and climate-related challenges.

REFERENCES

Ahamed V. P. A., A. Joshi, A. Mudey, S. Choudhari, J. Raut, and S. Ahmed. 2024. Unlocking the potential: Millets and their impact on diabetes management. *Cureus*. Apr 29;16(4): e59283. https://doi.org/10.7759/cureus.59283

Akbar, A., and A.P. Shreenath. 2023. High Fiber Diet. In *StatPearls*. Updated May 1, 2023. Treasure Island, FL: StatPearls Publishing. Accessed January 2025. https://www.ncbi.nlm.nih.gov/books/NBK559033/

Alshwaiyat, N.M., A. Ahmad, W. Wan Hassan, and H.A. Al-Jamal. 2021. Association between obesity and iron deficiency (Review). *Experimental and Therapeutic Medicine* 22: 1268. https://doi.org/10.3892/etm.2021.10703

Alzahrani, N. S., G.M. Alshammari, A. El-Ansary, A.E.A. Yagoub, M. Amina, A. Saleh, and M.A. Yahya. 2022. Anti-hyperlipidemia, hypoglycemic, and hepatoprotective impacts of pearl millet (*Pennisetum glaucum* L.) grains and their ethanol extract on rats fed a high-fat diet. *Nutrients* 14(9): 1791. https://doi.org/10.3390/nu14091791

Amadou, I., E.M. Gounga, and G. Le. 2013. Millets: Nutritional composition, some health benefits and processing – A review. *Emirates Journal of Food and Agriculture* 25(7): 501–508.

Ambati, K., and K.V. Sucharitha. 2019. Millets – Review on nutritional profiles and health benefits. *International Journal of Recent Scientific Research* 10(07I): 33943–33948.

American Diabetes Association. 2022. High blood sugar and hunger. *Diabetes Food Hub*. Retrieved July 14, 2025. https://diabetesfoodhub.org/blog/high-blood-sugar-and-hunger

Anderson, G. H., and D. Woodend. 2003. Effect of glycemic carbohydrates on short-term satiety and food intake. *Nutrition Reviews* 61(5 Pt 2): S17–26. https://doi.org/10.1301/nr.2003.may.s17-s26

Andrade, A. M., G.W. Greene, and K.J. Melanson. 2008. Eating slowly led to decreases in energy intake within meals in healthy women. *Journal of the Academy of Nutrition and Dietetics* 108(7): 1186–1191. https://doi.org/10.1016/j.jada.2008.04.026

Anitha, S., Kane-Potaka, J, Botha, R., Givens, D. I., Rajendran, A., Tsusaka, T. W., & Bhandari, R. K. 2021a. Can millet consumption help manage hyperlipidemia and obesity? A systematic review and meta-analysis. *Frontiers in Nutrition* 8: 703041.

Anitha, S., Kane-Potaka, J., Tsusaka, T. W., Botha, R., Rajendran, A., Givens, D. I., Parasannanavar, D. J., Subramaniam, K., Prasad, K. D. V., Vetriventhan, M., & Bhandari, R. K. 2021b. A systematic review and meta-analysis of the potential of millets for managing and reducing the risk of developing diabetes mellitus. *Frontiers in Nutrition* 8: 687428.

Anitha S., S. Upadhyay, and J. Kane-Potaka. 2024. Millets have the potential to increase satiety and reduce the feeling of hunger: A systematic review. *Frontiers in Sustainable Food Systems* 8: 1348068.

Anushia, K., J. Uma Mageshwari, P. Trueman, and V. Viswanathan. 2019. The effect of millet supplementation on weight and lipid profile. *TAPI Journal* 13 (3): 1–7.

Asritha, V. 2021. A review on role of millets in weight loss. *Indian Journal of Nutrition* 8(3): 239.

Beard, J., and B. Tobin. 2000. Iron status and exercise. *American Journal of Clinical Nutrition* 72(2 Suppl): 594S–7S. https://doi.org/10.1093/ajcn/72.2.594s

Bojarczuk, A., S. Skąpska, A.M. Khaneghah, and K. Marszałek. 2022. Health benefits of resistant starch: A review of the literature. *Journal of Functional Foods* 93: 105094. https://doi.org/10.1016/j.jff.2022.105094

Bornet, F. R. J., A.E. Jardy-Gennetier, N. Jacquet, and J. Stowell. 2007. Glycaemic response to foods: Impact on satiety and long-term weight regulation. *Appetite* 49(3): 535–553. https://doi.org/10.1016/j.appet.2007.04.006

Cava, E., N.C. Yeat, and B. Mittendorfer. 2017. Preserving healthy muscle during weight loss. *Advances in Nutrition* 8(3): 511–519. https://doi.org/10.3945/an.116.014506

Dalgaard, L. B., D.Z. Kruse, K. Norup, B.V. Andersen, and M. Hansen. 2024. A dairy-based, protein-rich breakfast enhances satiety and cognitive concentration before lunch in overweight to obese young females: A randomized controlled crossover study. *Journal of Dairy Science* 107(5): 2653–2667. https://doi.org/10.3168/jds.2023-24152

Dayakar Rao, B., K. Bhaskarachary, G.D. Arlene Christina, G. Sudha Devi, and A. Vilas Tonapi. 2017. *Nutritional and Health Benefits of Millets*. Hyderabad: ICAR_Indian Institute of Millets Research (IIMR).

Dhaniya, D., V. Verma, and E. Rani. 2024. Millets: The nutri-cereals crop trends in India. *International Journal of Humanities Social Science and Management (IJHSSM)* 4(1): 278–286.

Drummen, M., L. Tischmann, B. Gatta-Cherifi, T. Adam, and M. Westerterp-Plantenga. 2018. Dietary protein and energy balance in relation to obesity and co-morbidities. *Frontiers in Endocrinology* 9, 443. https://doi.org/10.3389/fendo.2018.00443

Duraiswamy, A., A. Sneha, K.S. Jebakani, S. Selvaraj, J.L. Pramitha, R. Selvaraj, K.I. Petchiammal, S.K. Sheriff, J. Thinakaran, S. Rathinamoorthy, and P.R. Kumar. 2023. Genetic manipulation of anti-nutritional factors in major crops for a sustainable diet in future. *Frontiers in Plant Science* 13:1070398. https://doi.org/10.3389/fpls.2022.1070398

Facchin, S., L. Bertin, E. Bonazzi, G. Lorenzon, C. De Barba, B. Barberio, F. Zingone, D. Maniero, M. Scarpa, C. Ruffolo, I. Angriman, and E.V. Savarino. 2024. Short-chain fatty acids and human health: From metabolic pathways to current therapeutic implications. *Life 14*(5): 559. https://doi.org/10.3390/life14050559

Fu, Y., Z. Zhu, Z. Huang, R. He, Y. Zhang, Y. Li, W. Tan, and S. Rong. 2023. Association between vitamin B and obesity in middle-aged and older Chinese adults. *Nutrients* 15(3):483. https://doi.org/10.3390/nu15030483

Geetha, K., M.G. Yankanchi, and N. Hiremath. 2019. Effect of high fibre food mix on lipid profile and body weight in obese subjects. *Biomedical Research* 30(4). https://doi.org/10.35841/biomedicalresearch.30-19-257

Gorin, A. A., S. Phelan, R.R. Wing, and J.O. Hill. 2004. Promoting long-term weight control: Does dieting consistency matter? *International Journal of Obesity and Related Metabolic Disorders* 28(2): 278–281. https://doi.org/10.1038/sj.ijo.0802550

Gowda, N.A., V. Kambhampati, M.K. Pulivarthi, *et al.* 2025. Thermal and non-thermal bioprocessing: A comprehensive review on millet starch properties and digestibility. *Food Measure* 19: 806–832. https://doi.org/10.1007/s11694-024-02998-6

Gowda, N.A.N., K. Siliveru, P.V.V. Prasad, Y. Bhatt, B.P. Netravati, and C. Gurikar. 2022. Modern processing of Indian millets: A perspective on changes in nutritional properties. *Foods* 11(4):499. https://doi.org/10.3390/foods11040499

Hawton, K., D. Ferriday, P. Rogers, P. Toner, J. Brooks, J. Holly, K. Biernacka, J. Hamilton-Shield, and E. Hinton. 2018. Slow down: Behavioural and physiological effects of reducing eating rate. *Nutrients* 11(1):50. https://doi.org/10.3390/nu11010050

Hou, D., J. Chen, X. Ren, C. Wang, X. Diao, X. Hu, Y. Zhang, and Q. Shen. 2018. A whole foxtail millet diet reduces blood pressure in subjects with mild hypertension. *Journal of Cereal Science* 84: 13–19. https://doi.org/10.1016/j.jcs.2018.09.003

ICMR. 2024. *Dietary Guidelines for Indians* – 2024: *ICMR-NIN Expert Committee*. Hyderabad: National Institute of Nutrition.

ICMR-NIN. 2018. *My Plate for the Day*. Hyderabad: Department of Health Research, Ministry of Health & Family Welfare, Govt of India.

IIMR (Indian Institute of Millets Research). 2025. Millets information. ICAR-IIMR. Accessed July 14, 2025. https://www.millets.res.in/millets_info.php

Jacob, J., V. Krishnan, C. Antony, M. Bhavyasri, C. Aruna, K. Mishra, T. Nepolean, C.T. Satyavathi, and K.B.R.S Visarada. 2024. The nutrition and therapeutic potential of millets: An updated narrative review. *Frontiers in Nutrition* 11:1346869. https://doi.org/10.3389/fnut.2024.1346869

Kalam Azad, M.O., D.I. Jeong, M. Adnan, T. Salitxay, J.W. Heo, M.T. Naznin, J.D. Lim, D.H. Cho, B.J. Park, and C.H. Park. 2019. Effect of different processing methods on the accumulation of the phenolic compounds and antioxidant profile of broomcorn millet (*Panicum miliaceum* L.) flour. *Foods* 8(7): 230. https://doi.org/10.3390/foods8070230

Kaur, N., B. Ray, and C.V. Kalyani. 2024. Millets: Ancient grains for modern nutrition – A comprehensive review. *Indian Journal of Community Medicine* 49(5): 665–668. https://doi.org/10.4103/ijcm.ijcm_765_23

Khaing, I.K., Y. Tahara, O. Chimed-Ochir, S. Shibata, and T. Kubo. 2025. Effect of breakfast protein intake on muscle mass and strength in adults: A scoping review. *Nutrition Reviews* 83(1): 175–199. https://doi.org/10.1093/nutrit/nuad167

Kim, J.Y. 2021. Optimal diet strategies for weight loss and weight loss maintenance. *Journal of Obesity and Metabolic Syndrome* 30(1): 20–31. https://doi.org/10.7570/jomes20065

Kreft, S., and B. Štrukelj. 2021. Influence of magnesium sulphate on cholecystokinin, hunger, and obesity. *Progress in Nutrition* 23(3): e2021312

Kristeller, J. L., and R.Q. Wolever. 2010. Mindfulness-based eating awareness training for treating binge eating disorder: The conceptual foundation. *Eating Disorders 19*(1): 49–61. https://doi.org/10.1080/10640266.2011.533605

Kumar, A., N.N. Shah, M.R. Chorawala, R. Kaushik, B. Prajapati, and R. Mehra. 2025. Exploring the molecular pathways underlying the anti-diabetic effects of millets. *Food Safety and Health* 00: 1–15.

Lee, C.Y. 2023. Effects of dietary vitamins on obesity-related metabolic parameters. *Journal of Nutritional Science* 12: e47. https://doi.org/10.1017/jns.2023.30

Leidy, H. J., L.C. Ortinau, S.M. Douglas, and H.A. Hoertel. 2013. Beneficial effects of a higher-protein breakfast on the appetitive, hormonal, and neural signals controlling energy intake regulation in overweight/obese, "breakfast-skipping," late-adolescent girls. *The American Journal of Clinical Nutrition* 97(4): 677–688. https://doi.org/10.3945/ajcn.112.053116

Liu, K., M. Luo, and S. Wei. 2019. The bioprotective effects of polyphenols on metabolic syndrome against oxidative stress: Evidences and perspectives. *Oxidative Medicine and Cellular Longevity* 2019: 6713194. https://doi.org/10.1155/2019/6713194

Longvah, T., R. Ananthan, K. Bhaskarachary, and K. Venkaiah. 2017. *Indian food composition tables.* Hyderabad: National Institute of Nutrition, Indian Council of Medical Research.

Mamun, M.A.A., A. Rakib, M. Mandal, S. Kumar, B. Singla, and U.P. Singh. 2024. Polyphenols: Role in modulating immune function and obesity. *Biomolecules* 14(2): 221. http://dx.doi.org/10.3390/biom14020221

Marreiro, D.D., K.J. Cruz, J.B. Morais, J.B. Beserra, J.S. Severo, and A.R. de Oliveira. 2017. Zinc and oxidative stress: Current mechanisms. *Antioxidants (Basel)* 6(2): 24. https://doi.org/10.3390/antiox6020024

Masud, T., T. Mahmood, A. Latif, S. Sammi, and T. Hameed. 2007. Influence of processing and cooking methodologies for reduction of phytic acid content in wheat (*Triticum aestivum*) varieties. *Journal of Food Processing and Preservation 31*(5): 583–594. https://doi.org/10.1111/j.1745-4549.2007.00147.x

Maurya, R., T. Boini, L. Misro, T. Radhakrishnan, A.P. Sreedharan, and D. Gaidhani. 2023. Comprehensive review on millets: Nutritional values, effect of food processing and dietary aspects. *Journal of Drug Research in Ayurvedic Sciences* 8(Suppl 1): S82–S98. https://doi.org/10.4103/jdras.jdras_123_23

Mikkelsen, P.B., S. Toubro, and A. Astrup. 2000. Effect of fat-reduced diets on 24-h energy expenditure: Comparisons between animal protein, vegetable protein, and carbohydrate. *American Journal of Clinical Nutrition* 72(5): 1135–1141. https://doi.org/10.1093/ajcn/72.5.1135

Millet Cultivation History and Trends – India Data Insights. 2023. Millet cultivation in India: History and trends. March 24, 2023. Retrieved July 16, 2025, from Millet cultivation in India: History and trends | IDR

Mohapatra, D., A.S. Patel, A. Kar, S.S. Deshpande, and M.K. Tripathi. 2019. Effect of different processing conditions on proximate composition, antioxidants, anti-nutrients and acid profile of grain sorghum. *Food Chemistry 271*: 129–135. https://doi.org/10.1016/j.foodchem.2018.07.196

Nagashree, V., N. Rumana, and M.L. Revathi Devi. 2015. Relationship between basal metabolic rate and body fat percentage in obese and non-obese females: A comparative study. *International Physiology* 3(2). https://doi.org/10.21088/ip.2347.1506.3215.1

National Research Council. 1989. *Diet and Health: Implications for Reducing Chronic Disease Risk.* Committee on Diet and Health. Washington, DC: National Academies Press (US). Available from: https://www.ncbi.nlm.nih.gov/books/NBK218735/

Olechnowicz, J., A. Tinkov, A. Skalny, and J. Suliburska. 2018. Zinc status is associated with inflammation, oxidative stress, lipid, and glucose metabolism. *Journal of Physiological Sciences* 68(1): 19–31. https://doi.org/10.1007/s12576-017-0571-7

Pesta, D.H., and V.T. Samuel. 2014. A high-protein diet for reducing body fat: Mechanisms and possible caveats. *Nutrition & Metabolism (London)* 11(1):53. https://doi.org/10.1186/1743-7075-11-53

Popova, A., and D. Mihaylova. 2019. Antinutrients in plant-based foods: A review. *Open Biotech Journal* 13: 13–68.

Rajakumar, R., U. Ammal, S. Ramasamy, J. Chinnadurai, U. Maruthanayagam, and V. Pai. 2023. Antinutritional factors in millets and their reduction strategies. In *Sensitizing the millet farming, consumption and nutritional security – Challenges and opportunities*, 323–328. Pandit Jawaharlal Nehru College of Agriculture & Research Institute, Karaikal.

Ren, X., R. Yin, D. Hou, Y. Xue, M. Zhang, X. Diao, Y. Zhang, J. Wu, J. Hu, X. Hu, and Q. Shen. 2018. The glucose-lowering effect of foxtail millet in subjects with impaired glucose tolerance: A self-controlled clinical trial. *Nutrients 10*(10): 1509. https://doi.org/10.3390/nu10101509

Rolls, B.J. 2014. What is the role of portion control in weight management? *International Journal of Obesity (London)*38 (Suppl 1): S1–S8. https://doi.org/10.1038/ijo.2014.82

Romano, B.C., I.M. de Araújo I.M., M.S.P Ribeiro, L.T. Parreiras E Silva, I. Dick-de-Paula, S.Y. Fukada, F.M. Porto, V. Jorgetti, F. de Assis Pereira, L.L.K Elias, and F.J.A. de Paula. 2024. Low-calorie and high-protein diet has diverse impacts on the muscle, bone, and bone marrow adipose tissues. *JBMR Plus 9*(1). https://doi.org/10.1093/jbmrpl/ziae150

Sabuz, A. A., M.R. Rana, T. Ahmed, M.M. Molla, N. Islam, H.H. Khan, G.F. Chowdhury, Q. Zhao, and Q. Shen. 2023. Health-promoting potential of millet: A review. *Separations 10*(2): 80. https://doi.org/10.3390/separations10020080

Sacks, F.M., and M. Katan. 2002. Randomized clinical trials on the effects of dietary fat and carbohydrate on plasma lipoproteins and cardiovascular disease. *American Journal of Medicine* 113 (Suppl 9B):13S–24S. https://doi.org/10.1016/s0002-9343(01)00987-1

Sadh, P.K., A. Kamboj, S. Kumar, *et al.* 2024. Perspectives of millets for nutritional properties, health benefits and food of the future: A review. *Discover Food* 4: 187.

Salim, R., I.B. Nehvi, R.A. Mir, A. Tyagi, S. Ali, and O.M. Bhat. 2023. A review on anti-nutritional factors: unraveling the natural gateways to human health. *Frontiers in Nutrition* 10: 1215873. https://doi.org/10.3389/fnut.2023.1215873

Samra, R.A. 2010. Fats and Satiety… In *Fat Detection: Taste, Texture, and Post Ingestive Effects*, edited by J. P. Montmayeur and J. le Coutre. Boca Raton, FL: CRC Press/Taylor & Francis. Available from: https://www.ncbi.nlm.nih.gov/books/NBK53550/

Samtiya, M., K. Soni, S. Chawla, A. Poonia, S. Sehgal, and T. Dhewa. 2021. Key anti-nutrients of millet and their reduction strategies: An overview. *Acta Scientific Nutritional Health* 5(12), 68–80.

Sarte, A. E., and E.J.M. Quinto. 2024. Understanding the importance of weight management: A qualitative exploration of lived individual experiences. *International Journal of Qualitative Studies on Health and Well-Being 19* (1). https://doi.org/10.1080/17482631.2024.2406099

Sheethal, H. V., C. Baruah, K. Subhash, A. Rajendran, and T. Longvah. 2022. Insights of nutritional and anti-nutritional retention in traditionally processed millets. *Frontiers in Sustainable Food Systems* 5, 735356. https://doi.org/10.3389/fsufs.2021.735356

Shenkin, A. 2006. Micronutrients in health and disease. *Postgraduate Medical Journal* 82 (971): 559–67. https://doi.org/10.1136/pgmj.2006.047670

Shi, J., S. Shan, H. Li, G. Song, and Z. Li. 2017. Anti-inflammatory effects of millet bran derived-bound polyphenols in LPS-induced HT-29 cell via ROS/miR-149/Akt/NF-κB signaling pathway. *Oncotarget* 8 (43):74582–74594.

Singh, R.B., J. Fedacko, V. Mojto, et al. 2020. Effects of millet based functional foods rich diet on coronary risk factors among subjects with diabetes mellitus: A single arm real world observation from hospital registry. *MOJ Public Health* 9(1):18–25. https://doi.org/10.15406/mojph.2020.09.00318

Singh, S.B., A.K. Meena, B.S. Sisodia, S. Sharma, M.M. Sharma, and P. Mansoria. 2023. From farm to gut: Unraveling the role of millets in promoting metabolic well-being via gut microbiota. *Journal of Drug Research in Ayurvedic Sciences* 8(Suppl 1): S50–S54. https://doi.org/10.4103/jdras.jdras_192_23

Singh, S. M., J.T. Joshi, S. Sivaranjani, N. Puja, M. Nagarajan, P. Kumar, and P.S. Rao. 2025. Comprehensive review of anti-nutrients in millets: Thermal and non-thermal reducing techniques. *Food Bioscience* 69: 106949. https://doi.org/10.1016/j.fbio.2025.106949

Singh, T. B., and R. Kaushik. 2025. Mitigation of anti-nutrients from millet by employing traditional to cutting-edge processing's to enhance nutrition profile. *Journal of Food Composition and Analysis* 143: 107605. https://doi.org/10.1016/j.jfca.2025.107605

Snijders, T., P.T. Res, J.S.J. Smeets, S. van Vliet, J. van Kranenburg, K. Maase, A.K. Kies, L.B. Verdijk, and L.J.C. van Loon. 2015. Protein ingestion before sleep increases muscle mass and strength gains during prolonged resistance-type exercise training in healthy young men. *Journal of Nutrition* 145(6): 1178–1184. https://doi.org/10.3945/jn.114.208371

Sobhana, P.P., B. Kandlakunta, R. Nagaraju, *et al.* 2020. Human clinical trial to assess the effect of consumption of multigrain Indian bread on glycemic regulation in type 2 diabetic participants. *Journal of Food Biochemistry* e13465. https://doi.org/10.1111/jfbc.13465

Sukumaran, S. A. D., P. Anbukkani, A. Singh, B.D. Rao, and G.K. Jha. 2022. Millet production and consumption in India: Where do we stand and where do we go? *National Academy Science Letters* 46(1): 65–70. https://doi.org/10.1007/s40009-022-01164-0

Surekha, N., B.V. Chimmad, and R.S. Naik. 2013. Hypoglycaemic and hypolipidemic efficacy of barnyard millet (*Echinochloa frumentacea* link) based health food. *Asian Journal of Home Science* 8 (2): 383–387.

Suryawan, A., R. A. Orellana, M. L. Fiorotto, and T. A. Davis. 2011. Triennial growth symposium: leucine acts as a nutrient signal to stimulate protein synthesis in neonatal pigs. *Journal of Animal Science* 89 (7): 2004–2016. https://doi.org/10.2527/jas.2010-3400

Teng, K.T., C.Y. Chang, L.F. Chang, and K. Nesaretnam. 2014. Modulation of obesity-induced inflammation by dietary fats: mechanisms and clinical evidence. *Nutrition Journal* 13:12. https://doi.org/10.1186/1475-2891-13-12

Ugare, R., B. Chimmad, R. Naik, P. Bharati, and S. Itagi. 2014. Glycemic index and significance of barnyard millet (*Echinochloa frumentacea*) in type II diabetics. *Journal of Food Science and Technology* 51(2):392–5. https://doi.org/10.1007/s13197-011-0516-8

Vissapragada, A. 2021. A case study on using millets in daily diet for weight loss. *International Journal of Nutrition Sciences* 6(3): 1057.

Wong, S. K., K.-Y. Chin, F.H. Suhaimi, F. Ahmad, and S. Ima-Nirwana. 2017. Vitamin E as a potential interventional treatment for metabolic syndrome: Evidence from animal and human studies. *Frontiers in Pharmacology* 8: 444. https://doi.org/10.3389/fphar.2017.00444

Wu, S., W. Jia, H. He, J. Yin, H. Xu, C. He, Q. Zhang, Y. Peng, and R. Cheng. 2023. A new dietary fiber can enhance satiety and reduce postprandial blood glucose in healthy adults: A randomized cross-over trial. *Nutrients* 15(21):4569. https://doi.org/10.3390/nu15214569

Zhang, W., G. Zhang, W. Liang, J. Tian, S. Sun, X. Zhang, X. Lv, P. Guo, A. Qu, and Z. Wu. 2024. Structure, functional properties, and applications of foxtail millet prolamin: A review." *Biomolecules* 14 (8):913. https://doi.org/10.3390/biom14080913

Zhou, J., R.J. Martin, R.T. Tulley, A.M. Raggio, K.L. McCutcheon, L. Shen, S.C. Danna, S. Tripathy, M. Hegsted, and M.J. Keenan. 2008. Dietary resistant starch upregulates total GLP-1 and PYY in a sustained day-long manner through fermentation in rodents. *American Journal of Physiology- Endocrinology and Metabolism* 295(5): E1160–E1166. https://doi.org/10.1152/ajpendo.90637.2008

9 Anti-Diabetic Potential of Millets

Ayushi Joshi, Krati Goel, and Archana Kushwaha
Department of Food and Nutrition, College of Community Sciences, G. B. Pant University of Agriculture and Technology, Pantnagar, Uttarakhand, India

9.1 INTRODUCTION

Diabetes is a major global public health issue that negatively affects socioeconomic development, mortality, and disability (Liu et al 2020). High blood glucose levels are a hallmark of this chronic metabolic disease, which is brought on by either inadequate insulin production or the body's poor utilization of insulin (IDF 2022; WHO 2022). Type 2 diabetes mellitus (T2DM), which causes hyperglycemia due to insulin resistance or insufficient insulin production, is the most common form of this illness (Gong et al 2020; WHO 2022). According to Carvalho et al (2023), it can seriously damage vital organs.

In India, a major epicenter of the disease, the prevalence of diabetes has sharply increased over the past 40 years due to socioeconomic changes and increased vulnerability (Mathur et al 2021). The World Diabetes Atlas (2021) estimates that 74.2 million Indians have diabetes, and by 2045, this number is predicted to increase to 124.9 million. According to the National Non-Communicable Disease Monitoring Survey (NNMS) (2017–18), 24.5% of individuals have impaired fasting glucose, and 9.3% have diabetes (Mathur et al 2021). According to a recent study by the Indian Council of Medical Research (ICMR), over 101 million Indians have diabetes, and another 136 million are at risk for pre-diabetes (Anjana et al 2023).

These health projections necessitate providing for this ailment and, therefore, more attention should be given to its management strategies. Diabetes mellitus (DM) is manageable through a set of interventions that include blood glucose control achieved through a combination of diet, exercise, and, if necessary, medication, as recommended by the **ICMR (2018) and WHO (2022)**.

9.1.1 Need for Functional Foods in Diabetes Management

The rising incidence of complications in diabetic patients should scare healthcare professionals enough to consider alternate management approaches alongside pharmaceutical treatments which include insulin and oral hypoglycemic agents (Mirmiran et al 2014; Li et al 2022). Nevertheless, the management of diabetes is still dominated by medical nutrition therapy (MNT), which focuses on dietary lipids, glycemic index (GI), carbohydrate counting, and energy and nutrient requirements (Mirmiran et al 2014). In addition, the use of supplements such as fiber, omega-3 fatty acids, antioxidant vitamins, and other botanicals is also being explored for glycemic control.

The concept of functional foods, i.e., foods that provide health benefits beyond basic nutrition, has become popular in the diabetes management regime. Both human and animal studies have shown that the protective effects of functional foods, which are rich in bioactive components, exist against diabetes. By virtue of their possible health benefits and ease of access, they therefore represent a feasible option for dietary control and a way of promoting disease prevention (Mirmiran et al 2014; Alkhatib et al 2017).

DOI: 10.1201/9781003686668-9

9.2 MILLETS: AN OVERVIEW AND ITS RELATION TO DIABETES

Millets are a diverse group of small-seeded grains. They have been a part of our life, as they were grown and eaten for a long time, particularly in Asia and Africa, where they were considered the main food sources that provided essential nutrients to the consumers (Goron and Raizada 2015; Mansoria and Singh 2023). However, increased urbanization, industrialization, and the development of modern food systems decreased the consumption of millets. As a result, staples such as rice, wheat, and maize occupied the portion of the meal that was earlier held by millets. Lately, millets have again come into the picture and received significant attention because of their unique nutritional composition and health-promoting properties, especially in the case of chronic diseases like DM.

The high dietary fiber (6–12%) content, micronutrient density, and wide array of phytochemicals in millets have drawn the attention of the scientific fraternity, leading to studies on their possible application as a food alternative for managing diabetes. Dietary fiber, which comprises both soluble and insoluble fiber components, slows down the digestion and absorption of carbohydrates and thereby helps in glycemic management by lowering postprandial glucose spikes. Apart from that, iron (0.8–6.4 mg/100 g), zinc (1.4–3 mg/100 g), and magnesium (81–153 mg/100 g) are also very important minerals in millets that maintain optimal metabolic function and improve the insulin action (Longvah 2017; Rao et al 2018). The bioactive compounds in millets, such as flavonoids and phenolic compounds, are anti-inflammatory and antioxidant agents that, in theory, may prevent the occurrence of diabetes complications.

While some researchers have examined the glycemic response to millet consumption, the understanding of the mechanisms and the long-term effects of diabetes management by millet requires further investigation. Millets are a group of Dhanya Varga in ancient medicine, particularly in Ayurveda, and are highly praised for their health benefits. Ayurvedic texts refer to millets by a number of designations such as Trina Dhanya (grains made from grass), Kshudra Dhanya (small-sized cereals), and Kudhanya (considered the lowest in the cereal family) (Kaiyadeva 2009; Bhavamishra 2011; Charaka 2011). These grains, due to their Kapha Pittahara, Vaatala, and Rakta-Shamak qualities, are considered ideal for treating metabolism-related diseases like diabetes. Besides that, they also have properties like Madhura (sweet) and Kashaya (astringent) (Kaiyadeva 2009; Bhavamishra 2011). Therefore, millet's role as a functional food is very promising in health conditions like diabetes.

9.3 NUTRITIONAL AND BIOACTIVE PROFILE OF MILLETS IN RELATION TO DIABETES MANAGEMENT

9.3.1 Dietary Fiber

Millets are very popular because they contain a lot of fiber, which is very necessary in the management and prevention of diabetes. Millet contains both soluble and insoluble fibers, and both aid in the regulation of blood sugar. The soluble fiber hinders the absorption of glucose as it forms a gel-like substance in the digestive tract; thus, it helps to improve glycemic control and the maintenance of more stable blood glucose levels. By slowing down the glucose release, diabetic individuals may have the opportunity to keep their blood sugar levels under control by avoiding sudden postprandial peaks.

At the same time, the insoluble fiber increases the volume of the stool, which facilitates digestion and keeps constipation away. Besides that, by giving a feeling of fullness, the fiber present in millets helps to stop hunger and thus the tendency to overeat, especially the consumption of high-glycemic foods, may be reduced. People with diabetes may become more proficient in blood glucose control and at the same time reduce the risk of health complications linked to poorly controlled diabetes by consuming millets in their diet (Mansoria and Singh 2023).

9.3.2 Carbohydrates

Carbohydrates are a broad group of substances with varying physical and chemical properties. They play a vital role in energy metabolism, glycemic regulation, insulin secretion, lipid metabolism, and colonic function (Bonsembiante et al 2021; Mansoria and Singh 2023). According to WHO, carbohydrates can be categorized into two main groups based on their digestibility, i.e., glycemic (available) and nonglycemic (unavailable) carbohydrates (Bonsembiante et al 2021).

Glycemic carbohydrates upon hydrolysis yield monosaccharides that are readily absorbed in the small intestine and thus increase the amount of glucose available in the blood. In this group are starches of the likes of potatoes, rice, corn, and wheat and sugars (all except alcohol sugars). The glycemic carbohydrates may also be subdivided into two groups: slowly absorbed glucose (from starches) and quickly absorbed glucose (from sugars), both of which influence blood glucose levels and glycemic management depending on their rate of absorption. However, nonglycemic carbohydrates might get fermented in the large intestine instead of being digested with human digestive enzymes. The members of this group are non-starch polysaccharides (present in fruits and vegetables), resistant starch (found in whole grains, legumes, and green bananas), sugar alcohol, and resistant short-chain carbs (non-digestible oligosaccharides).

Since their absorption is slow or almost negligible, these carbohydrates hardly raise blood glucose levels. The body's metabolic and endocrine responses, glucose homeostasis, and in particular, the glycemic carbohydrate's digestion and absorption, are very much affected by this, especially in diabetics. The severity of blood glucose fluctuations and hence the overall glycemic control greatly depend on the speed with which glucose is made available from glycemic foods. Non-digestible carbohydrates may also attenuate postprandial glucose peaks and contribute to long-term glucose control by not causing rapid increases in blood glucose levels (Bonsembiante et al 2021).

9.3.3 Phytochemicals

Millets are loaded with a plethora of phytochemicals, to name a few, polyphenolic compounds, flavonoids, lignans, and other antioxidants, in which, anti-inflammatory and antioxidant capabilities are the main ones attributed to these bioactive compounds, and these are the main factors in the proper controlling of diabetes. Both oxidative stress and chronic inflammation, the main promoters of diabetes and also its sequelae (nephropathy, neuropathy, and cardiovascular disease), are among the most outstanding factors of the disease. By capturing radicals, the antioxidant characters of flavonoids and phenolics reduce oxidative injury to the tissues and cells. In addition, these compounds have been implicated in modulating inflammatory pathways and thereby could decrease chronic low-grade inflammation which is typical of diabetic patients (Rao et al 2018; Mansoria and Singh 2023).

Millets are fortified with a variety of phenolic acids and other phenolic compounds, which are excellent radical scavengers and enzyme inhibitors that are connected with oxidative stress. The flavonoids such as quercetin and catechins are highly effective antioxidant agents and may also impact glucose metabolism, thereby improving insulin sensitivity (Ofosu et al 2020). Moreover, lignans present in millet are another group of phytochemicals that are proven responsible for improved lipid profiles and decreased inflammatory markers, and hence, have the potential to manage diabetes and complications associated with the disease.

Along with that, the anti-inflammatory and antioxidant effects of bioactive components present in millets, their potential as a remedy for diabetes increases. These phytochemicals present in millets may act on glycemic control, decrease insulin resistance, and prevent diabetic complications by imparting their anti-inflammatory and antioxidative effects (Ofosu et al 2020; Mansoria and Singh 2023).

9.3.4 Minerals

Millets are bundled with several micronutrients such as magnesium, potassium, phosphorus, and iron that play a significant role in the management of diabetes. These nutrients, with magnesium being the most prominent, are the main factors for insulin sensitivity and glucose metabolism (Saini et al 2021).

Magnesium performs a number of functions in metabolism, one of which is the regulation of insulin receptor activity and the enzymes that are responsible for insulin secretion. Besides that, it elevates insulin sensitivity by stimulating muscle and adipose tissue to take up glucose. As a result, keeping glucose at normal levels in the body depends on the intake of a sufficient amount of magnesium.

Low magnesium levels have been associated with an increased risk of developing type 2 diabetes. It is possible that low magnesium levels may hinder insulin action and cause insulin resistance (Barbagallo and Dominguez 2015). Research works also found that low levels of magnesium resulted in poor glycemic control, which makes it very important for people with diabetes to consume magnesium-rich foods such as millet (Mansoria and Singh 2023).

Besides magnesium, millets are loaded with other minerals such as potassium, phosphorus, and iron that, together, promote a healthy general metabolism. Potassium is a necessary component of the electrolyte that maintains the insulin mechanism by balancing the cell functions. Phosphorus acts as one of the contributors to the synthesis of high-energy phosphate bonds and, therefore, energy production, while iron is involved in cellular metabolism and oxygen transport. So, the presence of all these micronutrients in millets makes them a potential dietary source of the functional diet for diabetics, thus providing a comprehensive way to both improve glucose management and reduce the risk of diabetes complications (Barbagallo and Dominguez 2015; Saini et al 2021).

9.3.5 Proteins and Amino Acids

One of the focal points has been on proteins, particularly those coming from functional foods like millets, for their role in the management of diabetes through mechanisms such as trypsin inhibition and the presence of specific amino acids that promote insulin secretion (Kanetro 2018; Wojdyło et al 2020). In this regard, the amino acids phenylalanine, methionine, leucine, and isoleucine, among others, that have been singled out as influential factors for insulin production and release, are well represented in millets. A number of these free amino acids such as leucine, arginine, alanine, phenylalanine, isoleucine, lysine, and methionine, which are known to facilitate insulin secretion, do so by participating in the creation of phosphatidylinositol-3-kinase (PI3K), the component of the insulin receptor/tyrosine kinase pathway responsible for glucose metabolism; thus, they should be simply considered as key players in this process (Wojdyło et al 2020).

There are a number of different ways by which amino acids influence insulin secretion. One of the several cellular events such as membrane depolarization and mitochondrial function enhancement that are induced by amino acids and that together might explain how amino acids act as metabolic coupling factors resulting in the increased insulin release is certainly one of them (Kanetro 2018). It is the mitochondria of pancreatic β-cells that play a decisive role in the unification of the metabolism of nutrients and exocytosis of insulin, the latter being triggered by both glucose and amino acids. When certain amino acids bind with potassium (K^+) and calcium (Ca^{2+}) channels, they cause a stimulation of mitochondrial metabolism which is followed by insulin secretion by the β-cells (Kanetro 2018).

Millet proteins can become more bioactive through bioprocessing means such as germination which besides that also produces bioactive peptides. The peptides thus produced have been proven to produce the highest level of insulin release from pancreatic cells by impeding the action of enzyme dipeptidyl peptidase IV (DPP-IV), which is responsible for the degradation of incretin hormones (de Souza Rocha et al 2015; Kanetro 2018). This highlights the dietary potential of millets not only as a functional food capable of directly stimulating β-cells, but also as a source of bioactive peptides, offering a convenient approach to improving glycemic control in individuals with diabetes.

9.4 BIO-DIGESTIBILITY AND BIO-ACCESSIBILITY OF BIOACTIVE COMPOUNDS

The metabolism and health benefits of millets are dependent on their bio-digestibility and bio-accessibility of biologically active components like dietary fiber and polyphenols. Bio-accessibility represents the fraction of bioactive compounds that are released from the food matrix through gastrointestinal digestion, while bio-digestibility refers to their subsequent absorption and metabolism in the body (Hithamani and Srinivasan 2014). Some bioactive compounds, e.g., phenolic acids, are released and become bio-accessible after digestion; thus, they are able to accomplish their beneficial effects. On the other hand, the formation of complexes between phenolic acids and dietary fibers such as arabinoxylan may prevent the release of these substances from millets by decreasing their bio-accessibility (Devi et al 2014).

Moreover, the anti-nutritional components in millets, such as tannins and phytic acid, hinder nutrient availability to the body since the presence of these components can bind essential proteins and minerals and reduce the overall protein and starch digestibility. These factors not only affect starch and protein components but may also affect the overall nutritional value of millets as they limit the bioavailability of several other nutrients as well (Mitharwal et al 2021). However, millet-based foods generally have a lower GI than those based on other grains, such as wheat, which implies that they can be used as nutraceutical foods for glycemic control. As an example, the GI of millet flour is in the range of 42.24–49.28, while that of wheat flour is 62.59, which is mainly due to the presence of anti-nutritional factors that slow down the starch digestion and glucose absorption process (Sharma et al 2017).

Especially millets, particularly finger millet, are rich in polyphenolic compounds, which also contribute to their health benefits. Finger millet contains around 22 different polyphenolic compounds, 13 of which are bioavailable. Roasting of finger millet does not significantly alter its bio-accessible polyphenol and flavonoid contents which are about 2.65 and 1.09 mg/g, respectively, was the conclusion of Hithamani and Srinivasan (2014). However, it is the gut microbiota that plays a vital role in making high-molecular-weight polyphenols more available by converting them into more easily absorbable forms. Various studies suggest that the polyphenolic and antioxidant content of finger millet can be significantly elevated through gut fermentation. For example, it is found that the gut microbiota in the colon is finger millet fermenter; thus, it is responsible for the increase of antioxidants and polyphenols and subsequently, the health benefits of finger millet (Chandrasekara and Shahidi 2012; Mena et al 2015). Moreover, the study results indicate that the level of polyphenolic compounds and the antioxidant activity in finger millet flour is greatly enhanced due to fermentation (Mutshinyani et al 2020), thus, it can be inferred that fermentation is indispensable for the release of the medicinal potential of a millet-based diet.

If the millet polyphenols are fermented in the colon, this could lead to the production of certain gut microorganisms with anti-diabetic properties, thereby resulting in a lowered risk of diabetes. With the help of the gut microbiota, millets can be an excellent dietary source for the treatment of diabetes and for improving metabolic health as the gut microbiota is the key player in the bio-accessibility and the therapeutic effects of the bioactive components.

9.5 GLYCEMIC INDEX AND GLYCEMIC LOAD OF MILLETS

The GI of a food shows how fast the blood glucose levels increase when food is eaten in comparison to a standard food, usually white bread or glucose. GI figures serve for food classification: a low GI is ≤55, and a high GI is ≥70 (Atkinson et al 2021). Blood glucose levels increase very fast if one is eating high-GI meals such as rice, breakfast cereals, and some types of bread, while they increase more slowly and gradually if one is eating low-GI foods such as different types of legumes, pasta, fruits, and milk products. By and large, millets have a lower GI than refined cereals such as maize, wheat, and rice. The lower GI of millets demonstrates their slower rate of digestion and absorption, which results in a steady and continuous release of glucose into the blood. This gradual glucose disposal may help in the prevention of glycemic spikes and allow better glycemic control (Mansoria and Singh 2023).

Besides GI, glycemic load (GL) is another important parameter to evaluate the impact of a food on blood glucose concentration. GL takes into account both the carb content and the quality of a food (GI). The equation is GL = GI × available carbohydrate content per serving size in grams, followed by division by 100 (Willett and Liu 2019). When consuming foods with a high GL (≥20), blood glucose levels increase significantly, whereas, if foods with a low GL (≤10) are consumed, the increase is much lower. Foods are classified as having a medium GL if their GL is between 10 and 20 (Veit et al 2022).

Millets possess low GI and almost double the fiber content of the regular cereals; thus they yield a low to moderate GL. Both soluble and insoluble fibers in millets, which delay the digestion and absorption of carbohydrates, help the bloodstream to release glucose more slowly and, thereby, maintain its level under control. Due to the presence of bioactive fiber components which reduce the overall glycemic response after a meal and thus might improve the long-term glycemic control, millets are quite beneficial for diabetic individuals. Substituting millet for refined grains could alleviate the demand for insulin production and thus minimize the risk of insulin resistance among people (Mansoria and Singh 2023).

Therefore, millets are good glycemic profile foods because of their moderate-to-high dietary fiber content and decreased GI that allows the blood glucose level to be controlled in a better way, hence, making them a reasonable dietary option for those who want to manage or prevent T2DM.

9.6 MECHANISM OF ACTION: HOW MILLETS HELP MANAGE DIABETES?

9.6.1 Regulation of Postprandial Blood Glucose Levels

Before the pharmacologic therapies, people with early-stage diabetes should strictly follow nutritional methods that will improve postprandial glycemia and, in particular, lower the absorption of glucose from digestible carbohydrates (Ch'ng et al 2019). The enzymes digesting carbohydrates which should be focused on are those in particular α-amylase (1,4-α-D-glucan-glucanohydrolase) and α-glucosidase that can play a major role in controlling blood glucose levels after a meal. When it comes to starch and other carbohydrates, α-amylase, the enzyme, initiates the hydrolysis of α-1,4-glucan linkages, whereas the role of α-glucosidase is to convert maltose into glucose. These enzymes are the main agents in the digestion of carbohydrates (Gong et al 2020; Li et al 2022).

A practical method to slow down the food carbohydrate digestion to the last phases and to reduce the glucose absorption rate is the inhibition of these enzymes. It is a method of preventing sudden jumps of blood glucose levels after eating. Food polymeric carbohydrates such as starch and maltodextrins are first depolymerized by α-amylase into short oligosaccharides, and then these oligosaccharides are further depolymerized by α-glucosidase to monosaccharides, mainly glucose (Gong et al 2020). Postprandial hyperglycemia is the consequence of the sequential digestion process when glucose is released rapidly into the bloodstream (Figure 9.1).

Hence one important measure to regulate blood sugar after a meal can be considered the activity of α-amylase and α-glucosidase enzymes, i.e., their blockage. When these enzyme inhibitors are taken, the steps where carbohydrates are broken down are slowed, so less glucose enters the bloodstream. As a result, the level of glucose in the blood is better controlled and the rise of blood glucose is slower. The mechanism is in agreement with the idea of enzyme inhibitors as a first line of defense in the diabetic continuum, most notably, in early stages. So, diet interventions that alter enzyme activity in relation to carbohydrate digestibility provide a measure of non-pharmacological intervention in the control of postprandial glycemia and in reducing the risk of diabetes complications (Gong et al 2020; Li et al 2022).

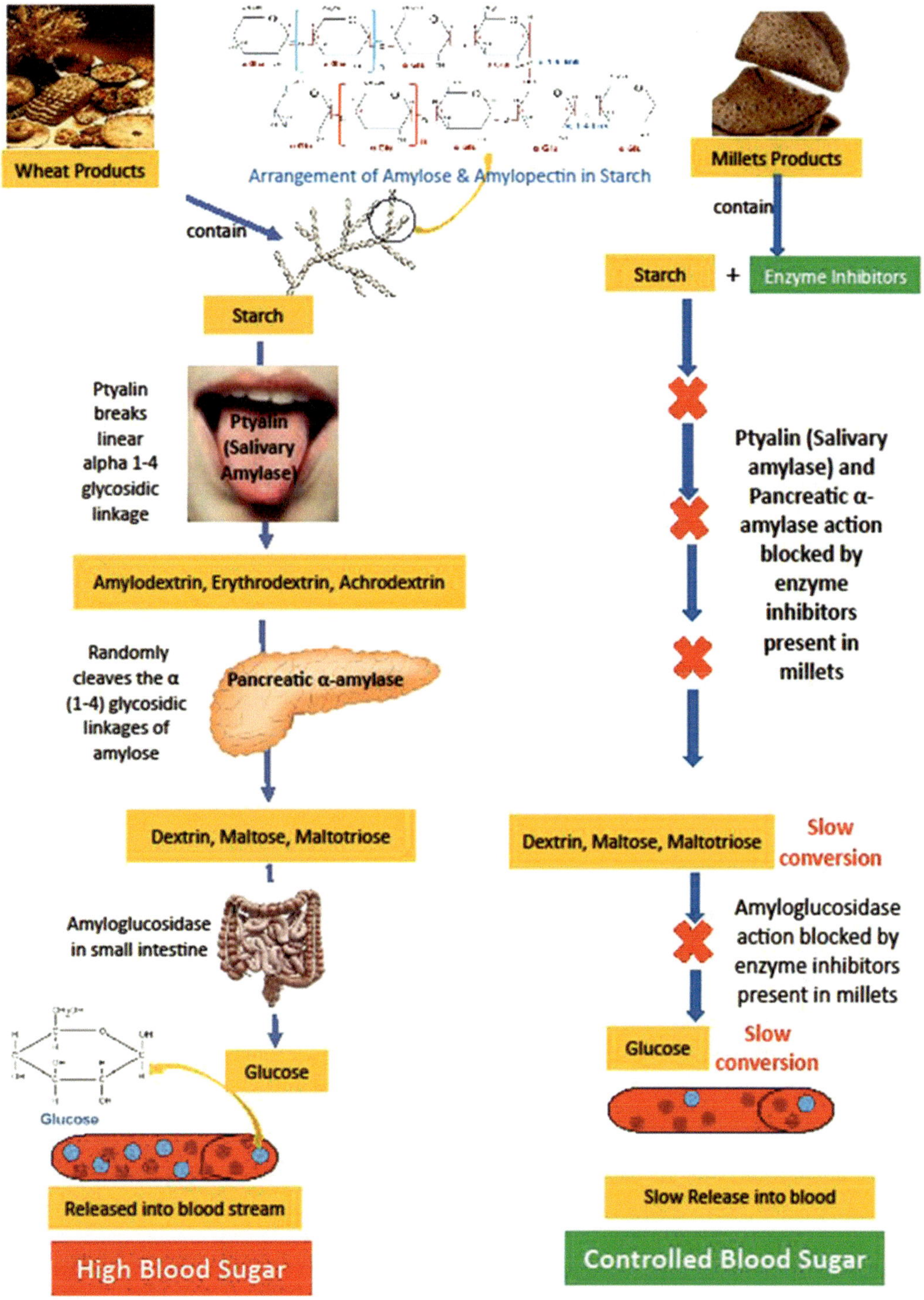

FIGURE 9.1 Potential mechanisms of α-amylase and α-glucosidase inhibitors from whole cereal foods in preventing hyperglycemia.

9.6.2 Enhancing Insulin Sensitivity

It is highly likely that millets may improve their ability to become sensitized to insulin with which insulin will better lower blood glucose levels (Sharma and Niranjan 2018; Majid and Priyadarshini 2020). While a lot of research is being done to pinpoint the components responsible, it is generally considered that the fiber content and bioactive phytochemicals of millets play a major role in raising insulin sensitivity.

The insoluble dietary fiber (IDF) in millet has a very significant influence on the improvement of insulin sensitivity. By maintaining a healthy gut, reducing inflammation, and controlling insulin release, the unique structural and physicochemical characteristics of IDs help to enhance glucose uptake by cells (both muscle and fat cells) and lower insulin resistance. One of the fundamental mechanisms through which IDF exerts its insulin-sensitizing effect is its porous structure. This structure of IDF enhances not only the capillary action but also the affinity for glucose molecules.

IDF contributes to the regulation of postprandial blood glucose levels through glucose adsorption on its surface leading to lower glucose concentrations in the small intestine. The large surface area of IDF is also that which secures glucose molecules by slowing down their rapid diffusion and absorption through the bloodstream. When the particle size of IDF and glucose molecules is smaller, their interaction becomes more significant because their surface area is larger and more polar and non-polar functional groups, among which free hydroxyl, ether linkages, phenolic, and carboxylic groups become exposed. The amount of glucose entering the bloodstream is further decreased by this better glucose adsorption (Zhang et al 2024).

The water-related properties, especially the swelling capacity (SC) and water holding capacity (WHC) of IDF, are very important in the regulation of blood sugar level. The higher the WHC, the more glucose adsorption may increase as it makes it easier for the hydrophilic glucose molecules to find the fiber. The functional groups in IDF, among which are hydrated hydroxyl, carboxyl, and uronic acid groups, assist water molecules in adsorbing by hydrogen bonding and capillary action. By improving water retention, dietary fiber is able to slow the rate of glucose absorption thus enhancing its ability of blood glucose regulation (Zhang et al 2024).

Besides the fiber content, many of the phytochemicals present in the millets such as flavonoids and phenolic compounds, were attributed to the improvement of glucose metabolism and insulin signaling (Mansoria and Singh 2023). These substances are anti-inflammatory and antioxidant in nature and therefore, their presence may alleviate inflammation and oxidative stress, which are the main culprits in insulin resistance. Accordingly, by elevating insulin sensitivity and facilitating effective glucose metabolism, these phytochemicals may be indispensable ones in the regulation of blood sugar (Sharma and Niranjan 2018; Mansoria and Singh 2023; Zhang et al 2024).

9.6.3 Reduction of Oxidative Stress and Inflammation

Chronic inflammation and oxidative stress are major causes, consequences, and complications of diabetes (Rochette et al 2014). Millets have shown powerful anti-inflammatory and antioxidant effects to alleviate such harmful consequences. They are loaded with bioactive components such as flavonoids, lignans, and phenolic acids. These bioactive compounds help in reducing inflammation and oxidative stress as they scavenge free radicals and inhibit the production of pro-inflammatory molecules.

The cellular signaling pathways, especially the NF-κB (nuclear factor kappa-light-chain-enhancer of activated B cells) and Nrf2 (nuclear factor erythroid 2-related factor 2) pathways, are the major responsible factors for antioxidative effects of millet polyphenols. Nrf2, a key transcription factor, is indispensable for the activation of antioxidant genes; thus, it helps to strengthen the body's antioxidative defense system. On the other hand, NF-κB is a protein complex that plays a significant role in the regulation of genes associated with inflammation and immune responses. By regulating the pathways, millet polyphenols might entail a very little presence of inflammatory responses and oxidative stress in diabetic tissue; thus, the development and progression of diabetes can be significantly slowed down or even prevented (Balkrishna et al 2024).

In addition, the interplay of gut microbiota with polyphenols appears to enhance the antioxidant and anti-inflammatory properties of millets. However, compositional and metabolic changes imparted by millets in the activity of gut microbiota, the intestinal milieu can be balanced, which thereby helps in providing prerequisite for adequate metabolic support. This millet–gut interaction may also lead to the diminution of chronic low-grade inflammation that is a hallmark of metabolic disorders, including T2DM (Balkrishna et al 2024).

Millets have the potential to manage post-meal glycemia and consolidate insulin sensitivity by a variety of mechanisms. By doing so, they can help prevent the occurrence of diabetic complications usually manifested as renal impairment, neuropathy, and cardiovascular diseases, which is achieved through the attenuation of inflammatory and oxidative stress states (Mansoria and Singh 2023). The existence of such proof provides the rationale for the dietary intervention of millet to act as a potent agent in the diabetes therapeutic regimen and a promoter of general metabolic health.

9.6.4 Gut Microbiota Modulation and Its Impact on Glucose Metabolism

Recent research reveals that the gut microbiota plays a crucial role in regulating glucose metabolism and insulin sensitivity. The homeostasis of glucose and other metabolic processes of the host can be significantly influenced by the composition and metabolic activity of the gut microbiota. Millets are packed with dietary fiber that acts as prebiotics and hence, better gut bacteria get the food they need (Sarita and Singh 2016). The high dietary fiber in millets is particularly important as it brings about the proliferation of fiber-fermenting microbes which in return release bioactive metabolites such as short-chain fatty acids (SCFAs) that have insulin-sensitizing and glucose metabolism-stimulating effects.

The production of SCFAs, such as butyrate, acetate, and propionate, results from the fermentation of millet-derived fiber by the gut bacteria. The available evidence confirms that SCFAs improve glucose metabolism, gut health as well as insulin sensitivity and in addition to these, they have very few positive effects on metabolic health. One of the main mechanisms through which SCFAs exert their positive effects is by the induction of the release of gut hormones that regulate satiety and blood glucose levels. In particular, SCFAs lead to the secretion of two crucial intestinal hormones that not only regulate glucose homeostasis but also control satiety: glucagon-like peptide-1 (GLP-1) and peptide YY (PYY) (Portincasa et al 2022).

The role of GLP-1 in increasing insulin secretion in a glucose-dependent way, thereby enhancing insulin sensitivity and lowering postprandial blood glucose levels, is beyond any doubt. Furthermore, by slowing gastric emptying and reducing appetite, GLP-1 assists patients in controlling their body weight and, thus, decreases their chances of developing obesity which is the main risk factor for type 2 diabetes. On the other hand, PYY, apart from helping to promote satiety, thus contributing to better appetite control and possibly reducing the risk of overeating which can subsequently cause insulin resistance as well as weight gain, has some other functions as well. In addition, SCFAs, by maintaining the gut lining's integrity and at the same time, preventing the entry of harmful bacteria and endotoxins, thus, contributing to the strengthening of the intestinal barrier and at the same time, relief from systemic inflammation, which in turn is a dominant factor of insulin resistance and metabolic diseases, are doing so.

The gut microbiota-derived fermentable millet fibers lead to the production of SCFAs, which are positive metabolites that promote not only gut health but also overall metabolic homeostasis. Such health-promoting interventions may confer a lower risk of diabetes and improved glycemic control (Mansoria and Singh 2023). The interaction between the gut bacteria and millet fiber underscores the significance of diets rich in fiber in regulating the gut flora's composition and activity. By stimulating the proliferation of beneficial bacteria that produce SCFAs, millets may well turn out to be an effective dietary strategy for enhancing insulin sensitivity, increasing glucose metabolism, and preventing as well as alleviating T2DM.

9.7 SCIENTIFIC EVIDENCE ON THE ANTI-DIABETIC PROPERTIES OF MILLETS

9.7.1 In Vitro Studies on Millets and Glucose Metabolism

It is very important to those with T2DM to allow the blood sugar to be within the normal range after meals. Besides being excellent antioxidant compounds, polyphenols in the diet have significantly shown that they can control hyperglycemia through several mechanisms one of which is the interaction with glucose transporters and competitive inhibition of digestive enzyme (Lacroix and Li-Chan 2014). Alpha-amylase and alpha-glucosidase are enzymes that postprandial blood glucose levels are increased by. In fact zymases, starch, and oligosaccharides are hydrolyzed by these enzymes and are converted to glucose in raise of blood glucose levels. Thus, blocking these enzymes is considered a necessary step toward the therapy of the condition of T2DM.

One of the main themes in the literature has been the anti-diabetic nature of the components of millet, singularly the aspect of the ability to block enzymes that hydrolyze carbohydrates. The anti-diabetic effect by which the finger millet and barnyard millet extracts work can be traced is their potent antioxidant activity. A research was conducted on biochemical characteristics of different extracts of barnyard millet (*Echinochloa utilis*), and their potential to suppress α-glucosidase enzyme activity was the focus of the study by Seo et al (2015). The ethyl acetate extract was considered a very effective natural antihyperglycemic drug as it showed the lowest IC50 value (70.2 μg/mL) in oxidizing *Saccharomyces cerevisiae* α-glucosidase. Millet grains can help a person keep well, and that potential is due to both the free and bound phenolic compounds present.

For instance, in the case of millet cultivars, two bound phenolic acids, namely, ferulic and p-coumaric acid, were the major ones and had potent antioxidant properties. Moreover, α-amylase and α-glucosidase activities were significantly reduced by both the soluble and the bound phenolic fractions thus pointing to the potential of the millet-based diet to lower the postprandial glucose levels (Pradeep and Sreerama 2018). Ofosu et al (2020) found that polyphenols from millet can provide an excellent dietary condition for the management of postprandial hyperglycemia. The prolamins from foxtail millet have also been investigated for their anti-diabetic effects besides the polyphenols. Prolamins from both raw and cooked foxtail millet were able to demonstrate α-amylase inhibition; however, the cooked prolamins had more activity (Fu et al 2023). This work is a good example of how important food processing is in enhancing bioactivity of millet-derived ingredients. These in vitro findings identify millets – especially their phenolic compounds and prolamins – as valuable resources for addressing hyperglycemia and its subsequent complications through enzyme inhibition and metabolic pathway modification.

9.7.2 Animal Studies Demonstrating Anti-Diabetic Effects

According to various researchers, millets have been proven to be beneficial to diabetic rats. One can thus consider the inclusion of millets in the diet to be a blood glucose-lowering strategy and subsequently lay down several diabetes management strategies based on that. Early research of diabetic mice by Hegde and Chandra (2005) revealed that diets composed of finger millet and kodo millet significantly lowered blood glucose levels (36–42%). Besides reduced lipid peroxidation levels, the inhibition of collagen glycation was also indicative of lowered glycemic and oxidative stress in these rats, thus implying a protective effect both on glucose metabolism and oxidative damage.

The findings were corroborated by experiments with a number of millet cultivars. The inhibition of hepatic gluconeogenesis was the major route through which the hypoglycemic effect was achieved by the ethanolic extracts of sorghum and foxtail millet in diabetic rats; hence, the effect was similar to that of conventional anti-diabetic drugs (Kim and Park 2012; Qi et al 2019). In the models of diabetic rats, Geetha et al (2020) also observed that millet-based diets led to the decrease of glycemic responses (FBS from 120.50 ± 18.73 to 97.81 ± 20.00 and HbA1c from 6.14 ± 0.30 to 5.67 ± 0.40). The effect was mainly attributed to the dietary fiber components of millets, which most likely delayed the digestion and absorption of carbohydrates.

Moreover, the peptides present in the millets have been proven responsible for the management of glycemia. In the study on diabetic rats, proteins and starch components from foxtail millet have been proven to manage lipid profiles, enhance glucose tolerance, and generally, manage glucose metabolism (Wang et al 2023). In addition, peptides derived from millet grains have been demonstrated as a very effective component that is responsible for the blood glucose-lowering effect (Fu et al 2023). Beyond these general discoveries, the studies have further leveled up to study the influence of the particular varieties of millets on glucose metabolism and the coinciding disorders associated with it. Nishizawa et al (2009) in their research found that the protein present in Japanese barnyard millet showed improvement in glucose control in diabetic mice. The consumption of barnyard millet bran led to a significant decrease in water intake, diabetic polyuria, and HbA1c levels in diabetic rats, thus giving more evidence to the therapeutic potential of millets (Ito et al 2022).

Moreover, proteins contained in millets seem to be having an impact on liver function as well as insulin resistance. Foxtail millet prolamin supplementation in diabetic rats led to the reduction of insulin resistance and glucose intolerance besides improvement in liver function and changes in serum metabolic profiles, particularly those associated with retinol and riboflavin metabolism (Fu et al 2021). A diet of whole grain proso millet through the interaction with the PI3K/AKT signaling pathway, probably modulated by miRNA regulation, resulted in less liver and kidney damage, increased glucose tolerance, and lowered insulin resistance in diabetic mice (Deng et al 2023).

The effect of millets on gut microbiota in relation to diabetes has also been a subject of research. The importance of millets in the regulation of the gut microbiota to alleviate hyperglycemia and improve general metabolic health has been substantiated by studies that found protein isolates from both raw and cooked foxtail millet to be effective in the relief of gut dysbiosis induced by diabetes (Fu et al 2021). Besides that, Wang et al (2023) reported that the protein and starch fractions of foxtail millet were responsible for the proliferation of *Lactobacillus* sp. which, in turn, led to the alleviation of liver dysfunction and gut microbiota dysbiosis in diabetic rats. Besides that, in non-alcoholic fatty liver disease (NAFLD), which is a common diabetes side effect, foxtail millet helped in the condition in the rat model of high-fat-diet-induced gut microbiota dysgenesis.

Moreover, millets exhibited the potential for management of diabetes-induced hepatic steatosis, cataracts, and dermal wound complications. According to Jacob et al (2024), finger millet consumption hastens the rate of cutaneous wound healing in diabetic rats. This speedy recovery was attributed to factors such as higher expression of nerve growth factor (NGF), altered antioxidant enzyme activities, and increased collagen synthesis. In addition, phenolics present in the seed of finger millet have the potential to delay the onset of cataracts in diabetic rats through a decrease in blood glycosylated hemoglobin levels, serum advanced glycation end products (AGEs), and lens aldose reductase (AR) activity.

In addition to it, the protein-enriched diet of Korean foxtail millet fed to the genetically diabetic KK-Ay mice showed a significant reduction in insulin levels and an improvement in insulin sensitivity (Jacob et al 2024). The adiponectin intervention was responsible for this effect, thus implying that millet proteins might enhance glucose metabolism and insulin signaling pathways in diabetics.

Those animal experiments, taken together, present strong evidence of the anti-diabetic effects of millets owing to their unique special bioactive components like dietary fiber, peptides, starch, and proteins. Millets are an excellent candidate as a food source in the intervention of diabetes and comorbidities. The mechanism of their actions includes raising insulin sensitivity, altering gut microbiota, and lessening the complications related to diabetes.

9.7.3 Human Clinical Trials and Observational Studies

One of the most convincing pieces of evidence for the anti-diabetic properties of millets came from human clinical trials, which showed significant improvements in various metabolic parameters such as blood sugar levels, insulin sensitivity, and even markers of glycemic control over time like HbA1c. A 12-week foxtail millet meal plan was able to significantly lower the fasting blood sugar level of pre-diabetic patients (impaired glucose tolerance) from 102.6 ± 16.2 to 95.4 ± 12.6 mg/dL (Ren et al 2018). The research points out that millet intake can be an effective means of preventing and even reversing early glucose intolerance; thus, it not only improves glycemic control in pre-diabetics but also stops the progression of the disease.

Apart from that, a clinical trial reported that type 2 diabetes patients who ate more millet-based foods had excellent glycemic control, showed reduction in their plasma lipid levels, and were less likely to suffer from hyperinsulinemia – a condition of high insulin levels usually associated with insulin resistance. The findings may indicate that diets rich in millet might be viable means of managing cholesterol and glucose levels in diabetics (Jali et al 2012). Further to that Liu et al (2022) revealed that intake of foxtail millet (fermented and germinated) could alleviate diabetic kidney damage, which is a common and severe complication arising from prolonged diabetes, therefore, offering more evidence regarding the therapeutic potential of millets for the treatment of diabetic complications. It points to the fact that the bioactive compounds in millet can, particularly when they undergo fermentation or germination, have a protective effect on kidney function in diabetics.

Besides that, diabetic patients on a millet-based diet that included foxtail millet, finger millet, and sorghum were found to have better blood glucose management, especially postprandial glucose levels than those on non-millet diets. This is additional evidence to support the role of millets in glycemic control among diabetics (Vedamanickam et al 2020). In addition, Scottish oat porridge (SOP)- and pearl millet porridge (PMP)-dependent breakfast revealed that PMP generated a larger incremental area under the curve (AUC) for stomach volume, and lower glucose-dependent insulinotropic polypeptide (GIP) response than SOP (Alyami et al 2019). The results are indicative of the potential of pearl millet in regulating gastrointestinal and insulin responses, thereby helping in the management of diabetes. Yet, more research is required to fully unfold the mechanisms involved.

Prolonged consumption of millet-based diets has been proven beneficial in managing HbA1c levels, which is an important factor for defining the state of glycemic control over time. Studies have shown that the consumption of millet-based diets for more than three months resulted in a 15% reduction of HbA1c figures (Geetha et al 2020). Eminently, in the case of pre-diabetics, the level of HbA1c further went down, leveling with that of normal value (from 6.65 ± 0.4 to $5.67 \pm 0.4\%$). The reduction was attributed to the dietary fiber component of millets and its low GI, both of which help to manage the glycation process. This way, glucose release is slowed down and its availability for HbA1c formation is also lowered. Based on the findings, millet-based diets can be suggested as a viable nutritional strategy for pre-diabetes management as well as hindering or preventing the onset of type 2 diabetes.

As per human clinical trials, millet-based diets, if consumed regularly, can bring numerous health benefits to persons with diabetes or at risk of developing the disease. Among other benefits, these include improved insulin sensitivity, lowered fasting blood glucose, better long-term glycemic control as measured by HbA1c, improved postprandial glucose management, and even possible alleviation of diabetic complications such as kidney disease. Given their high dietary fiber, low GI, and bioactive components that appear to be mostly responsible for the observed effects, millets are well placed as a valuable dietary intervention for diabetes management and prevention.

9.8 INCORPORATION OF MILLETS IN DIABETIC DIETS

9.8.1 Millet-Based Recipes and Products for Diabetics

Millets are highly flexible grains that can be effortlessly introduced into a diet suitable for diabetics. Millets' nutritional value, when combined with their ability to survive environmental hardships such as drought, has made them popular among people around the world. In response to this, various research considering different aspects of millets, such as better varieties and utilization of millets in food products, have been conducted (Kumar et al 2018). Millets have been an important part of Indian food culture that has its roots in ancient times. This can be seen in several regional cuisines such as ragi roti, mudde, and jhangora kheer that are not only very popular in Uttarakhand and Uttar Pradesh but also all over India (Rao et al 2018). The versatility of these grains—ranging from savory preparations like khichdi to crispy snacks and even sweet dishes—demonstrates their ability to meet diverse nutritional needs across different life stages (Thathola and Srivastava 2002).

Excellent health benefits are making millets popular worldwide. They are also seen as preventive and management agents for non-communicable diseases such as cancer, diabetes, and cardiovascular diseases (Anitha et al 2021; WHO 2022). Millets have a low GI, they are rich in dietary fiber, and they contain bioactive compounds that may improve insulin sensitivity and help regulate blood glucose levels, which together make them extremely beneficial to diabetics. Such a balanced diet, including millet, can not only make glucose management better but also enhance overall metabolic health.

Scientifically different possibilities of transforming millets into various products for food use have been thoroughly explored. Studies have been emphasizing the different methods of processing that can lead to the enhanced nutritional value and increased content of bioactive compounds in millets which are germination, fermentation, and milling (Table 9.1). The health benefits of millets can be further enhanced through the above-mentioned procedures so that they constitute a healthy food choice for diabetic patients as well as health-conscious individuals.

Millets are increasingly being recognized as a valuable contributor to dietary diversification and chronic disease prevention as consumer demand for nutritious, sensory-rich foods grows. Millets have the potential to become a significant part of future dietary guidelines with the extension of research and development work, particularly for diabetics.

9.9 FUTURE RESEARCH DIRECTIONS AND POTENTIAL AREAS OF STUDY

In the future, researches on millets have unlimited possibilities to contribute to their nutritional and medicinal utilization, particularly considering the escalating global health issues. Various millet species such as finger millet and pearl millet have received considerable attention, while foxtail millet and sorghum have been focused on for more comprehensive therapeutic study. The small millets such as little millet, kodo millet, brown top millet, and fonio are still largely unknown, and proso millet and barnyard millet have even less research on their potential as medicines. The lesser-known millet species with the richest nutritional profiles and possible medicinal advantages deserve more scientific study and investigation.

Development of millet breeding programs not only for high yields but also for health-beneficial specialty compounds could be one of the main points of future research. These breeding programs should aim to improve the nutrient content and medicinal value so as to help prevent the metabolic and chronic diseases, such as T2DM, cardiovascular diseases, and obesity, which are increasing in prevalence. The development of millet cultivars that not only provide high productivity but also

TABLE 9.1
Health-Promoting Components in Value-Added Millet Products Suitable for Diabetics as Impacted by Processing Method

Product/Type	Formulation	Health-Promoting Components	Reference
Processing method: Baking			
Waffles/RTE	30:30:40::FM:PM:WF	↑ Dietary fiber, resistant and slowly digestible starch ↑ Total polyphenols, flavonoids, and antioxidant activity ↓ caloric value	Chaitra et al (2020)
Cake/RTE	40: 60::FM:WF	↑ Protein and dietary fiber	Adanse et al (2021)
Buns/RTE	10:82.5:7.5::FM:RWF:ML	↑ Total polyphenols and dietary fiber content	Boria et al (2021)
Muffins/RTE	50:50::FM:RWF	↑ Total polyphenols and dietary fiber content ↓ Glycemic response and insulin response	Almaski et al (2023)
Cooking and dehydration			
Instant khichdi mix	22-28:28-35:3.59-6.41::FoM: GGD: Oats	Improved nutritional quality	Negi et al (2021)
Cooking/Roasting (gelatinization)			
Papad	100::FoM	↑ Resistant starch ↓ pGI (<55)	Arora et al (2023)
Papad	70:15:10:5::PM:BG:PH:RF	↑ Protein and dietary fiber ↓ Caloric value	Akshatha et al (2024)
Extrusion (cold)			
Vermicelli	64.25:22.32:2.36::BMF:RF:XG	↑ Protein, iron, beta-carotene	Goel et al (2021)
Vermicelli	40:58:2::BMF:WF:ERBP	↑ Protein, calcium, iron, potassium, and magnesium	Chandraprabha et al (2017)
Noodles	50:50::FM:WF	Improved nutritional quality	Gull et al (2014)
Fermentation			
Pizza base	25:25:50::FoM:BMF:RWF	↑ Protein and dietary fiber ↓ Carbohydrate content	Veena et al (2020)
Dhokla mix powder	55:35:10::FoM & BMF:LM:FS	↓ pGI (<55)	Pathak et al (2000)
Fermentation and Germination			
Idli mix	33:33:33::GMMF: RF:DBG	↑ Protein, calcium, and iron ↓ Phytic acid and tannins	Krishnamoorthy et al (2013)
Dosa mix	33:33:33::GMMF: RF:DBG	↑ Protein, calcium, and iron ↓ Phytic acid and tannins	Krishnamoorthy et al (2013)
Rabadi-beverage	SM-GPMF (5.3% of skim milk by weight) and 72.3% water by weight of set curd	Improved nutritional quality	Modha and Pal (2011)
Frying			
Doughnuts	50:50::FMF & QF:WF	↑ Protein and crude fiber ↓ Caloric value	Joshi et al (2023)
Germination and Baking			
Biscuits	40:10:50::NFMF:GFMF:WF	Improved nutritional quality	Shimray et al (2012)
Germination			
Porridge	100% GPM	↑ Protein and crude fiber ↓ Phytic acid content	Ocheme and Chinma (2008)

(Continued)

TABLE 9.1 *(Continued)*
Health-Promoting Components in Value-Added Millet Products Suitable for Diabetics as Impacted by Processing Method

Product/Type	Formulation	Health-Promoting Components	Reference
Milling and Roasting			
Chapatti	70:30::WF:FM	Improved nutritional quality	Gull et al (2014)
Chapatti	70-90:10-30::WF:FM	Improved nutritional quality	Panghal et al (2019)
Chapatti with spices	75:15:10::WF:BF:FM	Improved nutritional quality	Walde et al (2021)
Puffing			
Puffed millet	100% FM	Improved nutritional quality	Gull et al (2014)
Roasting			
Chapatti	10:90::RBMF:WF And 10:90::PCBMF:WF	↑ Polyphenol content and antioxidant activity	Devi and Nazni (2016)
Roasted and pressure-cooked			
Khichdi	70:25::LM:PuM	↑ Protein, dietary fiber, and micronutrient content	Chhabra and Kaur (2022)
Upma	85:8::FoM:BeG	↑ Protein, dietary fiber, and micronutrient content	Chhabra and Kaur (2022)
Laddu	60:40::FM:BeGF	↑ Calcium, phosphorus, iron, and fiber	Sharma and Yamer (2022)
Soaking			
Porridge	100% SPM	↑ Protein and crude fiber ↓ Phytic acid content	Ocheme and Chinma (2008)

Note: FM = Finger millet; WF = Wheat flour; RWF = Refined wheat flour; ML = Moringa leaf; FoM = Foxtail millet; GGD = Green gram dal; PMF = Pearl millet flour; BG = Black gram; RF = Rice flour; PH = Psyllium husk; BMF = Barnyard millet flour; XG = Xanthan gum; GMMF = Germinated millet mix flour comprising equal proportions of germinated finger millet, foxtail millet, proso millet, little millet, and kodo millet; DBG: Dehusked black gram; SM-GPMF = Skim milk and germinated pearl millet flour; LM = Legumes mix; FS = Fenugreek seeds: QF = Quinoa flour; GFMF = Germinated finger millet flour; NFMF = Native finger millet flour; GPM = Germinated pearl millet; BeGF = Bengal gram flour; SPM = Soaked pearl millet: BeG = Bengal gram: PuM = Mix of pulses comprising equal proportions of Green gram, yellow and red lentils: RBMF = Roasted barnyard millet flour; PCBMF = Pressure cooked barnyard millet flour: ERBP = Ekanayakam root bark powder.

impart improved medicinal and nutritional profiles may be a viable strategy to alleviate the escalating burden of these disorders.

9.10 CONCLUSION

DM remains one of the leading health problems worldwide. India is facing a major epidemic, which is expected to get worse by 2045. It is a proven fact that lifestyle changes are necessary for the management of diabetes; however, pharmacological treatments hardly ever succeed in preventing and controlling the onset of complications. Functional foods, with an emphasis on millet, are the next big thing in dietary interventions. Being loaded with both macro- and micronutrients, and bioactive compounds such as antioxidants, millets not only help in managing the blood glucose levels but also help in preventing complications associated with diabetes.

The reason for the high fiber content in millet is that the latter is the main one among the foods that slow glucose absorption, whereas their low GI and anti-inflammatory properties are the factors responsible for improved glycemic control. Millets also have significant minerals such as magnesium and phytochemicals that enhance the sensitivity of insulin receptors and thus facilitate insulin secretion from the pancreas. One of the studies revealed that millets have the potential to bring about the least activity of digestive enzymes such as α-amylase and α-glucosidase, thereby lessening glucose spikes after meals. Research on humans has brought about evidence of improvements in fasting glucose, insulin sensitivity, and long-term glycemic control (HbA1c), thus suggesting the use of foxtail millet as a possible prophylactic agent for kidney diseases.

Indeed, the advantages of millets in improving insulin sensitivity, glucose metabolism, and alleviation of inflammation and oxidative stress are further evidenced by studies on animals. Furthermore, millets are associated with beneficial gut flora that produces SCFAs which in turn help in glucose metabolism. Thanks to their nutritional benefits and versatility, millets can easily serve as part of diabetic dietary plans, thus providing a natural means of diabetes management and prevention.

Millets are mainly processed into various food products and hence are often referred to as substitutes of conventional staples such as rice, wheat, and maize, whose processing methods are limited to a few forms. The Indian Institute of Millets Research (ICAR-IIMR) situated in Hyderabad, India, is well-equipped with advanced technologies for the production of millet-based products, inclusive of ready-to-cook (RTC) and ready-to-eat (RTE) foods. The extent of the decortication of millet grains has a major impact on the determination of their ultimate uses; a less processed one might contain more bioactive compounds for therapeutic purposes, while grains are generally decorticated to a higher level for food utilization. Therefore, it is advisable to adjust millet processing in accordance with its intended use. This would not only help maximize but also optimize their health benefits.

Another focus area that requires prior attention is the millet's bioactive peptides that are already present in them. These peptides have been identified as a potential source of functional food ingredients due to their potent antioxidant, anti-inflammatory, and antihyperglycemic effects. Nevertheless, the biological impact and health benefits of these peptides have yet to be confirmed through scientific evidence of in vivo studies. Despite the current ensemble of studies, much remains to be known about the health benefits of millets. Therefore, subsequent studies should put their focus on unraveling the exact modus operandi of various nutrient components of millets such as polyphenols, fiber, proteins, and micronutrients. Comprehending these mechanisms to a greater extent will be of vital importance in optimizing millets' consumption for therapeutic purposes.

So far, millets have not been studied in the burgeoning field of nutrigenomics, which studies the interaction between diet and the genome. Studying deeper into the aspects of how millet consumption influences gene expression, particularly in relation to metabolic pathways and chronic disease prevention, might provide significant insights into the molecular mechanisms underlying millet's health benefits. Thus, it could lead to nutrition precision strategies that aim at improving health outcomes of individuals, especially those who are prone to chronic diseases.

The potential entrepreneurial ventures linked with the rising demand for specialized millet-based food products are enormous, in addition to the benefits already discussed. Millet-based products with added values of nutritional/dietary features such as gluten-free, high-fiber, or low-GI are created to meet the dietary requirements, as well as serve the growing number of health-conscious consumers. These products also provide a good source of income to farmers, self-help groups (SHGs), industrialists as well as contributing to the developing economy from the growing global market for functional foods and nutraceuticals.

To sum up, the present scientific literature on millets has set a reliable base; however, the focus of the subsequent investigations should be on uncovering more about millets' therapeutic and nutritional properties, thus addressing the existing gaps in knowledge. The subsequent research could unlock full potential of millets as an environmentally friendly source of healthy food by looking into bioactive compounds, facilitating breeding programs, and further study of less-known millet species. Besides, the emerging research on millet-based functional foods is a source of excitement for entrepreneurs and, therefore, strengthens the argument for sustained research and development in this field.

REFERENCES

Adanse, J., Bıgson, K., Maureen, N. A., and Dorothy, A. 2021. Quality characteristics and sensory evaluation of cakes produced from composite blends of wheat (*Titricum aestivum* L.) and finger millet (*Pennisetum glaucum*) flour. *Eurasian J Sci Technol* 5, no. 2: 190–204.

Akshatha, Rohitha, T., and Zabia, A. 2024. Evolution of fiber-rich papad from psyllium husk: A comparative study. *Int J Innovative Sci Res* 2, no.1: 6–13.

Alkhatib, A., Tsang, C., Tiss, A., Bahorun, T., Arefanian, H., Barake, R., Khadir, A., and Tuomilehto, J. 2017. Functional foods and lifestyle approaches for diabetes prevention and management. *Nutrients* 9, no. 12: 1310.

Almaski, A., Coe, S., Lightowler, H., Clegg, M. E., and Thondre, P. S. 2023. Finger millet-based muffin decreases insulin response in individuals with prediabetes in a randomised controlled trial. *Br J Nutr* 129, no. 4: 650–659.

Alyami, J., Whitehouse, E., Yakubov, G. E., Pritchard, S. E., Hoad, C. L., Blackshaw, E., Heissam, K., Cordon, S. M., Bligh, H. F. J., Spiller, R. C., and Macdonald, I. A. 2019. Glycaemic, gastrointestinal, hormonal and appetitive responses to pearl millet or oats porridge breakfasts: A randomised, crossover trial in healthy humans. *Br J Nutr* 122, no. 10: 1142–1154.

Anitha, S., Kane-Potaka, J., Tsusaka, T. W., Botha, R., Rajendran, A., Givens, D. I., and Bhandari, R. K. 2021. A systematic review and meta-analysis of the potential of millets for managing and reducing the risk of developing diabetes mellitus. *Front Nutr* 8: 687428.

Anjana, R. M., Unnikrishnan, R., Deepa, M., Pradeepa, R., Tandon, N., Das, A. K., Joshi, S., Bajaj, S., Jabbar, P. K., Das, H. K., and Kumar, A. 2023. Metabolic non-communicable disease health report of India: The ICMR-INDIAB national cross-sectional study (ICMR-INDIAB-17). *Lancet Diabetes Endocrino* 11, no. 7: 474–489.

Arora, L., Aggarwal, R., Dhaliwal, I., Gupta, O. P., and Kaushik, P. 2023. Assessment of sensory and nutritional attributes of foxtail millet-based food products. *Front Nutr* 10: 1146545.

Atkinson, F. S., Brand-Miller, J. C., Foster-Powell, K., Buyken, A. E., and Goletzke, J. 2021. International tables of glycemic index and glycemic load values 2021: A systematic review. *Am J Clin Nutr* 114, no. 5: 1625–1632.

Balkrishna, A., Verma, S., Singh, S. K., Dobhal, V., and Arya, V. 2024. Exploring the antioxidant mechanisms of millet polyphenols: Regulation of Nrf2 and NF-κB and their impact on gut microbiota. *Discov Food* 4, no. 1: 123.

Barbagallo, M., and Dominguez, L. J. 2015. Magnesium and type 2 diabetes. *World J Diabetes* 6, no. 10: 1152.

Bhavamishra. 2011. Dhanya Varga. In: Srikantha Murthy, K.R (ed.) *Bhavaprakasha*. Varanasi: Chowkhamba Krishna Das Academy, p. 374.

Bonsembiante, L., Targher, G., and Maffeis, C. 2021. Type 2 diabetes and dietary carbohydrate intake of adolescents and young adults: What is the impact of different choices? *Nutrients* 13, no. 10: 3344.

Boria, A., Gour, S., Dubey, A. D., and Shukla, S. S. 2021. Chemical composition and shelf-life of burger buns from ragi and moringa leaf powder. *Pharma Innov* 10, no. 10: 2179–2185.

Carvalho, F., Lahlou, R. A., Pires, P., Salgado, M., and Silva, L. R. 2023. Natural functional beverages as an approach to manage diabetes. *Int J Mol Sci* 24, no. 23: 16977.

Ch'ng, L. Z., Barakatun-Nisak, M. Y., Zukiman, W. Z. H. W., Abas, F., and Wahab, N. A. 2019. Nutritional strategies in managing post-meal glucose for type 2 diabetes: A narrative review. *Diabetes Metab Syndr Clin Res Rev* 13, no. 4: 2339–2345.

Chaitra, U., Abhishek, P., Sudha, M. L., Vanitha, T., and Crassina, K. 2020. Impact of millets on wheat based Belgian waffles: Quality characteristics and nutritional composition. *LWT* 124: 109136.

Chandraprabha, L. S., Sharon, C. L., Panjikkaran, S. T., Aneena, E. R., and Beena, C. 2017. Development and nutritional qualities of vermicelli prepared from barnyard millet and Ekanayakam root bark. *J Pharmacogn Phytochem* 6, no. 6: 2359–2362.

Chandrasekara, A., and Shahidi, F. 2012. Bioaccessibility and antioxidant potential of millet grain phenolics as affected by simulated in vitro digestion and microbial fermentation. *J Funct Foods* 4, no. 1: 226–237.

Charaka, A. 2011. Sutrasthana, Annapanavidhi Adhyaya. In: Vaidya Jadavaji Trikamji Acharya (ed.) *Charaka Samhitha*. Delhi: Chaukhamba Prakashan, p. 154.

Chhabra, I., and Kaur, A. 2022. Development of a convenient, nutritious ready to cook packaged product using millets with a batch scale process development for a small-scale enterprise. *J Food Sci Technol* 59, no. 2: 488–497.

Deng, X., Liang, J., Wang, L., Niu, L., Xiao, J., Guo, Q., Liu, X., and Xiao, C. 2023. Whole grain proso millet (*Panicum miliaceum* L.) attenuates hyperglycemia in type 2 diabetic mice: Involvement of miRNA profile. *J Agric Food Chem* 71, no. 24: 9324–9336.

de Souza Rocha, T., Hernandez, L. M. R., Mojica, L., Johnson, M. H., Chang, Y. K., and de Mejía, E. G. 2015. Germination of Phaseolus vulgaris and alcalde hydrolysis of its proteins produced bioactive peptides capable of improving markers related to type-2 diabetes in vitro. *Food Res Int* 76: 150–159.

Devi, P. B., Vijayabharathi, R., Sathyabama, S., Malleshi, N. G., and Priyadarisini, V. B. 2014. Health benefits of finger millet (*Eleusine coracana* L.) polyphenols and dietary fiber: A review. *J Food Sci Technol* 51: 1021–1040.

Devi, R. S., and Nazni, P. 2016. Sensory characteristics, total polyphenol content and in vitro antioxidant activity of value added processed barnyard millet flour chapattis. *JFPT* 7, no. 6.

Fu, Y., Liu, Z., Wang, H., Zhang, F., Guo, S., and Shen, Q. 2023. Comparison of the generation of α-glucosidase inhibitory peptides derived from prolamins of raw and cooked foxtail millet: *In vitro* activity, de novo sequencing, and in silico docking. *Food Chem* 411: 135378.

Fu, Y., Yin, R., Guo, E., Cheng, R., Diao, X., Xue, Y., and Shen, Q. 2021. Protein isolates from raw and cooked foxtail millet attenuate development of type 2 diabetes in streptozotocin-induced diabetic mice. *Mol Nutr Food Res* 65, no. 6: 2000365.

Fu, Y., Zhang, F., Liu, Z., Zhao, Q., Xue, Y., and Shen, Q. 2021. Improvement of diabetes-induced metabolic syndrome by millet prolamin is associated with changes in serum metabolomics. *Food Biosci* 44: 101434.

Geetha, K., Yankanchi, G. M., Hulamani, S., and Hiremath, N. 2020. Glycemic index of millet-based food mix and its effect on pre diabetic subjects. *J Food Sci Tech* 57: 2732–2738.

Goel, K., Goomer, S., and Aggarwal, D. 2021. Formulation and optimization of value-added barnyard millet vermicelli using response surface methodology. *Asian J Dairy Food Res* 40, no. 1: 55–61.

Gong, L., Feng, D., Wang, T., Ren, Y., Liu, Y., and Wang, J. 2020. Inhibitors of α-amylase and α-glucosidase: Potential linkage for whole cereal foods on prevention of hyperglycemia. *Food Sci Nutr* 8, no. 12: 6320–6337.

Goron, T. L., and Raizada, M. N. 2015. Genetic diversity and genomic resources available for the small millet crops to accelerate a New Green Revolution. *Front Plant Sci* 6: 157.

Gull, A., Jan, R., Nayik, G. A., Prasad, K., and Kumar, P. 2014. Significance of finger millet in nutrition, health and value-added products: A review. *Magnesium (mg)* 130, no. 32: 120.

Hegde, P. S., and Chandra, T. S. 2005. ESR spectroscopic study reveals higher free radical quenching potential in kodo millet (*Paspalum scrobiculatum*) compared to other millets. *Food Chem* 92, no. 1: 177–182.

Hithamani, G., and Srinivasan, K. 2014. Effect of domestic processing on the polyphenol content and bioaccessibility in finger millet (*Eleusine coracana*) and pearl millet (*Pennisetum glaucum*). *Food Chem* 164: 55–62.

ICMR 2018. *ICMR Guidelines for Management of Type 2 Diabetes*. New Delhi: Indian Council of Medical Research, p. 16–21.

International Diabetes Federation (IDF). 2022. *About Diabetes*. Available at: https://diabetesatlas.org (accessed [20042026]).

Ito, Y., Suzuki, A., Nasukawa, H., Miyaki, K., Yano, A., and Nagasawa, T. 2022. Ameliorative effects of Japanese barnyard millet (*Echinochloa esculenta* H.Scholz) bran supplementation in streptozotocin-induced diabetic rats. *Food Sci Technol Res* 28, no. 5: 431–439.

Jacob, J., Krishnan, V., Antony, C., Bhavyasri, M., Aruna, C., Mishra, K., Nepolean, T., Satyavathi, C. T., and Visarada, K. B. 2024. The nutrition and therapeutic potential of millets: An updated narrative review. *Front Nutr* 11: 1346869.

Jali, M. V., Kamatar, M. Y., Jali, S. M., Hiremath, M. B., and Naik, R. K. 2012. Efficacy of value added foxtail millet therapeutic food in the management of diabetes and dyslipidamea in type 2 diabetic patients. *Recent Res Sci Technol* 4, no. 7: 3–4.

Joshi, A., Srivastava, S., Shahi, N. C., Kushwaha, A., and Acharya, R. 2023. Formulation and numerical optimization of finger millet and quinoa incorporated eggless doughnuts. *Asian J Dairy Food Res* 44, no. 6: 931–939.

Kaiyadeva, A. 2009. *Dhanyavarga. Kaiyadeva Nighantu (Pathyaapthyavibhodika)*. Varanasi: Choukambha Orientalia, p. 318.

Kanetro, B. 2018. Amino acid profile of soybean (Glycine max) sprout protein for determining insulin stimulation amino acids. *Int Food Res J* 25, no. 6: 2497–2502.

Kim, J., and Park, Y. 2012. Anti-diabetic effect of sorghum extract on hepatic gluconeogenesis of streptozotocin-induced diabetic rats. *Nutr Metab* 9: 1–7.

Krishnamoorthy, S., Kunjithapatha, S., and Manickam, L. 2013. Traditional Indian breakfast (Idli and Dosa) with enhanced nutritional content using millets. *Nutr Diet* 70, no. 3: 241–246.

Kumar, A., Tomer, V., Kaur, A., Kumar, V., and Gupta, K. 2018. Millets: A solution to agrarian and nutritional challenges. *Agric Food Secur* 7, no. 1: 1–15. https://doi.org/10.1186/s40066-018-0183-3

Lacroix, I. M., and Li-Chan, E. C. 2014. Overview of food products and dietary constituents with antidiabetic properties and their putative mechanisms of action: A natural approach to complement pharmacotherapy in the management of diabetes. *Mol Nutr Food Res* 58, no. 1: 61–78.

Li, X., Bai, Y., Jin, Z., and Svensson, B. 2022. Food-derived non-phenolic α-amylase and α-glucosidase inhibitors for controlling starch digestion rate and guiding diabetes-friendly recipes. *LWT* 153: 112455.

Liu, J., Ren, Z. H., Qiang, H., Wu, J., Shen, M., Zhang, L., and Lyu, J. 2020. Trends in the incidence of diabetes mellitus: Results from the Global Burden of Disease Study 2017 and implications for diabetes mellitus prevention. *BMC Public Health* 20: 1–12.

Liu, X., Qiu, B., Liu, W., Zhang, Y., Wang, X., Li, X., and Zhang, D. 2022. The preventive effects of fermented and germinated foxtail millet whole grain on kidney damage in a diabetic mouse model. *Front Nutr* 9: 940404.

Longvah, T., Ananthan, R., Bhaskarachary, K., and Venkaiah, K. 2017. Indian Food Composition Tables. *National Institute of Nutrition*, Indian Council of Medical Research, Hyderabad, India, Pp. 2–58.

Majid, A., and Priyadarshini, C. G. P. 2020. Millet derived bioactive peptides: A review on their functional properties and health benefits. *Crit Rev Food Sci Nutr* 60, no. 19: 3342–3351.

Mansoria, P., and Singh, S. B. 2023. Unlocking the therapeutic potential of millets: A path to diabetes control. *J Ayurveda Integr Med Sci* 8, no. 6: 152–157.

Mathur, P., Kulothungan, V., Leburu, S., Krishnan, A., Chaturvedi, H. K., Salve, H. R., and Garg, S. 2021. National non-communicable disease monitoring survey (NNMS) in India: Estimating risk factor prevalence in adult population. *PloS One* 16, no. 3: e0246712.

Mena, P., Calani, L., Bruni, R., and Del Rio, D. 2015. Bioactivation of High-Molecular-Weight Polyphenols by the Gut Microbiome. In: *Diet-Microbe Interactions in the Gut.* Amsterdam: Academic Press, pp. 73–101.

Mirmiran, P., Bahadoran, Z., and Azizi, F. 2014. Functional foods-based diet as a novel dietary approach for management of type 2 diabetes and its complications: A review. *World J Diabetes* 5, no. 3: 267.

Mitharwal, S., Kumar, S., and Chauhan, K. 2021. Nutritional, polyphenolic composition and in vitro digestibility of finger millet (*Eleusine coracana* L.) with its potential food applications: A review. *Food Biosci* 44: 101382.

Modha, H., and Pal, D. 2011. Optimization of Rabadi-like fermented milk beverage using pearl millet. *J Food Sci Technol* 48, no. 2: 190–196.

Mutshinyani, M., Mashau, M. E., and Jideani, A. I. O. 2020. Bioactive compounds, antioxidant activity and consumer acceptability of porridges of finger millet (*Eleusine coracana*) flours: Effects of spontaneous fermentation. *Int J Food Propert* 23: 1692–710.

Negi, N., Srihari, S. P., Wadikar, D. D., Sharma, G. K., and Semwal, A. D. 2021. Optimization of instant foxtail millet based khichdi by using response surface methodology and evaluation of its shelf stability. *J Food Sci Technol* 58: 4478–4485. https://doi.org/10.1007/s13197-020-04929-x

Nishizawa, N., Togawa, T., Park, K. O., Sato, D., Miyakoshi, Y., Inagaki, K., Ohmori, N., Ito, Y., and Nagasawa, T. 2009. Dietary Japanese millet protein ameliorates plasma levels of adiponectin, glucose, and lipids in type 2 diabetic mice. *Biosci Biotechnol Biochem* 73, no. 2: 351–360.

Ocheme, O. B., and Chinma, C. E. 2008. Effects of soaking and germination on some physicochemical properties of millet flour for porridge production. *J Food Technol* 6, no. 5: 185–188.

Ofosu, F. K., Elahi, F., Daliri, E. B. M., Chelliah, R., Ham, H. J., Kim, J. H., and Oh, D. H. 2020. Phenolic profile, antioxidant, and antidiabetic potential exerted by millet grain varieties. *Antioxidants* 9, no. 3: 254.

Panghal, A., Khatkar, B. S., Yadav, D. N., and Chhikara, N. 2019. Effect of finger millet on nutritional, rheological, and pasting profile of whole wheat flat bread (chapatti). *Cereal Chem* 96, no. 1: 86–94.

Pathak, P., Srivastava, S., and Grover, S. 2000. Development of food products based on millets, legumes and fenugreek seeds and their suitability in the diabetic diet. *Int J Food Sci Nutr* 51, no. 5: 409–414.

Portincasa, P., Bonfrate, L., Vacca, M., De Angelis, M., Farella, I., Lanza, E., Khalil, M., Wang, D. Q. H., Sperandio, M., and Di Ciaula, A. 2022. Gut microbiota and short chain fatty acids: Implications in glucose homeostasis. *Int J Mol Sci* 23, no. 3: 1105.

Pradeep, P. M., and Sreerama, Y. N. 2018. Phenolic antioxidants of foxtail and little millet cultivars and their inhibitory effects on α-amylase and α-glucosidase activities. *Food Chem* 247: 46–55.

Qi, W., Wang, Y., Song, G., Sun, H., Pang, S., and Li, A. 2019. Effects of four coarse cereals on blood glucose levels in rats with STZ-induced hyperglycemia. *Food Agric Immunol* 30, no. 1: 487–496.

Rao, B. D., Bhat, B. V., and Tonapi, V. A. 2018. *Nutri Cereals for Nutritional Security.* Hyderabad: Indian Institute of Millets Research, p. 148.

Ren, X., Yin, R., Hou, D., Xue, Y., Zhang, M., Diao, X., Zhang, Y., Wu, J., Hu, J., Hu, X., and Shen, Q. 2018. The glucose-lowering effect of foxtail millet in subjects with impaired glucose tolerance: A self-controlled clinical trial. *Nutrients* 10, no. 10: 1509.

Rochette, L., Zeller, M., Cottin, Y., and Vergely, C. 2014. Diabetes, oxidative stress, and therapeutic strategies. *Biochim Biophys Acta* 1840, no. 9: 2709–2729.

Saini, S., Saxena, S., Samtiya, M., Puniya, M., and Dhewa, T. 2021. Potential of underutilized millets as Nutri-cereal: An overview. *J Food Sci Tech* 58:4465–4477.

Sarita, E. S., and Singh, E. 2016. The potential of millets: Nutrients composition and health benefits. *J Sci Innov Res* 5, no. 2: 46–50.

Seo, K. H., Ra, J. E., Lee, S. J., Lee, J. H., Kim, S. R., Lee, J. H., and Seo, W. D. 2015. Anti-hyperglycemic activity of polyphenols isolated from barnyard millet (*Echinochloa utilis* L.) and their role inhibiting α-glucosidase. *Korean Soc Appl Biol Chem* 58: 571–579.

Sharma, B., Gujral, H. S., and Solah, V. 2017. Effect of incorporating finger millet in wheat flour on mixolab behavior, chapatti quality, and starch digestibility. *Food Chem* 231: 156–164. https://doi.org/10.1016/j.foodchem.2017.03.118

Sharma, D., and Yamer, P. 2022. Value addition of products from finger millet (*Eleusine coracana*). *J Postharvest Technol* 10, no. 2: 120–138.

Sharma, N., and Niranjan, K. 2018. Foxtail millet: Properties, processing, health benefits, and uses. *Food Rev Int* 34, no. 4: 329–363.

Shimray, C. A., Gupta, S., and Venkateswara Rao, G. 2012. Effect of native and germinated finger millet flour on rheological and sensory characteristics of biscuits. *Int J Food Sci Technol* 47, no. 11: 2413–2420.

Thathola, A., and Srivastava, S. 2002. Physicochemical properties and nutritional traits of millet-based weaning food suitable for infants of the Kumaon hills, Northern India. *Asia Pac J of Clin Nutr* 11, no. 1: 28–32.

Vedamanickam, R., Anandan, P., Bupesh, G., and Vasanth, S. 2020. Study of millet and non-millet diet on diabetics and associated metabolic syndrome. *Biomed* 40, no. 1: 55–58.

Veena, T., Nidoni, U., and Devi, G. S. 2020. Millet incorporated pizza base. *Int J Curr Microbiol App Sci* 9, no. 10: 2830–2837.

Veit, M., van Asten, R., Olie, A., and Prinz, P. 2022. The role of dietary sugars, overweight, and obesity in type 2 diabetes mellitus: A narrative review. *Eur J Clin Nutr* 76, no. 11: 1497–1501.

Walde, S. G., Agrawal, S., and Mittal, S. 2021. Development of multigrain chapatti with spices mix to enhance the nutritional values and their storage study. *J Food Sci Technol* 58, no. 3: 1132–1142.

Wang, H., Zhao, Q., Fu, Y., Liu, Z., Zhu, Y., Wang, C., and Shen, Q. 2023. Foxtail millet (*Setaria italica*) alleviates non-alcoholic fatty liver disease in high-fat diet/streptozotocin-induced diabetic mice through gut microbiota modulation. *Food Biosci* 53: 102797.

WHO 2022. https://www.who.int/health-topics/diabetes#tab=tab_1

Willett, W. C., and Liu, S. 2019. Carbohydrate quality and health: Distilling simple truths from complexity. *Am J Clin Nutr* 110, no. 4: 803–804.

Wojdyło, A., Nowicka, P., Tkacz, K., and Turkiewicz, I. P. 2020. Sprouts vs. microgreens as novel functional foods: Variation of nutritional and phytochemical profiles and their in vitro bioactive properties. *Molecules* 25, no. 20: 4648.

World Diabetes Atlas 2021. Diabetes Atlas – International Diabetes Federation. https://diabetesatlas.org/atlas/tenth-edition/

Zhang, G., Wang, D., Ding, Y., Zhang, J., Ding, Y., and Lyu, F. 2024. Effect and mechanism of insoluble dietary fiber on postprandial blood sugar regulation. *Trends Food Sci Technol* 146: 104354.

10 Cardioprotective and Anti-Cancer Effects of Millets

Alpana Joshi[1] *and Ayushi Joshi*[2]
[1] Department of Hospitality Management, Amrapali University, Haldwani, Uttarakhand, India
[2] College of Community Sciences, G. B. Pant University of Agriculture and Technology, Pantnagar, Uttarakhand, India

10.1 INTRODUCTION

Millets are taken into account as "wholesome grains," are becoming increasingly popular for their nutritional benefits and potential role in preventing different lifestyle diseases. Millets, a diverse group of small-seeded grasses, including species like *Eleusine coracana* (finger millet), *Pennisetum glaucum* (pearl millet), *Setaria italica* (foxtail millet), and *Panicum miliaceum* (proso millet), have been cultivated for thousands of years in Asia and Africa. These grains are not only prized for their ability to thrive in harsh climates and poor soil conditions but are also gaining recognition for their potential health benefits, particularly their roles in the prevention and management of cardiovascular diseases (CVDs) and cancer (Devi et al 2014; Nithiyanantham et al 2019).

According to World Health Organization (WHO), CVDs are the leading cause of death globally, approximately 17.9 million deaths per year due to CVD (WHO 2021). Dietary habits play a vital role in the pathological process of CVDs, and there is mounting evidence that whole grains, especially millets, can noteworthy reduce cardiovascular risk factors (Aune et al 2016). Millets are inherently gluten-free and are rich in dietary fiber, complex carbohydrates, polyunsaturated fatty acids, and bioactive phytochemicals, all of which contribute to their cardioprotective properties (Saleh et al 2013).

Studies have shown that regular intake of millets in regular diet can help lower total cholesterol (TC), low-density lipoprotein (LDL) (bad cholesterol), and triglycerides (TG), while also increasing high-density lipoprotein (HDL) (good cholesterol) levels, as demonstrated by Shobana et al (2010) in their extensive research on finger millet. Millets are notably rich in magnesium and potassium, minerals that have been found to hold up healthy blood pressure (BP) and reduce the risk of stroke, according to Singh et al (2023). Additionally, millets have a low glycemic index, which helps in managing blood glucose levels and, in turn, contributes to better cardiovascular health, as noted by Ahamed et al (2024).

Millets contain bioactive compounds like phenolic acids and flavonoids, which function as antioxidants and anti-inflammatory agents. These substances help neutralize harmful free radicals, lower oxidative stress, and block inflammatory pathways, thereby shielding cardiovascular tissues from damage (Jacob et al 2024). In addition, millets are rich in lignans and phytosterols, which play a leading role in regulating lipid metabolism and enhancing endothelial function, supporting overall vascular health (Awasthi et al 2025).

Alongside their cardiovascular benefits, millets are also being studied for their anti-cancer properties. According to GLOBOCAN (2021), there were about 19.3 million new cancer cases and nearly 10 million deaths worldwide in 2020. The anti-cancer potential of millets is linked to their rich content of phenolic compounds, dietary fiber, and specific micronutrients, which have been shown to interfere with carcinogenesis at various stages (Pradeep and Sreerama 2015; Tripathi et al 2023). These bioactive components may help inhibit cancer cell growth, promote apoptosis, and support gut health, making millets a promising area of research in cancer prevention.

DOI: 10.1201/9781003686668-10

Research has shown that millet extracts rich in polyphenols can effectively diminish the proliferation of cancer cells, trigger apoptosis (programmed cell death), and prevent the formation of new blood vessels (angiogenesis) in various cancer cell types, including those from colon, breast, and liver cancers (Nithiyanantham et al 2019). Moreover, the dietary fiber in millets supports gut health by promoting the production of short-chain fatty acids (SCFAs), especially butyrate, which has been demonstrated to inhibit tumor growth and decrease inflammation in the colon (Ragaee et al 2006; Jacob et al 2024).

Millets also play a significant role in immunoregulation. Research has indicated that millet-based diets may influence cytokine profiles, reduce systemic inflammation, and enhance the immune system's ability to suppress tumor progression and cardiovascular inflammation (Sachdev et al 2023; Mohanan et al 2025).

Although there is strong scientific evidence highlighting the health benefits of millets, these grains are still not widely used in global food systems. Limited awareness of consumer, inadequate industrial processing, and the dominance of staple cereals like wheat and rice have hindered their broader adoption. However, with the growing burden of non-communicable diseases and the urgent need for climate-resilient crops, millets offer a sustainable and health-promoting alternative that deserves greater attention. Integrating millets into public health strategies could help address both health and environmental challenges, making them a valuable choice for the future of nutrition.

This chapter comes up with a detailed look at the heart-protective and cancer-fighting qualities of millets, combining insights from biochemical, clinical, and population-based research. It aims to show how these traditional grains can offer real benefits in modern diets, helping to prevent chronic diseases and support overall health. Millets are packed with nutrients, fiber, and bioactive compounds that help lower cholesterol, regulate BP, and maintain stable blood sugar levels, all of which are important for reducing the risk of heart disease and certain cancers. By exploring the latest scientific evidence, this chapter highlights how millets can be a powerful tool for improving public health and making nutrition more sustainable and effective.

10.2 PREVALENCE OF CARDIOVASCULAR DISEASES (CVDs) AND CANCER: GLOBAL AND INDIAN PERSPECTIVES

CVDs remain a major public health challenge around the world, with the WHO reporting that CVDs are the leading cause of death globally. In 2022 alone, approximately 19.8 million people died from CVDs, accounting for about 32% of all global deaths—over three-quarters of which occurred in low- and middle-income countries (LMICs). The rising burden is driven by factors such as population growth, aging, urbanization, and unhealthy lifestyle habits, including poor diet, lack of physical activity, and tobacco use. This trend is observed in both developed and developing regions, highlighting the urgent need for preventive strategies and improved healthcare policies.

Similarly, cancer continues to be a leading cause of mortality, significantly impacting life expectancy worldwide (Obafemi and Umahi-Ottah 2023). According to WHO data from 2019, cancer ranks as the leading or second-leading cause of death before the age of 70 in 112 out of 183 countries. It is one of the top causes of adult deaths globally, underscoring its role as a major public health concern that requires sustained attention and action.

10.2.1 Cardiovascular Diseases (CVDs)

CVDs—such as heart disease, stroke, and conditions linked to high BP—are becoming increasingly common around the world. This rise is largely driven by the growing number of older adults and the rapid pace of urbanization, both of which contribute to higher rates of these health problems.

10.2.1.1 Global Prevalence of CVDs

Globally, CVDs are the key player of death, responsible for approximately 17.9 million deaths annually, which accounts for 32% of all global deaths (WHO 2021). The majority of these deaths occur in LMICs, a result of a combination of unhealthy lifestyles, inadequate healthcare access, and the rising prevalence of risk factors such as hypertension, diabetes, obesity, and smoking.

Vaduganathan et al (2022) revealed that CVDs are the leading contributor to the global disease burden, with ischemic heart disease (IHD) and cerebrovascular diseases (stroke) accounting for the greatest share of these deaths. The study also highlighted an alarming increase in the incidence of CVDs in LMICs, which is expected to continue rising due to changing diets, urbanization, and the lack of health infrastructure (Roth et al 2020).

One of the main factors of this global burden is the epidemic of hypertension, which remains underdiagnosed and undertreated in many countries, leading to a high incidence of strokes and heart failure. According to the American Heart Association (AHA), the global prevalence of hypertension is estimated to be around 30–45% of the adult population; the prevalence and absolute burden of hypertension are increasing globally, especially in LMICs. In 2010, an estimated 1.39 billion adults worldwide had hypertension of whom 1.04 billion were in LMICs and 349 million in HICs (Mills et al 2020).

10.2.1.2 Cardiovascular Diseases in India

India is experiencing a rise in CVD cases. The annual number of deaths from CVD in India is estimated to rise from 2.26 million (1990) to 4.77 million (2020) (Huffman et al 2011). Hypertension is primarily driven by urbanization, lifestyle changes, and a predominance of risk factors like diabetes and obesity. Studies suggest that hypertension alone affects 30–35% of Indian adults, with CVDs accounting for approximately 25–30% of all deaths in the country (Raghupathy et al 2014).

A key factor contributing to the rising incidences of CVDs in India is poor adherence to lifestyle changes, with sedentary lifestyles and high-fat diets becoming more common, especially in urban populations. In 2016, CVDs accounted for 28.1% (95% UI: 26.5–29.1) of all deaths and 14.1% (12.9–15.3) of total Disability-Adjusted Life Years (DALYs) in India. This marks a significant increase from 1990, when these figures were 15.2% (13.7–16.2) for deaths and 6.9% (6.3–7.4) for DALYs. That year, the burden of IHD varied ninefold across Indian states, while stroke and rheumatic heart disease showed sixfold and fourfold differences, respectively, in DALY rates (Prabhakaran 2018). Moreover, India's rapidly growing diabetes epidemic, with approximately 8–9% of the population affected, further exacerbates the risk for cardiovascular conditions (Sharma and Gujral 2019).

The Indian Heart Association (IHA) and different other studies have revealed that the urban–rural divide in CVD prevalence in India is significant. While urban regions have higher rates of IHD, rural areas are also facing challenges due to the lack of awareness, late detection, and fewer treatment options, leading to more severe outcomes once diagnosed (Jan et al 2024).

10.2.2 Cancer: Prevalence and Global Trends

Globally, it was found that cancer is the second leading cause of death, responsible for more or less 10 million deaths in 2020 (Sung et al 2021). It seems that the number of cancer cases is expected to rise, driven by factors such as aging populations, changing lifestyles, and advances in diagnostic technologies that increase detection rates.

10.2.2.1 Global Prevalence of Cancer

The different types of cancers worldwide include lung cancer, colorectal cancer, breast cancer, and prostate cancer. According to the report of the International Agency for Research on Cancer (IARC), there are more than 18 million new cancer cases annually, with lung cancer seeming the most prevalent, pursued by breast cancer and colorectal cancer (IARC 2020). While high-income countries have better probability of survival due to early detection and advanced treatment options, LMICs face an imbalanced burden of both incidence and mortality due to limited healthcare resources and lack of screening infrastructure.

One of the most noteworthy issues globally is the increasing burden of cancers linked to infectious agents such as human papillomavirus (HPV), hepatitis B virus (HBV), and hepatitis C virus (HCV), which account for a significant proportion of cancers in developing regions. Cervical cancer is a serious issue in many parts of sub-Saharan Africa, South Asia, and Latin America, where vaccination and screening programs are less widespread (IARC 2019).

The existence risk of developing cancer between the ages of 0 and 74 is 20.2%, with men facing a higher risk (22.4%) than women (18.2%) (Mattiuzzi and Lippi 2019). In 2018, there were around 18 million new cancer cases emerged globally, with lung and breast cancers each accounting for 2.09 million cases, and prostate cancer for 1.28 million cases. For most cancers, it was observed that the incidence is higher in men than women, except for cancer of thyroid, which is more common in women, with a male-to-female ratio of 0.30. Cancer is the second leading cause of death globally, causing 8.97 million deaths, following IHD. However, estimation suggests cancer may become the leading cause of death by 2060, with an average of 18.63 million deaths. Lung, liver, and stomach cancers are the majorly fatal, while lung cancer is the peak cause of cancer-related mortality in men and breast cancer in women. Prostate and thyroid cancers have the highest survival rates, with five-year survival close to 100%, whereas oesophageal, liver, and pancreatic cancers have the poorest prognosis, with five-year survival rates typically below 20% (Mattiuzzi and Lippi 2019).

10.2.2.2 Cancer in India: A Growing Challenge

Cancer incidence in India is rising gradually, with an approximately 1,461,427 new cases reported in 2022 (crude rate: 100.4 per 100,000 population). On an average, one in nine people in India is prone to develop cancer during their lifetime (Sathishkumar et al 2022). Lung cancer is the leading type of cancer among males, while breast cancer is the most common among females. In children (0–14 years), lymphoid leukemia is the most frequent cancer, affecting 29.2% of boys and 24.2% of girls. The National Cancer Registry Programme Report 2020, released by Indian Council of Medical Research (ICMR) and National Centre For Disease Informatics and Research (NCDIR), projected that cancer cases in India would increase from 13.9 lakh in 2020 to 15.7 lakh by 2025, representing a 12.8% rise (Sathishkumar et al 2022). The most common cancers observed among Indian women are breast, cervical, and ovarian cancer, while Indian men are most prone to be affected by oral, lung, and stomach cancers.

India is confronting a dual cancer burden, with an increasing rate of lifestyle-related cancers (such as breast cancer and colorectal cancer) adjacent to cancers linked to infections (such as cervical cancer, oral cancer, and liver cancer) (Rahmat and He 2024). Studies reveal that oral cancer is particularly high in tobacco-consuming populations, with India contributing to more than 50% of the global burden of oral cancer (Borse et al 2019).

The urban–rural divide is also noticeable in cancer prevalence in India. While urban populations have exposure to higher rates of breast, prostate, and colorectal cancers, rural populations have a the higher incidence of cervical cancer due to limited access to screening and vaccination programs (Sinha and Gupta 2020). Moreover, the lack of awareness about early detection and prevention contributes to delayed diagnosis and poor survival rates, especially in rural areas.

A particularly alarming trend is the rise in cervical cancer. Cervical cancer is ranked as the most common cancer in women in India. India has a population of approximately 365.71 million women above 15 years of age, who are at risk of developing cervical cancer. The current estimates suggest approximately 132,000 new cases diagnosed and 74,000 deaths annually in India, accounting for nearly 1/3 of the global cervical cancer deaths (WHO/ICO 2007).

10.3 CAUSES/RISK FACTORS FOR CVD AND CANCER

10.3.1 Factors Contribute to the Development of Cardiovascular Diseases

- *Unhealthy Diet*: A diet high in cholesterol, saturated fats, trans fats, and sodium can contribute to the development of CVDs. The risk of CVD increased according to dietary habits, with a higher risk of CVD observed in high-income countries, characterized by higher intake of sugar, trans fatty acids, and sugar-sweetened beverages, while a lower consumption of fruits and vegetables. Consuming large amounts of sugars and fats, particularly trans and saturated fats, raises the risk of atherosclerosis, while excessive sodium intake elevates the risk of hypertension, both of which are major contributors to CVD (Timmis et al 2022).
- *Physical Inactivity*: A sedentary lifestyle is a significant risk factor for CVD as it leads individuals to hypertension, dyslipidemia (high TG and low HDL), insulin resistance, type 2 diabetes, and obesity (Wilkins et al 2017). Physical inactivity contributes to a chronic lopsidedness between intake of calories and expenditure of energy. This imbalance fosters visceral fat accumulation, leading to overweight and obesity, which are well-established forerunner to metabolic disturbances. A sedentary lifestyle is also independently associated with the forming of the core components of metabolic syndrome (Booth et al 2012). Additionally, chronic inactivity contributes to systemic inflammation and hepatic steatosis, further promoting non-alcoholic fatty liver disease (NAFLD). These metabolic disturbances not only increase the risk of CVD but also contribute to liver-related morbidity and mortality.
- *Obesity*: Excess body weight is related to high BP, diabetes, and dyslipidemia. Excess body weight, particularly central or abdominal obesity, is a key contributor to the global rise in hypertension, type 2 diabetes mellitus (DM) (T2DM), and dyslipidemia. Overweight and obesity are major risk agents for a number of chronic diseases, including CVD, diabetes, and musculoskeletal disorders (WHO 2021a). Hypertension, or high BP, is closely linked to obesity through a process such as increased renin–angiotensin–aldosterone system (RAAS) activity, heightened sympathetic nervous system stimulation, and insulin resistance, all of which elevate blood volume and vascular resistance (Hall et al 2015). The National Heart, Lung, and Blood Institute confirms that "as body weight increases, so does blood pressure" (National Heart, Lung, and Blood Institute (NHLBI) 2022). Obesity is strongly associated with dyslipidemia, often characterized by increased TG, reduced HDL cholesterol (HDL-C), and elevated LDL particles. This lipid imbalance stems from an increase in free fatty acid flux to the liver and altered lipoprotein metabolism (Després 2012). According to the American Diabetes Association, "dyslipidaemia in obesity is often atherogenic, contributing significantly to cardiovascular complications" (American Diabetes Association (ADA) 2022). Recent meta-analyses have strengthened the evidence linking high Body Mask Index (BMI) to chronic diseases. Afshin et al (2017) reported that "high BMI was significantly associated with increased risk of diabetes and cardiovascular disease in both high- and low-income countries." These related metabolic disorders, collectively known as metabolic syndrome, are now considered a major global health challenge, primarily driven by increasing obesity rates (Grundy 2008). As a result, achieving and maintaining a healthy weight through balanced nutrition and regular physical activity is vital for the prevention and management of these conditions.
- *Smoking and Alcohol Consumption*: Both are major contributors to vascular damage and atherosclerosis. Smoking is a significant modifiable risk factor for CVD. It can elevate the risk of IHD by promoting blood clot formation, increasing BP, and accelerating atherosclerosis through its inflammatory effects on arterial walls. Additionally, smoking is associated with reduced plasma HDL-C levels and diminished exercise capacity (Wilkins

et al 2017). Smoking in moderation (one to four cigarettes per day) or on non-consecutive days has been found to increase the risk of myocardial infarction (Teo et al 2006) or mortality (Zhu et al 2021) compared to non-smokers. Whereas smoking cessation sustained for ≥5 years significantly lowers the risk of all-cause mortality compared to current smokers (Zhu et al 2021). Moreover, excessive alcohol intake—particularly binge drinking—heightens the risk of CVD by elevating BP and increasing serum triglyceride levels (Wilkins et al 2017).

- *Chronic Diseases*: Conditions like diabetes and hypertension significantly elevate CVD risk. Hypertension is a leading factor contributing to the global incidence of CVD and associated deaths (del Pinto et al 2022). Diabetes is a key risk factor for CVD, particularly in older adults (Halter et al 2014). Diabetic cardiomyopathy (DCM) refers to heart disease that arises directly as a consequence of diabetes (Toedebusch et al 2018). Historically, adults with diabetes have shown a significantly higher prevalence of CVD compared to those without the condition. Furthermore, the risk of developing CVD progressively increases with elevated fasting plasma glucose levels—even before they reach the threshold for a diabetes diagnosis (Singh et al 2013).
- *Oxidative Stress and Inflammation*: These play a crucial role in endothelial dysfunction and plaque formation. Oxidative stress and inflammation are two interrelated processes that play central roles in the pathogenesis and progression of CVDs. Oxidative stress arises from an imbalance between the production of reactive oxygen species (ROS) and the antioxidant defenses of the body, leading to cellular and tissue damage. In the vascular system, excessive ROS can reduce the bioavailability of nitric oxide (NO), a critical vasodilator, resulting in endothelial dysfunction—a key early event in atherogenesis (Harrison et al 2003). ROS also promote lipid peroxidation and oxidation of LDLs, further exacerbating vascular injury and plaque formation (Dhalla et al 2000). Simultaneously, oxidative stress acts as a trigger for inflammatory responses, activating transcription factors such as nuclear factor-kappa B (NF-κB), which induces the expression of pro-inflammatory cytokines and adhesion molecules. This promotes the recruitment of leukocytes and perpetuates a chronic inflammatory state within the arterial wall (García et al 2017). Inflammatory cells, in turn, generate additional ROS, creating a vicious cycle that accelerates endothelial dysfunction and plaque instability. The significance of this interplay is evidenced by elevated markers of oxidative stress and inflammation in patients with coronary artery disease and heart failure (Pickering 2021). Recent research also emphasizes the therapeutic potential of targeting this oxidative stress-inflammation axis. While the efficacy of generic antioxidant supplements in reducing cardiovascular risk has shown inconsistent results, more targeted approaches—such as monoclonal antibodies against interleukin-1β or therapies modulating the NLRP3 inflammasome—have demonstrated beneficial cardiovascular outcomes (Leopold and Loscalzo 2008). Moreover, some pharmacological agents, including certain antidiabetic drugs like SGLT2 inhibitors and glucagon-like peptide-1 (GLP-1) receptor agonists, exhibit antioxidant and anti-inflammatory properties that contribute to their cardioprotective effects (Elrakybi et al 2022). These findings underscore the importance of oxidative stress and inflammation not only as contributors to cardiovascular pathology but also as potential targets for novel therapeutic strategies.

10.3.2 Factors Contribute to the Development of Cancer

- *Physical Factor*: Physical factors such as ionizing radiation, ultraviolet (UV) radiation, and chronic mechanical injury significantly contribute to the beginning and growth of various cancers. Ionizing radiation—including X-rays, gamma rays, and radioactive substances—can penetrate deep into body tissues and directly damage DNA by inducing double-strand breaks and chromosomal mutations, thereby increasing the risk of cancers such as leukemia, breast, and thyroid cancers (United Nations Scientific Committee on the Effects of Atomic Radiation (UNSCEAR) 2000; Hall and Giaccia 2012). Survivors of the atomic bombings in Hiroshima and Nagasaki exhibited increased cancer mortality decades later, exemplifying the long-term carcinogenic effects of radiation exposure (Preston et al 2007). Similarly, UV radiation—especially Ultraviolet B (UVB)—induces mutagenic DNA lesions such as cyclobutane pyrimidine dimers, which, if unrestored, can lead to mutations in critical genes like *TP53*, a hallmark of many skin cancers (Narayanan et al 2010). Chronic mechanical irritation or scarring can also promote cancer by stimulating sustained inflammation, oxidative stress, and cellular proliferation, creating a tumor-promoting microenvironment (Balkwill and Mantovani 2001; Coussens and Werb 2002). For instance, chronic irritation from schistosomiasis has been linked to bladder cancer, and long-standing scars have been associated with squamous cell carcinoma (Wallingford et al 2011). These physical factors function through multiple mechanisms, primarily by causing genomic instability, altering cellular signaling pathways, and compromising tissue homeostasis, thereby facilitating carcinogenesis.

- *Chemical Factor*: Tobacco smoking, alcohol, certain medications, and chemicals may also have carcinogenic effects like stilbestrol derivatives given in threatening abortions, aromatic benzene derivatives, chloro-organic substances, phenoxy acetic acid derivatives and myelosuppressive antibiotics (O'Mahony and Hegarty 2009; Fung et al 2011). Exposure to chemical agents is a major contributor to cancer development through mechanisms such as DNA damage, oxidative stress, and hormonal disruption. One of the most widely studied chemical carcinogens is tobacco smoke, which contains over 7000 compounds, of which more than 70 are known carcinogens, including benzo[a]pyrene, formaldehyde, and nitrosamines (Hecht 2003). These chemicals form DNA adducts and induce mutations in key genes like *TP53*, driving the development of cancers such as lung, oral, oesophageal, and bladder cancer (Smith et al 2016). As the IARC notes, "there is sufficient evidence in humans for the carcinogenicity of tobacco smoking" (IARC 2012). Occupational exposure to chemicals is another well-established risk. For instance, asbestos fibers, used historically in construction, are strongly linked to mesothelioma and lung cancer, with a latency period of decades (Straif et al 2009). Benzidine, once used in dye production, has been linked to bladder cancer, and vinyl chloride, used in plastics, causes hepatic angiosarcoma (Bosetti et al 2008). Aflatoxins, produced by *Aspergillus* species in contaminated grains and nuts, are among the most potent hepatocarcinogens, especially aflatoxin B1, which causes DNA mutations when combined with HBV (Wild and Gong 2010). In food, nitrosamines and heterocyclic amines (HCAs) are formed during high-heat cooking of meat and are associated with the increased risk of gastrointestinal and colorectal cancers (Sinha et al 1998; Zheng and Lee 2009). Pesticide exposure, particularly in agricultural settings, has also been linked to several cancers. Alavanja et al (2013) stated that "epidemiologic studies of agricultural populations show associations between pesticide exposure and cancers of the prostate, lung, and hematopoietic system." Additionally, endocrine-disrupting chemicals (EDCs) such as bisphenol A (BPA), phthalates, and dioxins, commonly found in plastics, food packaging, and industrial by-products, mimic natural hormones and disrupt signaling pathways, especially those involving estrogen and androgen receptors (Diamanti-Kandarakis et al 2009). These disruptions are associated with hormone-sensitive cancers like breast, prostate, and testicular cancers (Zhou et al 2014). WHO and United Nation Environment Programme (UNEP) report that EDCs may lead to "increased risk of hormone-related cancers and infertility" (WHO/UNEP 2013). Together, these chemical agents contribute to cancer risk through a variety of mechanisms, including genotoxicity, epigenetic alteration, oxidative stress, and receptor-mediated pathways, especially with chronic exposure and accumulation in tissues over time.

- *Biological Factor*: Biological factors such as diet, physical inactivity, food-derived mutagens, nitrosamines, infections, and hormonal imbalances significantly influence cancer development. Diets rich in red and processed meats, low in fiber, and high in saturated fats are strongly linked to colorectal, gastric, and pancreatic cancers (Bouvard et al 2015; WCRF/AICR 2018). Processed meats contain nitrates and nitrites, which under acidic stomach conditions form nitrosamines, classified as Group 1 carcinogens (IARC 2010). These compounds induce DNA alkylation, leading to mutations in oncogenes and tumor suppressor genes (Jakszyn and Gonzalez 2006). In addition, HCAs and polycyclic aromatic hydrocarbons (PAHs), formed during high-temperature cooking methods such as grilling and frying, have been shown to be mutagenic and linked to colorectal, prostate, and breast cancers (Sinha et al 1998; Cross et al. 2010). Sedentary behavior and obesity, often stemming from poor diet and lack of physical activity, increase cancer risk by promoting chronic inflammation, insulin resistance, and altered sex hormone metabolism (Calle and Kaaks 2004; Moore et al 2016). Physical inactivity is associated with higher incidence of endometrial, colon, and breast cancers, possibly through increased levels of circulating estrogens and insulin-like growth factors (Friedenreich et al 2010). Moreover, infections by certain viruses and bacteria play a major biological role in oncogenesis. For example, HPV infection is responsible for nearly 100% of cervical cancers (Walboomers et al 1999), H. pylori for approximately 90% of non-cardia gastric cancers (Peek and Blaser 2002), and hepatitis B and C viruses are strongly associated with hepatocellular carcinoma (El-Serag 2012). According to de Martel et al (2020), "nearly 13% of global cancer cases are attributable to infections."

  Dietary deficiencies, particularly of antioxidant vitamins (A, C, E) and minerals like selenium and zinc, weaken cellular defense against oxidative DNA damage, thereby facilitating carcinogenesis (Ames et al 1995; Ferguson 2010). Additionally, hormonal factors, especially prolonged exposure to estrogens (endogenous or through hormone replacement therapy), are associated with breast and endometrial cancers (Key et al 2001; Yager and Davidson 2006). Together, these biological elements act by modulating inflammation, DNA stability, immune response, and hormonal pathways—thereby significantly increasing cancer susceptibility.

10.3.3 Shared Risk Factors Between CVDs and Cancer

Several common risk factors contribute to both CVDs and cancer, and addressing these risk factors can significantly reduce the burden of both diseases:

- *Tobacco Use*: Smoking is the leading modifiable risk factor for both CVDs and cancer, particularly lung cancer. According to the American Cancer Society (ACS), smoking is responsible for 30% of cancer-related deaths and 11% of cardiovascular deaths globally (American Cancer Society (ACS) 2021). In India, smoking and tobacco use are the leading causes of oral cancer, and they contribute to CVD (Borse et al 2019).
- *Obesity and Physical Inactivity*: Both CVDs and cancer have strong links to obesity, sedentary lifestyles, and poor dietary habits. Rising rates of obesity in India, particularly among the urban population, have been associated with an increased risk of both CVDs and certain cancers such as colon cancer (Masoudkabir et al 2023).
- *Diet and Nutrition*: Diets rich in processed foods, sugary beverages, and saturated fats increase the risk of heart disease and cancer, particularly colon cancer. In India, dietary transitions toward high-calorie, nutrient-poor foods have contributed to the rise in both conditions (Zodpey and Subramanian 2018).
- *Chronic Inflammation*: Chronic low-grade inflammation is a shared pathophysiological mechanism that contributes to both CVDs and cancer. Inflammation, caused by factors

such as diet, obesity, and chronic infections, can accelerate atherosclerosis and promote tumor development (Coussens and Werb 2002).

10.4 MILLET COMPONENTS IN CVD AND CANCER MANAGEMENT

Millets have a unique nutritional profile that makes them suitable for managing cardiovascular health and cancer. Their cardioprotective effects are attributed to their rich content of dietary fiber, antioxidants, and essential minerals as well as the role millets play in scavenging cancerous cells.

10.4.1 Mechanism of Millets for Heart Health and Scavenging Cancerous Cells

Lipid Profile Improvement: Soluble fibers in millets promote bile acid excretion, reducing cholesterol levels. A systematic review and meta-analysis was carried out to assess the impact of millet consumption on lipid profiles, including TC, triacylglycerol, HDL-C, LDL-cholesterol (LDL-C), and very-LDL-C (VLDL-C) (Anitha et al 2021a). The findings from 19 studies revealed that consuming millets for as little as 21 days up to 4 months led to significant reductions in TC, triacylglycerol, LDL-C, and VLDL-C by 8.0, 9.5, 10, and 9.0%, respectively ($P < 0.01$). Four studies specifically showed that millet intake brought TC and triacylglycerol levels down to normal ranges (<200 mg/dL and <150 mg/dL, respectively). Additionally, eating millet-based meals resulted in a 6.0% increase in HDL-C, a 4.0% reduction in systolic BP, a 5.0% reduction in diastolic BP, and a 7.0% decrease in BMI. These results indicate that millet consumption helps lower hyperlipidemia and hypertension, while also increasing HDL-C (good cholesterol), which could help reduce the risk of hypertension and atherosclerotic CVDs in the future (Anitha et al 2021a).

Blood Pressure Regulation: High BP has now become a major public health problem and a leading cause of death and disability in many countries worldwide. It affects the quality of life among hypertensive patients in terms of physical, physiological, social, and environmental domains. High levels of magnesium and potassium in millets act as natural vasodilators, reducing hypertension. After screening, 45 subjects with untreated mild hypertension received a daily average of approximately 50 g of whole foxtail millet, replacing their partial regular staple food for the clinical intervention, and were included in the analyses. Measurements included BP, RAAS, blood lipids, fasting blood glucose, anthropometric indices, body composition, and bone density. After 12 weeks of whole foxtail millet diet intervention, significant reductions in the participants' SBP (4.13 mmHg, $P = 0.022$) and DBP (3.49 mmHg, $P = 0.002$) were observed (Hou et al 2018).The low sodium content further supports healthy BP.

Antioxidant Activity: Millets contain bioactive compounds like polyphenols and flavonoids that neutralize free radicals, thereby lowering oxidative stress and inflammation. These processes play a central role in regulating the onset and advancement of chronic conditions, including cancer, CVD, and autoimmune disorders (Chavda et al 2024). Ferulic acid boosts the activity of antioxidant enzymes that eliminate free radicals, acting as a direct scavenger itself. It effectively targets hydrogen peroxide, superoxide, hydroxyl radicals, and nitrogen dioxide. Compared to caffeic acid, ferulic acid shows superior scavenging of NO and ABTS + radicals (Maurya and Devasagayam 2010). At 250 mg/L, it nearly fully scavenges hydroxyl radicals in a Fenton reaction system (Ou et al 2003). These compounds further protect against lipid peroxidation and endothelial injury. Giri et al (2024) illustrate in Figure 10.1 how millets' anti-cancer bioactivities combat cancer development.

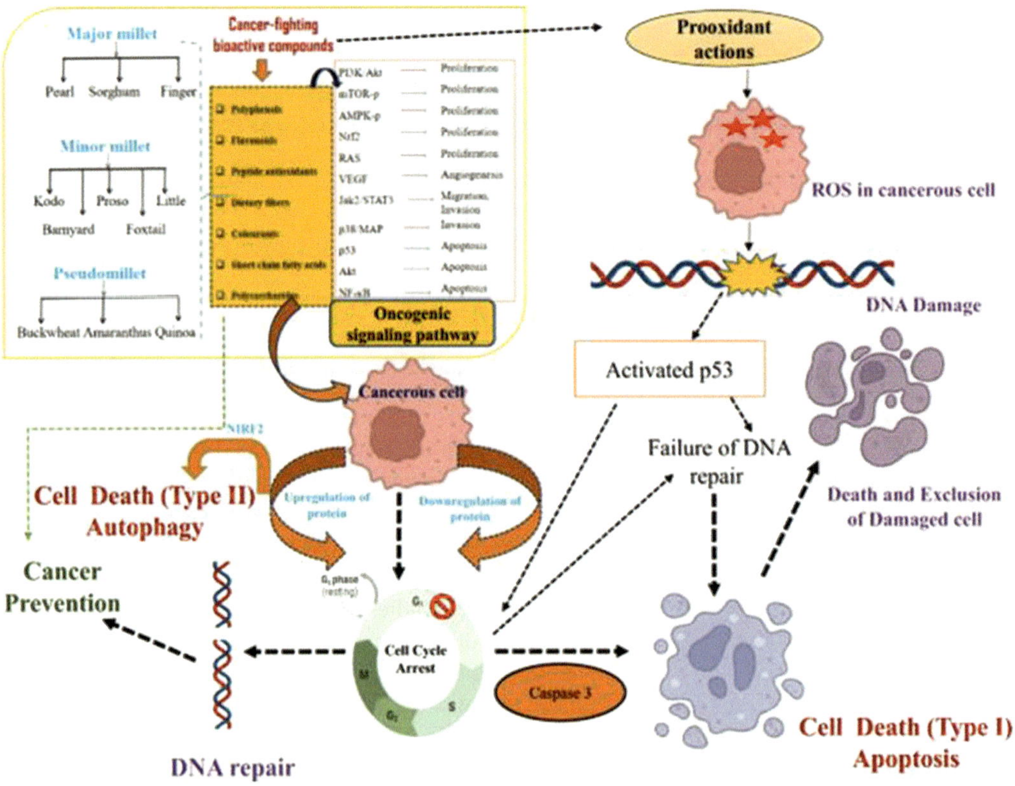

FIGURE 10.1 Mechanism of cancer prevention by cancer-fighting bioactive compounds of millets. (Source: Reprinted from "Potential therapeutic use of millet with broad spectrum anti-cancer properties: current trends and prospects" by Giri, A., Sultana, S., Roy, A., Ray, D., Barui, I., and Sengupta, S., 2024, *Discover Food*, *4*(1), 190).)

Glycemic Control: According to the WHO, "diabetes is a chronic disease that occurs either when the pancreas does not produce enough insulin or when the body cannot effectively use the insulin it produces" (WHO 2023). DM is a metabolic disorder characterized by hyperglycemic conditions resulting from inadequate insulin production or sensitivity. Millets' low glycemic index prevents spikes in blood sugar levels, reducing the risk of metabolic syndrome and type 2 diabetes (Tomar et al 2018). Millets provide rich amounts of protein, fiber, vitamins, minerals, and bioactive compounds. These nutrients can enhance insulin sensitivity by elevating adiponectin levels and blocking dipeptidyl peptidase-IV (DPP-IV) activity. They also suppress α-amylase and α-glucosidase, slowing glucose digestion and absorption. The other potential mechanisms may include the modulation of gluconeogenesis and glycolysis via the PI3K/AKT signaling pathway (increased glucose uptake and utilization), improving glucose transporters (increased glucose uptake by cells), increased leptin levels (appetite regulation), inhibition of NF-κB pathway, less production of cytokine, and mitigation of oxidative and nitrosative stress. The complex carbohydrate, fiber, and phenolic compounds may increase the abundance of probiotics and SCFAs concentration (Kumar et al 2025). Improved insulin sensitivity indirectly lowers cardiovascular risk.

Weight Management: The high fiber and protein content in millets promote satiety, aiding in weight management and reducing obesity-related CVD risk. Millets are emerging as a functional food in weight-management strategies due to their high fiber, low glycemic index, and plant-based protein content, which together promote satiety and metabolic health. The dietary fiber in millets slows digestion and prolongs fullness, thereby reducing total food intake. As noted by Taylor (2004), "the high fiber content in millets contributes to delayed gastric emptying and reduced postprandial blood glucose peaks." Moreover, proteins in millets increase satiety hormones such as peptide YY (PYY) and GLP-1, supporting energy balance and appetite control (Hall 2010). A study by Radha et al (2024) demonstrated that the intake of high-fiber food helps to improve bowel function and reduce the incidence of obesity by improving digestion and absorption in the body which is crucial for controlling weight and preventing obesity-related complications. The high-fiber content in millets helps in stimulating the satiety and helps in reducing obesity, constipation, abdominal cramps, and bloating. According to the International Crops Research Institute for the Semi-Arid Tropics (ICRISAT), "millets have a GI 30–50% lower than refined grains, making them suitable for weight management and diabetic diets" (ICRISAT 2020). Obesity is a major modifiable risk factor for CVDs, and millet-based diets have been associated with improved lipid profiles and reduced inflammation (Samtiya et al 2023). WHO recognizes that "whole grains high in dietary fiber, such as millets, can aid in body weight control and lower the risk of heart disease" (WHO 2021b). The regular consumption of millets, therefore, supports holistic weight management by addressing satiety, blood sugar control, lipid metabolism, and inflammation—factors intricately linked with CVD prevention. Figure 10.2 shows the mechanism of CVD prevention by bioactive components of millets.

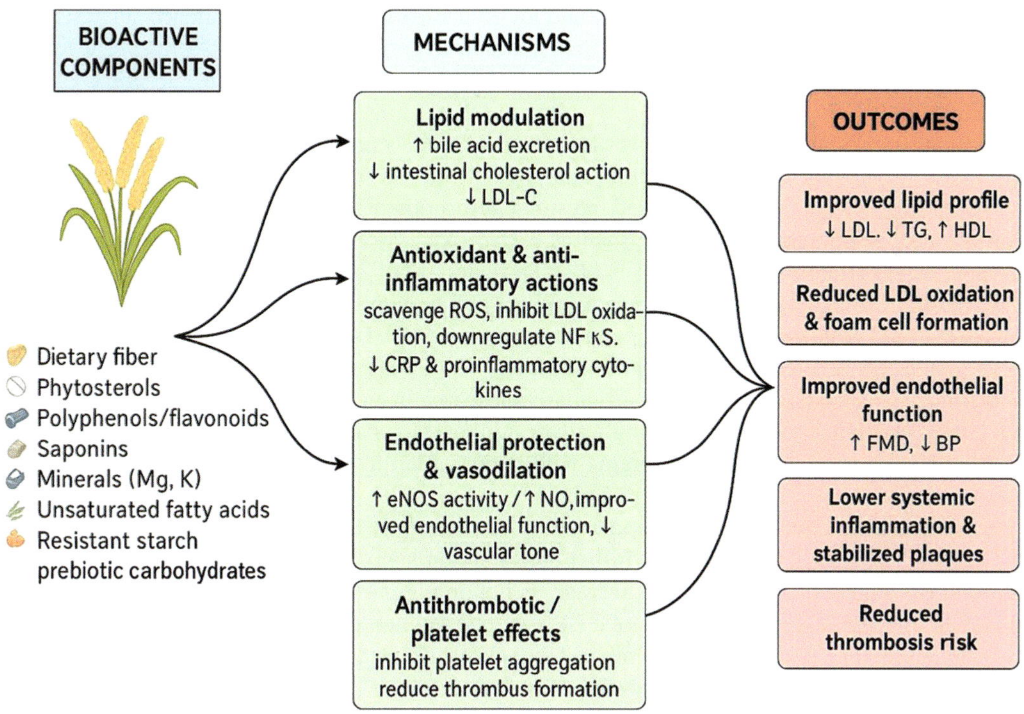

FIGURE 10.2 Mechanism of CVD prevention by bioactive components of millet.

10.4.2 Clinical Evidences of Effects of Millets on CVD

Studies have demonstrated significant reductions in LDL and TC among participants consuming millet-based diets. Consumption of proso millet protein concentrate resulted in an increase in the plasma HDL-C and adiponectin levels (Ambati and Sucharitha 2019). The role of dietary interventions in managing dyslipidemia is well-established, and millets have garnered increasing attention as functional foods with lipid-lowering properties. A growing body of clinical evidence supports the efficacy of millets in reducing serum cholesterol levels, particularly TC, LDL-C, and TG, while sometimes elevating HDL-C.

A meta-analysis by Anitha et al (2021b) comprising 19 human intervention studies reported significant reductions in TC (8.0%), LDL-C (10.0%), and TG (10.0%) among participants who consumed millet-based diets for durations ranging from 21 days to 4 months. Importantly, the studies involved various types of millets such as finger millet, pearl millet, foxtail millet, and little millet. The lipid-lowering effect was more pronounced in individuals with existing hyperlipidemia compared to normolipidemic individuals, suggesting a therapeutic role for millets in cardiovascular risk management.

One of the randomized controlled trials included in the meta-analysis examined the impact of finger millet on lipid profiles in T2DM patients. The results demonstrated a substantial reduction in LDL-C (12.8%) and TG (13.5%) levels after 12 weeks of intervention compared to a rice-based control group (Sudha et al 2018). The study attributed these effects to the high content of dietary fiber and polyphenols in finger millet, which may reduce cholesterol absorption and enhance bile acid excretion.

A notable study by Anitha et al (2021a) examined the effects of millet consumption on various lipid markers, including TC, triacylglycerol, HDL-C, LDL-C, and VLDL-C. The results from 19 studies indicated that consuming millets for 21 days to 4 months led to significant reductions in TC, triacylglycerol, LDL-C, and VLDL-C by 8.0, 9.5, 10, and 9.0%, respectively ($P < 0.01$). Four studies found that millet intake brought TC and triacylglycerol levels back to normal (<200 mg/dL and <150 mg/dL, respectively). Additionally, millet-based meals increased HDL-C by 6.0%, reduced systolic and diastolic BP by 4.0 and 5.0%, and lowered BMI by 7.0%. This evidence suggests that millet consumption helps manage hyperlipidemia and hypertension, while also raising levels of HDL-C (good cholesterol), which may lower the risk of hypertension and atherosclerotic CVDs in the future.

Mechanistically, the cholesterol-lowering effects of millets are thought to stem from their rich content of insoluble fiber, resistant starch, and phytochemicals such as ferulic acid and flavonoids. These components contribute to reduced intestinal absorption of lipids and improved lipid metabolism through modulation of enzymes such as 3-Hydroxy-3-Methylglutaryl Coenzyme A (HMG-CoA) reductase (Hadimani and Malleshi 1993; Develaraja et al 2016).

Given the compelling clinical evidence, millets can be considered a viable dietary option for improving lipid profiles, especially in populations at risk of CVDs.

Hypertension is a leading modifiable risk factor for CVDs and affects over a billion people worldwide. Nutritional interventions, particularly those rich in dietary fiber, magnesium, potassium, and bioactive compounds, are increasingly advocated for effective BP management. In this context, millets have emerged as functional grains with potential antihypertensive effects, owing to their rich nutritional profile and low glycemic index.

A comprehensive meta-analysis conducted by Anitha et al (2021b), which included 15 human clinical studies, revealed that regular millet consumption significantly reduced both systolic and diastolic BP among participants. The average reduction observed was approximately 4–6 mmHg in systolic BP and 2–4 mmHg in diastolic BP over intervention periods ranging from three weeks to four months. These changes, while modest, are clinically meaningful and contribute to reduced cardiovascular risk at the population level.

Hou et al (2018) reported that a 12-week intervention with a whole foxtail millet diet led to significant reductions in systolic and diastolic BP, BMI, and fat mass among participants ($P < 0.05$).

Additionally, in spontaneously hypertensive rats (SHRs), a four-week supplementation with raw and extruded foxtail millet peptide samples (200 mg peptides/kg body weight) effectively lowered serum angiotensin-converting enzyme (ACE) activity, angiotensin II levels, and BP compared to controls.

Mechanistically, millets are rich in magnesium, a mineral known for its vasodilatory and calcium-channel blocking properties. Furthermore, the polyphenols and peptides present in millets have shown ACE inhibitory activity in *in vitro* and animal studies, which may contribute to BP regulation (Nambiar et al 2011; Shobana et al 2013).

These findings collectively affirm that millets, when consumed regularly as part of a balanced diet, can contribute to the prevention and management of hypertension, particularly in populations with high cardiovascular risk. The incorporation of millets into traditional and modern dietary patterns could thus serve as an accessible and culturally acceptable strategy for BP control. The functional components of millets for prevention of CVD are shown in Table 10.1.

10.4.3 Clinical Evidences of Effects of Millets on Cancer

Increased levels of antioxidant enzymes such as superoxide dismutase and catalase were observed in individuals consuming millet-rich diets (Giri et al 2024).

TABLE 10.1
Functional Components of Millets for the Prevention of Cardiovascular Disease (CVD)

Functional Component	Where in Millets/Examples	Mechanisms Relevant to CVD	References
Dietary fiber (soluble + insoluble)	High in most millets (finger, foxtail, little, proso)	Lowers LDL and total cholesterol by reducing bile acid reabsorption, improves satiety and weight control.	Anitha et al (2021a)
Resistant starch/slowly digestible carbohydrates	Present in whole-grain millets and some processed forms	Lowers postprandial glucose and insulin excursions → reduces insulin resistance. Improves lipid profile indirectly.	Hou et al (2018)
Polyphenols and flavonoids (phenolic acids, tannins)	Especially high in finger millet, foxtail millet, and millet bran/shell	Antioxidant + anti-inflammatory actions reduce the oxidative modification of LDL and vascular inflammation.	Devi et al (2014)
Phytosterols	Present across millets (whole grain)	Compete with cholesterol for intestinal absorption → reduce LDL-cholesterol.	Jacob et al (2024)
Essential minerals (Mg, K, Ca)	Millets are good sources (finger millet: Ca, many millets: Mg, K)	Mg and K lower blood pressure; Ca supports vascular and metabolic health.	Hou et al (2018)
Tocopherols, carotenoids (lipid-soluble antioxidants)	Variable across millet types (whole grain > refined)	Protect lipids from oxidative damage; support endothelial health.	Balyatanda et al (2024)
Saponins, tannins and other phytochemicals	Found in outer layers and bran of millets	May reduce cholesterol absorption, exert anti-inflammatory effects, and inhibit foam-cell formation.	Liu et al (2023)
Bioactive peptides/protein fractions	Generated during processing (malt, fermentation)	Some peptides show ACE-inhibitory or vasodilatory effects → antihypertensive action.	Park et al (2021)

Recent scientific and medical research suggests that millet may play a significant role in cancer prevention and therapy through various mechanisms, including antioxidant activity, apoptosis induction, anti-inflammatory effects, and inhibition of cancer cell proliferation.

Oxidative stress, resulting from an imbalance between free radicals and antioxidants, is a known contributor to cancer development. Millets are rich in polyphenolic compounds such as ferulic acid, catechins, gallic acid, and quercetin. These compounds act as potent antioxidants, neutralizing free radicals and preventing oxidative DNA damage (Rudrapal et al 2022). Chandrasekara and Shahidi (2011) analyzed phenolic extracts from several millets and found strong radical scavenging abilities and inhibition of oxidative DNA scission, indicating their potential role in reducing mutagenesis and carcinogenesis.

Apoptosis, or programmed cell death, is essential for eliminating cells that have undergone malignant transformation. Millet-derived polyphenols have been shown to activate caspase pathways, modulate Bcl-2 family proteins, and promote mitochondrial dysfunction leading to apoptosis in cancer cells as shown in Figure 10.1. Devi et al (2014) demonstrated that finger millet extracts induced apoptosis in MCF-7 breast cancer cells by increasing caspase-3 activity and disrupting mitochondrial membrane potential.

Millet extracts have demonstrated anti-proliferative effects against various human cancer cell lines, including HT-29 (colon), HepG2 (liver), and HeLa (cervical) cells. This activity is often linked to the downregulation of proliferation markers and upregulation of tumor suppressor genes. Choi et al (2007) found that proso millet extract suppressed proliferation of HT-29 colon cancer cells by inhibiting cyclooxygenase-2 (COX-2) expression and enhancing apoptosis-related gene expression.

Dietary fiber in millet contributes to gut health and the production of SCFAs like butyrate through microbial fermentation. Butyrate has demonstrated the ability to inhibit colon cancer cell growth, induce apoptosis, and act as a histone deacetylase (HDAC) inhibitor. Ferguson and Harris (1996) outlined the role of dietary fiber and SCFAs in colon cancer prevention, emphasizing how fiber-rich diets reduce risk by modulating inflammation and improving gut microbiota.

Chronic inflammation is a significant contributor to tumorigenesis. Millet contains bioactive compounds that inhibit pro-inflammatory cytokines such as TNF-α, IL-6, and NF-κB, thereby reducing cancer-promoting inflammation. There are various functional factors present in the millets which help in reducing cancer cells as shown in Table 10.2. Amadou et al (2013) demonstrated that pearl millet polyphenolic extracts reduced inflammatory markers in LPS-stimulated macrophages.

Millets exhibit a range of anti-cancer properties, including antioxidant activity, apoptosis induction, anti-proliferative effects, and inflammation modulation. These actions are primarily attributed to their rich composition of bioactive compounds. While clinical data are still emerging, current medical and experimental evidence strongly supports the inclusion of millet in cancer-preventive diets. Further human trials are necessary to fully establish the therapeutic potential of millet against cancer.

10.5 MILLET-BASED FOOD PRODUCTS FOR CVD AND CANCER: AVAILABILITY AND OPPORTUNITIES

Millets are small grains that are packed with nutrients and offer many health benefits. Today, people are becoming more aware of what they eat. Instead of just eating to feel full, many now focus on foods that are rich in nutrients. Millets fit well into this shift in food habits, as they help in preventing and managing several NCDs like diabetes, CVD, and obesity. Millets are also farmer-friendly. They are cheap to grow, need very little water, and can be easily grown without using harmful chemicals. India grows many types of millets such as bajra (pearl millet), ragi (finger millet), jhangora (barnyard millet), jowar (sorghum), barri (proso or common millet), kangni (foxtail or Italian millet), and kodra (kodo millet) (Bhatt et al 2022).

TABLE 10.2
Functional Components of Various Millets and Their Roles in Inhibiting Cancer Cell Growth

Millets	Cancer	Functional Factor	References
Pearl millet	Colon cancer	Total Platelet Count (TPC), hydroxyl and peroxyl radical inhibition	Chandrasekara and Shahidi (2011)
Foxtail millet	Colon cancer	35 kDa protein Foxtail Millet Bran Protein (FMBP) extracted from foxtail millet bran	Shan et al (2014)
	Breast cancer	Bound Polyphenol of Inner Shell (BPIS) from foxtail millet bran (vitexin and syringic acid)	Kuruburu et al (2022a) and Zhang et al (2021)
	Breast cancer	Phytochemical rich fractions (free and bound phenolics)	Kuruburu et al (2022a)
	Liver cancer	TPC and peroxyl radical scavenging capacity	Zhang and Liu (2015)
Proso millet	Colon cancer	Vanillin (4-hydroxy-3 methoxybenzaldehyde)	Ramadoss and Sivalingam (2020)
	Breast cancer		Ramadoss and Sivalingam (2021)
	Colon cancer		Ramadoss and Sivalingam (2021)
Barnyard millet	Breast cancer	Vanillin (4-hydroxy-3 methoxybenzaldehyde), alpha-amino butyric acid	Ramadoss and Sivalingam (2021) and Sharma et al (2016b)
Finger millet	Brest cancer	Free phenolics (procyanidin B1, 3-O-methyl quercetin, and epigallocatechin)	Kuruburu et al (2022b)
Kodo millet	Colon cancer	TPC, hydroxyl and peroxyl radical inhibition	Chandrasekara and Shahidi (2011)

India is one of the largest producers and exporters of millets in the world. In 2020, India produced about 41% of the world's millets and was the fifth-largest exporter. In the year 2020–21, India exported millets worth about USD 26.97 million. The main countries that bought millets from India were Nepal, the United Arab Emirates (UAE), Saudi Arabia, Libya, Tunisia, Morocco, the United Kingdom (UK), Yemen, Oman, and Algeria. Among these, Nepal (USD 6.09 million), UAE (USD 4.84 million), and Saudi Arabia (USD 3.84 million) were the top importers. To promote the use of millets, the Government of India declared them as "Nutri-cereals" in April 2018. It also made new rules to allow easier movement of extra millet harvests from one state to another. Through the Food Corporation of India (FCI), these surplus grains can now be sent to states that request them in advance before the harvest begins (Bhatt et al 2022).

Millet-based food products are becoming increasingly available in the market due to their recognized health benefits. Millet-based food products such as flours, ready-to-eat (RTE) snacks, breakfast cereals, and fermented beverages are becoming increasingly available in the market due to their recognized health benefits, including their potential roles in reducing the risk of CVDs, diabetes, celiac disease, and certain cancers (Saleh et al 2013; Devi et al 2014; Srivastava et al 2020). The different millet-based food products developed are shown in Table 10.3.

Opportunities:

In the face of rising global health challenges, particularly the increasing prevalence of CVDs and cancer, the demand for functional foods with therapeutic potential is higher than ever. Among various dietary interventions, millet-based food products present a unique and underutilized opportunity to address these health burdens through nutrition. Millets are nutrient-dense, gluten-free, and rich in bioactive compounds with documented cardioprotective and anti-cancer effects. Transforming millets into

TABLE 10.3
Different Products Developed from Different Millets

Product	Ingredients	Reference
Flat bread	Pearl millet flour	Siroha et al (2016)
	Wheat flour and extruded finger millet flour	Kumar et al (2021)
	Wheat flour and different millets (finger, foxtail, barnyard, kodo, little, proso)	Sharma and Gujral (2019)
	Wheat, finger millet	Panghal et al (2019)
Bread	Pearl millet flour	Nehra et al (2021)
	Foxtail millet flour	Passi et al (2023)
Biscuit	Foxtail millet	Reaz et al (2023)
	Finger millet	Chinma et al (2022) and Saha et al (2011)
Cookies	Foxtail millet	Patimah et al (2019)
	Flour blends were prepared by mixing foxtail, barnyard, and kodo millet flour	Sharma et al (2016a)
	Pearl millet flour	Florence et al (2014)
Muffins	Barnyard millet, refined wheat flour	Goswami et al (2015)
Cake	Proso millet, corn meal, cake flour	Xiao et al (2023)
Dalia	Foxtail millet	Arora et al (2023)
Sattu	Foxtail millet	Arora et al (2023)

a variety of value-added food products offers a sustainable, culturally acceptable, and health-promoting strategy with broad-reaching implications for both public health and the functional food industry.

1. *Nutritional and Therapeutic Potential of Millets*

   Millets such as finger millet, pearl millet, foxtail millet, kodo millet, barnyard millet, and proso millet are rich in dietary fiber, resistant starch, polyphenols, flavonoids, and essential micronutrients like magnesium, potassium, and iron. These nutritional properties play a significant role in

   - Lowering BP
   - Regulating blood glucose
   - Improving lipid profiles
   - Neutralizing free radicals
   - Reducing chronic inflammation

   Given that oxidative stress and inflammation are key mediators of both, atherosclerosis and tumor development, millets offer a dual-action preventive mechanism that is ideal for incorporation into therapeutic diets.

2. *Innovations in Millet-Based Functional Foods*

   Millets have great potential to be used in making a wide variety of functional foods especially for people with heart disease and cancer. These foods can be developed in ways that preserve or even boost the natural health-promoting compounds found in millets. Some product categories include the following:

   - *RTE Foods*: These include millet flakes, puffed snacks, extruded products, and energy bars that are rich in natural antioxidants. They are convenient, tasty, and support heart and immune health.
   - *Fermented Foods*: Millet-based probiotic drinks and yogurts can improve digestion and strengthen the immune system, which is especially helpful in cancer prevention and care.

- *Bakery Items*: Products like cookies, breads, and cakes made with millet flour can be further enhanced by adding omega-3 fatty acids or plant-based proteins, making them healthier options for everyday use.
- *Meal Replacements and Porridges*: Millet-based porridges or gruels can be made more nutritious by adding ingredients like flaxseed, turmeric, or moringa. These are ideal for patients needing special diets, both at home and in clinical settings.
- *Beverages*: Millets can also be used to make healthy drinks such as smoothies, malted beverages, or herbal teas, often combined with medicinal herbs and natural antioxidants.

These millet-based innovations not only match today's growing demand for healthy and convenient food options but also provide specific health benefits. They can play an important role in preventing or managing chronic illnesses like CVD and cancer.

3. *Clinical and Market-Based Opportunities*

As more research highlights the health benefits of millets, there is growing interest in using them as part of medical nutrition therapy especially for people at risk of or living with CVD and cancer. Doctors and dietitians are now recommending whole grains and low-glycemic index foods more often, and millets are an excellent fit for these diets.

From a business and market perspective, the global demand for natural, organic, and health-focused foods is rising. This creates strong potential for millet-based products. In countries like India and regions of Africa, where millets have been part of traditional farming and food culture, promoting millet-based diets can bring both health and economic benefits. Around the world, the increasing popularity of plant-based and gluten-free foods also supports the growth of millet products.

Another area is personalized nutrition that is creating millet-based foods designed for specific health needs, age groups, or even based on a person's genetic background. This approach, known as *nutrigenomics*, is an emerging field where diet is customized to help prevent disease based on individual genetic makeup.

4. *Sustainable and Localized Solutions*

Making food products from millets is not just good for health, it also helps the environment and supports food security. Millets are strong crops that can grow in dry areas, need very little water, and help protect the environment by supporting plant and animal life. Growing more millets can reduce our need for crops like wheat and rice, which use a lot of water and other resources.

Also, using local traditions and old recipes in making millet foods can help people accept and enjoy them more. Bringing back dishes like ragi mudde, bajra khichdi, millet dosas, and upma connects our food traditions with modern healthy eating. This makes millet foods both tasty and familiar, while also being good for our health.

5. *Research and Innovation Pathways*

Although millets have great potential, there are still some challenges in making millet-based products more appealing. These include improving taste, shelf life, and how well the products hold up during processing. But ongoing research in areas like food technology, packaging, enzyme use, and nutrient fortification can help solve these problems and improve product quality.

To move forward, we need

- Clinical trials to prove how millet-based foods can help prevent or manage heart disease and cancer.
- Bioavailability studies to check if the beneficial compounds in millets are well absorbed and used by the body.
- Consumer education to help people understand the health benefits of millets and encourage them to include millets in their daily diet.

To make millet-based foods more common and popular, it's important for scientists, food makers, farmers, and health workers to work together.

10.6 CONCLUSION

Millets are powerful grains with great potential to improve health, especially in preventing and managing heart disease and different types of cancer. They are rich in fiber, antioxidants, and important minerals, which makes them a smart and healthy choice for daily diets. Including millets regularly in meals can help people take charge of their health in a natural way. Although some studies have explored the benefits of millets, especially lesser-known ones, more scientific research is still needed. This includes understanding how the nutrients in millets work in the body and how millet-based foods can be used in large-scale health programs.

Often called "*Nutri-cereals*," millets are gaining worldwide attention not only for their excellent nutrition but also for their health-boosting properties. With growing concerns about NCDs like heart disease and cancer, it is important to look at natural foods that can help prevent these illnesses. Millets are emerging as one such food with proven benefits backed by scientific studies.

The heart-health benefits of millets come from their unique nutrition profile. They are high in fiber, good fats, complex carbohydrates, and minerals like magnesium, potassium, and iron. These help lower bad cholesterol, control blood sugar, reduce stress in the body, and improve blood flow. Research has shown that millets help lower LDL (bad cholesterol), increase HDL (good cholesterol), and improve overall heart health. Their fiber also helps control BP and gives a feeling of fullness, which helps with weight management. Millets are also rich in natural plant chemicals like phenolic acids, flavonoids, and tannins, which have strong antioxidant effects. These help fight harmful molecules in the body, protect blood vessels, and lower the risk of heart attacks and strokes.

Besides heart health, millets have shown promise in preventing cancer. Their high antioxidant and polyphenol content supports cell repair, strengthens the immune system, and slows the growth of tumors. Some types of millets—like finger millet, foxtail millet, and pearl millet—have been found to kill cancer cells, stop them from spreading, and block the growth of blood vessels in tumors. These effects have been seen in cancers like breast, colon, liver, and cervical cancer. Millets also fight inflammation, which is known to play a major role in cancer development. By lowering inflammation, millets help create a healthier body environment that reduces cancer risk. While lab and animal studies support these findings, more human research is needed to confirm these effects.

On a larger scale, promoting millets in diets not only supports health but also environmental and food security goals. Millets grow very well in dry place, without much water and fertilizer, and are resistant to pests and climate changes. This makes them important for sustainable farming and feeding growing populations in tough conditions. Eating more millets can help fight both malnutrition and chronic diseases at the same time. Millets also have a low glycemic index, which means they raise blood sugar slowly. This makes them ideal for people with diabetes or those at risk of it a condition closely linked to heart problems and some cancers.

In summary, millets are amazing and truly natural gems, packed with abundant health benefits that make them an exceptional choice for preventing and managing lifestyle-related diseases such as diabetes, heart conditions, and obesity. For centuries people have known about how good millets are from ages, conventional knowledge has celebrated the nutritional and medicinal value of millets, but now modern scientific research is increasingly authenticating these age-old claims with factual proof.

To unlock the full potential of millets, more extensive research is essential, especially studies involving real people to better understand how millets impact health in real-world settings. Alongside this, raising public awareness about the benefits of millets, implementing supportive government policies, and promoting health education are all crucial steps. These efforts will help integrate millets into everyday diets, ensuring that more people can enjoy their nutritional advantages.

As globally people continue their search for healthier and more sustainable food sources, millets stand out as a promising solution. Their resilience, low environmental footprint, and rich nutrient profile position them well for a significant role in future nutrition and wellness worldwide. Embracing millets today could lay the foundation for healthier populations and a more incorporating planet tomorrow.

REFERENCES

ACS (American Cancer Society). 2021. *Cancer Facts and Figures 2021.* American Cancer Society. https://www.cancer.org/research/cancer-facts-statistics/all-cancer-facts-figures/cancer-facts-figures-2021.html

ADA (American Diabetes Association). 2022. Cardiovascular disease and risk management: Standards of medical care in diabetes. *Diabetes Care* 45, no. Supplement_1: S144–S174. https://doi.org/10.2337/dc22-S011

Afshin, A., Forouzanfar, M. H., Reitsma, M. B., Reitsma, M. B., Sur, P., Estep, K., Lee, A., and GBD Obesity Collaborators. 2017. Health effects of overweight and obesity in 195 countries over 25 years. *NEJM* 377, no. 1: 13–27. https://doi.org/10.1056/NEJMoa1614362

Ahamed, V. P. A., Joshi, A., Mudey, A., Choudhari, S., Raut, J., and Ahmed, S. 2024. Unlocking the potential: Millets and their impact on diabetes management. *Cureus* 16, no. 14: e59283. https://doi.org/10.7759/cureus.59283.

Alavanja, M. C. R., Ross, M. K., and Bonner, M. R. 2013. Increased cancer burden among pesticide applicators and others due to pesticide exposure. *CA: A Cancer Journal for Clinicians* 63, no. 2: 120–142. https://doi.org/10.3322/caac.21170

Amadou, I., Gounga, M. E., and Le, G. W. 2013. Millets: Nutritional composition, some health benefits and processing—A review. *EJFA* 25, no. 7: 501–508. https://doi.org/10.9755/ejfa.v25i7.12045

Ambati, K., and Sucharitha, K. V. 2019. Millets-review on nutritional profiles and health benefits. *International Journal of Recent Scientific Research* 10, no. 7: 33943–33948.

Ames, B. N., Shigenaga, M. K., and Hagen, T. M. 1995. Oxidants, antioxidants, and the degenerative diseases of aging. *Proceedings of the National Academy of Sciences* 90, no. 17: 7915–7922. https://doi.org/10.1073/pnas.90.17.7915

Anitha, S., Botha, R., Kane-Potaka, J., Givens, D. I., Rajendran, A., Tsusaka, T. W., and Bhandari, R. K. 2021a. Can millet consumption help manage hyperlipidemia and obesity?: A systematic review and meta-analysis. *Frontiers in Nutrition* 8: 700778. https://doi.org/10.3389/fnut.2021.700778

Anitha, S., Kane-Potaka, J., Tsusaka, T. W., Rajendran, A., Botha, R., and Givens, D. I. 2021b. A systematic review and meta-analysis of the potential of millets for managing and reducing the risk of developing diabetes mellitus and cardiovascular diseases. *Frontiers in Nutrition* 8: 687428. https://doi.org/10.3389/fnut.2021.687428

Arora, L., Aggarwal, R., Dhaliwal, I., Gupta, O. P., and Kaushik, P. 2023. Assessment of sensory and nutritional attributes of foxtail millet-based food products. *Frontiers in Nutrition* 10: 1146545. https://doi.org/10.3389/fnut.2023.1146545

Aune, D., Keum, N., Giovannucci, E., Fadnes, L. T., Boffetta, P., Greenwood, D. C., Tonstad, S., Vatten, L. J., Riboli, E., and Norat, T. 2016. Whole grain consumption and risk of cardiovascular disease, cancer, and all cause and cause specific mortality: systematic review and dose-response meta-analysis of prospective studies. *BMJ* 353. https://doi.org/10.1136/bmj.i2716

Awasthi, J., Mishra, A., Rathod, S., Verma, S., and Pandey, A. K. 2025. A review of the nutraceutical composition of milletsand their health benefits. *Current Functional Foods* 3, no. 2. https://doi.org/10.2174/01266686292987432403200352O3. ISSN: 2666–8629; E-ISSN: 2666-8637

Balkwill, F., and Mantovani, A. 2001. Inflammation and cancer: Back to Virchow? *The Lancet* 357, no. 9255: 539–545. https://doi.org/10.1016/S0140-6736(00)04046-0

Balyatanda, S. B., Gowda, N. A. N., Subbiah, J., Chakraborty, S., Prasad, P. V. V., and Siliveru, K. 2024. Physiochemical, bio, thermal, and non-thermal processing of major and minor millets: A comprehensive review on antinutritional and antioxidant properties. *Foods* 13 no. 22: 3684. https://doi.org/10.3390/foods13223684

Bhatt, S., Verma, P., Sharma, S., and Katnoriya, S. K. 2022. Millet products: Traditional medicinal diet for modern lifestyle health issues. *European Journal of Molecular & Clinical Medicine* 9, no. 7. https://www.researchgate.net/publication/369627236_Millet_Products_Traditional_Medicinal_Diet_For_Modern_Lifestyle_Health_Issues

Booth, F. W., Roberts, C. K., and Laye, M. J. 2012. Lack of exercise is a major cause of chronic diseases. *Comprehensive Physiology* 2, no. 2: 1143–1211. https://doi.org/10.1002/cphy.c110025

Borse, V., Kaur, J., and Sharma, R. 2019. Tobacco and its link to oral cancer: A review of current evidence in India. *Indian Journal of Cancer* 56, no. 4: 293–299. https://doi.org/10.4103/ijc.IJC_458_19

Bosetti, C., McLaughlin, J. K., Tarone, R. E., Pira, E., and La Vecchia, C. 2008. Cancer risk for workers exposed to vinyl chloride: A review of the epidemiologic literature. *European Journal of Cancer Prevention* 17, no. 5: 453–463.

Bouvard, V., Loomis, D., Guyton, K. Z., Grosse, Y., El Ghissassi, F., Benbrahim-Tallaa, L., and Straif, K. 2015. Carcinogenicity of consumption of red and processed meat. *The Lancet Oncology* 16, no. 16: 1599–1600. https://doi.org/10.1016/S1470-2045(15)00444-1

Calle, E. E., and Kaaks, R. 2004. Overweight, obesity and cancer: Epidemiological evidence and proposed mechanisms. *Nature Reviews Cancer* 4, no. 8: 579–591. https://doi.org/10.1038/nrc1408

Chandrasekara, A., and Shahidi, F. 2011. Antiproliferative potential and DNA scission inhibitory activity of phenolics from whole millet grains. *Journal of Functional Foods* 3, no. 3: 159–170. https://doi.org/10.1016/j.jff.2011.03.008

Chavda, V. P., Feehan, J., and Apostolopoulos, V. 2024. Inflammation: The cause of all diseases. *Cells* 13, no. 22: 1906. https://doi.org/10.3390/cells13221906

Chinma, C. E., Ibrahim, P. A., Adedeji, O. E., Ezeocha, V. C., Ohuoba, E. U., Kolo, S. I., and Adebo, O. A. 2022. Physicochemical properties, in vitro digestibility, antioxidant activity and consumer acceptability of biscuits prepared from germinated finger millet and Bambara groundnut flour blends. *Heliyon* 8, no. 10: 10849. https://doi.org/10.1016/j.heliyon.2022.e10849

Choi, Y., Jeong, H. S., Lee, J., and Sung, J. 2007. Effects of processing on the antioxidant activity of proso millet extracts. *Journal of Agricultural and Food Chemistry* 55, no. 23: 9044–9050.

Coussens, L. M., and Werb, Z. 2002. Inflammation and cancer. *Nature* 420, no. 6917: 860–867. https://doi.org/10.1038/nature01322

Cross, A. J., Ferrucci, L. M., Risch, A., Graubard, B. I., Ward, M. H., Park, Y., and Sinha, R. 2010. A large prospective study of meat consumption and colorectal cancer risk: An investigation of potential mechanisms underlying this association. *Cancer Research* 70, no. 6: 2406–2414. https://doi.org/10.1158/0008-5472.CAN-09-3929

Del Pinto, R., Grassi, G., Muiesan, M. L., Borghi, C., Carugo, S., Cicero, A. F., Di Meo, L., Iaccarino, G., Minuz, P., Mulatero, P., and Mulè, G. 2022. World hypertension day 2021 in Italy: results of a nationwide survey. *High Blood Pressure & Cardiovascular Prevention* 29, no. 4: 353–359. https://doi.org/10.1007/s40292-022-00519-4

de Martel, C., Georges, D., Bray, F., Ferlay, J., and Clifford, G. M. 2020. Global burden of cancer attributable to infections in 2018: A worldwide incidence analysis. *The Lancet Global Health* 8, no. 2: e180–e190. https://doi.org/10.1016/S2214-109X(19)30488-7

Després, J. P. 2012. Body fat distribution and risk of cardiovascular disease: An update. *Circulation Research* 126, no. 10: 1301–1313. https://doi.org/10.1161/CIRCULATIONAHA.111.067264

Develaraja, S., Reddy, A., Yadav, M., Jain, S., and Yadav, H. 2016. Whole grains in amelioration of metabolic derangements. *Journal of Nutrition Health and Food Science* 4, no. 4: 1–11. https://doi.org/10.15226/jnhfs.2016.00173

Devi, P. B., Vijayabharathi, R., Sathyabama, S., Malleshi, N. G., and Priyadarisini, V. B. 2014. Health benefits of finger millet (*Eleusine coracana* L.) polyphenols and dietary fiber: A review. *Journal of Food Science and Technology* 51, no. 6: 1021–1040. https://doi.org/10.1007/s13197-011-0584-9

Dhalla, N. S., Temsah, R. M., and Netticadan, T. 2000. Role of oxidative stress in cardiovascular diseases. *Journal of Hypertension* 18, no. 6: 655–673. https://doi.org/10.1097/00004872-200018060-00002

Diamanti-Kandarakis, E., Bourguignon, J. P., Giudice, L. C., Hauser, R., Prins, G. S., Soto, A. M., and Gore, A. C. 2009. Endocrine-disrupting chemicals: An Endocrine Society scientific statement. *Endocrine Reviews* 30, no. 4: 293–342. https://doi.org/10.1210/er.2009-0002

Elrakybi, A., Laubner, K., Zhou, Q., Hug, M. J., and Seufert, J. 2022. Cardiovascular protection by SGLT2 inhibitors – Do anti-inflammatory mechanisms play a role? *Molecular Metabolism* 64: 101549. https://doi.org/10.1016/j.molmet.2022.101549

El-Serag, H. B. 2012. Epidemiology of viral hepatitis and hepatocellular carcinoma. *Gastroenterol* 142, no. 6: 1264–1273.e1. https://doi.org/10.1053/j.gastro.2011.12.061

Ferguson, L. R. 2010. Meat and cancer. *Meat Science* 84, no. 2: 308–313. https://doi.org/10.1016/j.meatsci.2009.06.023

Ferguson, L. R., and Harris, P. J. 1996. Studies on the role of specific dietary fibres in protection against colorectal cancer. *Mutation Research* 350, no. 1: 173–184. https://doi.org/10.1016/0027-5107(95)00105-0

Florence, S. P., Urooj, A., Asha, M. R., and Rajiv, J. 2014. Sensory, physical and nutritional qualities of cookies prepared from pearl millet (*Pennisetum typhoideum*). *Journal of Food Processing & Technology* 5, no. 377: 2. https://doi.org/10.4172/2157-7110.1000377

Friedenreich, C. M., Neilson, H. K., and Lynch, B. M. 2010. State of the epidemiological evidence on physical activity and cancer prevention. *European Journal of Cancer* 46, no. 14: 2593–2604. https://doi.org/10.1016/j.ejca.2010.07.028

Fung, T. T., Hu, F. B., Hankinson, S. E., Willett, W. C., and Holmes, M. D. 2011. Low-carbohydrate diets, dietary approaches to stop hypertension-style diets, and the risk of postmenopausal breast cancer. *American Journal of Epidemiology* 174, no. 6: 652–660. https://doi.org/10.1093/aje/kwr148

García, N., Zazueta, C., and Aguilera-Aguirre, L. 2017. Oxidative stress and inflammation in cardiovascular disease. *Oxidative Medicine and Cellular Longevity* 2017: 5853238. https://doi.org/10.1155/2017/5853238

Giri, A., Sultana, S., Roy, A., Ray, D., Barui, I., and Sengupta, S. 2024. Potential therapeutic use of millet with broad spectrum anticancer properties: current trends and prospects. *Discover Food* 4, no. 1: 190.

GLOBOCAN. 2021. *Global Cancer Observatory.* International Agency for Research on Cancer. https://gco.iarc.fr

Goswami, D., Gupta, R. K., Mridula, D., Sharma, M., and Tyagi, S. K. 2015. Barnyard millet based muffins: Physical, textural and sensory properties. *Lebensmittel-Wissenschaft & Technologie* 64, no. 1: 374–380. https://doi.org/10.1016/j.lwt.2015.05.060

Grundy, S. M. 2008. Metabolic syndrome pandemic. *ATVB* 28, no. 4: 629–636. https://doi.org/10.1161/ATVBAHA.107.151092

Hadimani, N. A., and Malleshi, N. G. 1993. Studies on milling, physicochemical properties, nutrient composition and dietary fiber content of millets. *Journal of Food Science and Technology* 30, no. 1: 17–20. URI: http://ir.cftri.res.in/id/eprint/299

Hall, E. J., and Giaccia, A. J. 2012. *Radiobiology for the Radiologist* (7th ed.). Lippincott Williams and Wilkins.

Hall, J. E., do Carmo, J. M., da Silva, A. A., Wang, Z., and Hall, M. E. 2015. Obesity-induced hypertension: Interaction of neurohumoral and renal mechanisms. *Circulation Research* 116, no. 6: 991–1006. https://doi.org/10.1161/CIRCRESAHA.116.305697

Hall, W. L. 2010. Dietary protein and satiety. *British Journal of Nutrition* 104, no. S2: S132–S135.

Halter, J. B., Musi, N., McFarland Horne, F., Crandall, J. P., Goldberg, A., Harkless, L., Hazzard, W. R., Huang, E. S., Kirkman, M. S., Plutzky, J., and Schmader, K. E. 2014. Diabetes and cardiovascular disease in older adults: current status and future directions. *Diabetes* 63, no. 8: 2578–2589. https://doi.org/10.2337/db14-0020

Harrison, D., Griendling, K. K., Landmesser, U., Hornig, B., and Drexler, H. 2003. Role of oxidative stress in atherosclerosis. *American Journal of Cardiology* 91, no. 3A: 7A–11A. https://doi.org/10.1016/S0002-9149(02)03144-2

Hecht, S. S. 2003. Tobacco carcinogens, their biomarkers and tobacco-induced cancer. *Nature Reviews Cancer* 3, no. 10: 733–744. https://doi.org/10.1038/nrc1190

Hou, D., Chen, J., Ren, X., Wang, C., Diao, X., Hu, X., Zhang, Y., and Shen, Q. 2018. A whole foxtail millet diet reduces blood pressure in subjects with mild hypertension. *Journal of Cereal Science* 84: 13–19. https://doi.org/10.1016/j.jcs.2018.09.003

Huffman, M. D., Prabhakaran, D., Osmond, C., Fall, C. H., Tandon, N., Lakshmy, R., Ramji, S., Khalil, A., Gera, T., Prabhakaran, P., Biswas, S. K., Reddy, K. S., Bhargava, S. K., and Sachdev, H. S. 2011. New Delhi Birth Cohort. Incidence of cardiovascular risk factors in an Indian urban Cohort results from the New Delhi Birth Cohort. *Journal of the American College of Cardiology* 57, no. 17: 1765–74. https://doi.org/10.1016/j.jacc.2010.09.083. PMID: 21511113; PMCID: PMC3408699.

IARC. 2010. *Ingested Nitrate and Nitrite, and Cyanobacterial Peptide Toxins* (Vol. 94). IARC Monographs on the Evaluation of Carcinogenic Risks to Humans.

IARC. 2012. *A Review of Human Carcinogens: Personal Habits and Indoor Combustions (Vol. 100E).* International Agency for Research on Cancer.

IARC. 2019. *Global Cancer Statistics 2020.* IARC. Retrieved from https://gco.iarc.fr/today

IARC. 2020. *Global Cancer Statistics 2020.* International Agency for Research on Cancer.

ICRISAT. 2020. *Smart Food: Millets and Sorghum Are Good for You and the Planet.* International Crops Research Institute for the Semi-Arid Tropics. https://www.icrisat.org

Jacob, J., Krishnan, V., Antony, C., Bhavyasri, M., Aruna, C., Mishra, K., Nepolean, T., Satyavathi, C. T., and Visarada, K. B. 2024. The nutrition and therapeutic potential of millets: An updated narrative review. *Frontiers in Nutrition* 11: 1346869. https://doi.org/10.3389/fnut.2024.1346869. PMID: 38746941; PMCID: PMC11091339.

Jakszyn, P., and Gonzalez, C. A. 2006. Nitrosamine and related food intake and gastric and oesophageal cancer risk: A systematic review of the epidemiological evidence. *World Journal of Gastroenterology* 12, no. 27: 4296–4303. https://doi.org/10.3748/wjg.v12.i27.4296

Jan, B., Dar, M. I., Choudhary, B., Basist, P., Khan, R., and Alhalmi, A. 2024. Cardiovascular diseases among Indian older adults: A comprehensive review. *Cardiovascular Therapy*: 6894693. https://doi.org/10.1155/2024/6894693

Key, T. J., Verkasalo, P. K., and Banks, E. 2001. Epidemiology of breast cancer. *The Lancet Oncology* 2, no. 3: 133–140. https://doi.org/10.1016/S1470-2045(00)00254-0
Kumar, A., Shah, N. N., Chorawala, M. R., Kaushik, R., Prajapati, B., and Mehra, R., 2025. Exploring the Molecular Pathways Underlying the Anti-Diabetic Effects of Millets. *Food Safety and Health.* 3, no. 3: 300–314. https://doi.org/10.1002/fsh3.70007
Kumar, P., Kaur, C., and Jambh, H. K. 2021. Rheological, textural, and technological modifications in wheat unleavened flatbread substituted with extruded finger millet. *Journal of Texture Studies* 52, no. 3: 400–409. https://doi.org/10.1111/jtxs.12595
Kuruburu, M. G., Bovilla, V. R., Leihang, Z., and Madhunapantula, S. V. 2022a. Phytochemical-rich fractions from foxtail millet (*Setaria italica* (L.) P. Beauv) seeds exhibited antioxidant activity and reduced the viability of breast cancer cells in vitro by inducing DNA fragmentation and promoting cell cycle arrest. *Anti-Cancer Agents in Medicinal Chemistry* 22, no. 13: 2477–2493. https://doi.org/10.2174/1871520622666220215122141
Kuruburu, M. G., Bovilla, V. R., Naaz, R., Leihang, Z., and Madhunapantula, S. V. 2022b. Variations in the anticancer activity of free and bound phenolics of finger millet (*Eleusine Coracana* (L) Gaertn; variety KMR-301) seeds. *Phytomedicine Plus* 2, no. 2: 100276. https://doi.org/10.1016/j.phyplu.2022.100276
Leopold, J. A., and Loscalzo, J. 2008. Oxidative mechanisms and atherothrombotic cardiovascular disease. *Drug Discovery Today: Therapeutic Strategies* 5, no. 1: 5–13. https://doi.org/10.1016/j.ddstr.2008.02.001
Liu, F., Shan, F., Li, H., Shi, J., Yang, R., and Li, Z. 2023. Millet shell polyphenols ameliorate atherosclerosis. Millet shell polyphenols ameliorate atherosclerosis development by suppressing foam cell formation. *Journal of Nutritional Biochemistry* no. 115: 109271. https://doi.org/10.1016/j.jnutbio.2023.109271
Masoudkabir, F., Mohammadifard, N., Mani, A., Ignaszewski, A., Davis, M. K., Vaseghi, G., Mansourian, M., Franco, C., Gotay, C., and Sarrafzadegan, N. 2023. Shared lifestyle-related risk factors of cardiovascular disease and cancer: Evidence for joint prevention. *The Scientific World Journal* 2023: 2404806. https://doi.org/10.1155/2023/2404806. PMID: 37520844; PMCID: PMC10386903.
Mattiuzzi, C., and Lippi, G. 2019. Current cancer epidemiology. *Journal of Epidemiology and Global Health* 9, no. 4: 217–222. https://doi.org/10.2991/jegh.k.191008.001. ISSN 2210-6006; E-ISSN 2210-6014
Maurya, D. K., and Devasagayam, T. P. A. 2010. Antioxidant and prooxidant nature of hydroxycinnamic acid derivatives ferulic and caffeic acids. *Food and Chemical Toxicology* 48, no. 12: 3369–3373. https://doi.org/10.1016/j.fct.2010.09.006. Epub 2010 Sep 17. PMID: 20837085.
Mills, K. T., Stefanescu, A., and He, J. 2020. The global epidemiology of hypertension. *Nature Reviews Nephrology* 16, no. 4: 223–237. https://doi.org/10.1038/s41581-019-0244-2
Mohanan, M. M., Vijayakumar, A., Bang-Berthelsen, CH., Mudnakudu-Nagaraju, KK., and Shetty, R. 2025. Millets: Journey from an ancient crop to sustainable and healthy food. *Foods* 14, no. 10: 1733. https://doi.org/10.3390/foods14101733. PMID: 40428513; PMCID: PMC12111017.
Moore, S. C., Lee, I. M., Weiderpass, E., Campbell, P. T., Sampson, J. N., Kitahara, C. M., and Patel, A. V. 2016. Association of leisure-time physical activity with risk of 26 types of cancer in 1.44 million adults. *JAMA Internal Medicine* 176, no. 6: 816–825. https://doi.org/10.1001/jamainternmed.2016.1548
Nambiar, V. S., Dhaduk, J. J., Sareen, N., Shahu, T., and Desai, R. 2011. Potential functional implications of pearl millet (*Pennisetum glaucum*) in health and disease. *Journal of Applied Pharmaceutical Science* 1, no. 10: 62–67.
Narayanan, D. L., Saladi, R. N., and Fox, J. L. 2010. Ultraviolet radiation and skin cancer. *International Journal of Dermatology* 49, no. 9: 978–986. https://doi.org/10.1111/j.1365-4632.2010.04474.x
Nehra, M., Siroha, A. K., Punia, S., and Kumar, S. 2021. Process standardization for bread preparation using composite blend of wheat and pearl millet: Nutritional, antioxidant and sensory approach. *Current Research in Nutrition and Food Science* 9, no. 2: 511–520.
NHLBI (National Heart, Lung, and Blood Institute). 2022. *High Blood Pressure and Obesity.* https://www.nhlbi.nih.gov/health/high-blood-pressure
Nithiyanantham, S., Kalaiselvi, P., Mahomoodally, M. F., Zengin, G., Abirami, A., and Srinivasan, G., 2019. Nutritional and functional roles of millets—A review. *Journal of Food Biochemistry* 43, no. 7: 12859. https://doi.org/10.1111/jfbc.12859
O'Mahony, M., and Hegarty, J., 2009. Help seeking for cancer symptoms: A review of the literature. *Oncology Nursing Forum* 36, no. 4: 178–184. https://doi.org/10.1188/09.ONF.E178-E184
Obafemi, F. A., and Umahi-Ottah, G. J. J. C. R. T. P. 2023. A review of global Cancer prevalence and therapy. *Journal of Cancer Research, Treatment & Prevention* 1, no. 3: 128–47.

Ou, L., Kong, L. Y., Zhang, X. M., and Niwa, M. 2003. Oxidation of ferulic acid by *Momordica charantia* peroxidase and related anti-inflammation activity changes. *Biological and Pharmaceutical Bulletin* 26, no. 11: 1511–1516. https://doi.org/10.1248/bpb.26.1511

Panghal, A., Khatkar, B. S., Yadav, D. N., and Chhikara, N. 2019. Effect of finger millet on nutritional, rheological, and pasting profile of whole wheat flat bread (chapatti). *Cereal Chemistry* 96, no. 1: 86–94. https://doi.org/10.1002/cche.10111

Park, S. Y., Jeong, E. W., Yang, Y. S., Kim, H. J., Go, G. W., and Lee, H. G. 2021. Finger millet ethanol extracts prevent hypertension by inhibiting the angiotensin-converting enzyme level and enhancing the antioxidant capacity in spontaneously hypertensive rats. *Antioxidants (Basel)* 10, no. 11: 1766. https://doi.org/10.3390/antiox10111766

Passi, P., Kaur, K., Kaur, J., and Kaul, S. 2023. Quality characterization, bread making properties and storage stability of foxtail millet incorporated bread ready-mix. *Journal of Stored Products Research* 104: 102208. https://doi.org/10.1016/j.jspr.2023.102208

Patimah, S., Arundhana, A. I., Mursaha, A., and Syam, A. 2019. Development of foxtail millet and flying fish flour-based cookies as functional food. *Current Research in Nutrition and Food Science* 7, no. 2: 504–516.

Peek, R. M., and Blaser, M. J. 2002. *Helicobacter pylori* and gastrointestinal tract adenocarcinomas. *Nature Reviews Cancer* 2, no. 1: 28–37. https://doi.org/10.1038/nrc703

Pickering, R. J. 2021. Oxidative stress and inflammation in cardiovascular diseases. *Antioxidants* 10, no. 2: 171. https://doi.org/10.3390/antiox10020171

Prabhakaran, D. 2018. India state-level disease burden initiative CVD Collaborators. 2018 The changing patterns of cardiovascular diseases and their risk factors in the states of India: The global burden of disease study 1990–2016. *Lancet Global Health* 6, no. 12:1339–1351. https://doi.org/10.1016/S2214-109X(18)30407-8

Pradeep, P. M., and Sreerama, Y. N. 2015. Soluble and bound phenolics of two different millet genera and their milled fractions: Comparative evaluation of antioxidant properties and inhibitory effects on starch hydrolyzing enzyme activities. *Journal of Functional Foods* 14: 736–745. https://doi.org/10.1016/j.jff.2015.02.026

Preston, D. L., Shimizu, Y., Pierce, D. A., Suyama, A., and Mabuchi, K. 2007. Studies of mortality of atomic bomb survivors: Report 13. *Radiation Research* 167, no. 4: 379–406. https://doi.org/10.1667/RR0763.1

Radha, S., Mekala, A., Premkumar, K., Bhanu, S., Samraj, K., and Thilagavathi, R. 2024. Therapeutic potential of millets in the management of metabolic syndrome—A review. *Journal of Research in Siddha Medicine* 7, no. 1: S36–S43. https://doi.org/10.4103/jrsm.jrsm_18_23

Ragaee, S., Abdel-Aal, E. S. M., and Noaman, M. 2006. Antioxidant activity and nutrient composition of selected cereals for food use. *Food Chemistry* 98, no. 1: 32–38. https://doi.org/10.1016/j.foodchem.2005.04.039

Raghupathy, A., Nanda, K., Pant, H., Khan, H., Franco,OH., Emanuele, D. A., and Dorairaj, P. 2014. Hypertension in India: A systematic review and meta-analysis of prevalence, awareness, and control of hypertension. *Journal of Hypertension* 32, no. 6: 1170–1177.

Rahmat, S. A., and He, Y., 2024. Cancer Burden and attributable risk factors of cancers in China: epidemiological insights and comparisons with India. *Cancer Control* 31: 10732748241276674. https://doi.org/10.1177/10732748241276674

Ramadoss, D. P., and Sivalingam, N. 2020. Vanillin extracted from Proso and Barnyard millets induce apoptotic cell death in HT-29 human colon cancer cell line. *Nutrition and Cancer* 72, no. 8: 1422–1437. https://doi.org/10.1080/01635581.2019.1672763

Ramadoss, D. P., and Sivalingam, N. 2021. Vanillin extracted from proso and barnyard millets induces cell cycle inhibition and apoptotic cell death in MCF-7 cell line. *Journal of Cancer Research and Therapeutics* 17, no. 6: 1425–33.

Reaz, A. H., Abedin, M. J., Abdullah, A. T. M., Satter, M. A., and Farzana, T. 2023. Physicochemical and structural impact of CMC-hydrocolloids on the development of gluten-free foxtail millet biscuits. *Heliyon* 9, no. 6.https://doi.org/10.1016/j.heliyon.2023.e17176

Roth, G. A., Mensah, G. A., Johnson, C. O., Addolorato, G., Ammirati, E., Baddour, L. M., Barengo, N. C., Beaton, A. Z., Benjamin, E. J., Benziger, C. P., and Bonny, A. 2020. Global burden of cardiovascular diseases and risk factors, 1990–2019: update from the GBD 2019 study. *Journal of the American College of Cardiology* 76, no. 25: 2982–3021. https://doi.org/10.1016/j.jacc.2020.11.010

Rudrapal, M., Khairnar, S. J., Khan, J., Dukhyil, A. B., Ansari, M. A., Alomary, M. N., Alshabrmi, F. M., Palai, S., Deb, P. K., and Devi, R. 2022. Dietary polyphenols and their role in oxidative stress-induced human diseases: Insights into protective effects, antioxidant potentials and mechanism (s) of action. *Frontiers in Pharmacology* 13: 806470. https://doi.org/10.3389/fphar.2022.806470

Sachdev, N., Goomer, S., Singh, L. R., Pathak, V. M., Aggarwal, D., and Chowhan, R. K. 2023. Current status of millet seed proteins and its applications: A comprehensive review. *Applied Food Research* 3, no. 1: 100288. https://doi.org/10.1016/j.afres.2023.100288

Saha, S., Gupta, A., Singh, S. R. K., Bharti, N., Singh, K. P., Mahajan, V., and Gupta, H. S. 2011. Compositional and varietal influence of finger millet flour on rheological properties of dough and quality of biscuit. *LWT – Food Science and Technology* 44, no. 3: 616–621. https://doi.org/10.1016/j.lwt.2010.08.009

Saleh, A. S. M., Zhang, Q., Chen, J., and Shen, Q. 2013. Millet grains: Nutritional quality, processing, and potential health benefits. *Comprehensive Reviews in Food Science and Food Safety* 12, no. 3: 281–295. https://doi.org/10.1111/1541-4337.12012

Samtiya, M., Aluko, R. E., Dhaka, N., Dhewa, T., and Puniya, A. K. 2023. Nutritional and health-promoting attributes of millet: current and future perspectives. *Nutrition Reviews* 81, no. 6: 684–704. https://doi.org/10.1093/nutrit/nuac081

Sathishkumar, K., Chaturvedi, M., Das, P., Stephen, S., and Mathur, P. 2022. Cancer incidence estimates for 2022 & projection for 2025: result from National Cancer Registry Programme, India. *Indian Journal of Medical Research* 156, no. 4&5: 598–607. https://doi.org/10.4103/ijmr.ijmr_1821_22

Shan, S., Li, Z., Newton, I. P., Zhao, C., Li, Z., and Guo, M. 2014. A novel protein extracted from foxtail millet bran displays anti-carcinogenic effects in human colon cancer cells. *Toxicology Letters* 227, no. 2: 129–138. https://doi.org/10.1016/j.toxlet.2014.03.008

Sharma, B., and Gujral, H. S. 2019. Modulation in quality attributes of dough and starch digestibility of unleavened flat bread on replacing wheat flour with different minor millet flours. *International Journal of Biological Macromolecules* 141: 117–124. https://doi.org/10.1016/j.ijbiomac.2019.08.252

Sharma, S., Saxena, D. C., and Riar, C. S. 2016a. Nutritional, sensory and in-vitro antioxidant characteristics of gluten free cookies prepared from flour blends of minor millets. *Journal of Cereal Science* 72: 153–161. https://doi.org/10.1016/j.jcs.2016.10.012

Sharma, S., Saxena, D. C., and Riar, C. S. 2016b. Analysing the effect of germination on phenolics, dietary fibres, minerals and γamino butyric acid contents of barnyard millet (Echinochloa frumentaceae). *Food Bioscience* 13: 60–68. https://doi.org/10.1016/j.fbio.2015.12.007

Shobana, S., Harsha, M. R., Platel, K., Srinivasan, K., and Malleshi, N. G. 2010. Amelioration of hyperglycaemia and its associated complications by finger millet (*Eleusine Coracana* L.) seed coat matter in streptozotocin-induced diabetic rats. *British Journal of Nutrition* 104: 1787–1795.

Shobana, S., Harsha, M. R., Platel, K., Srinivasan, K., and Malleshi, N. G. 2013. Amelioration of hyperglycemia and its associated complications by finger millet diet in alloxan-induced diabetic rats. *Plant Foods for Human Nutrition* 68, no. 3: 233–239.

Singh, G. M., Danaei, G., Farzadfar, F., Stevens, G. A., Woodward, M., Wormser, D., Kaptoge, S., Whitlock, G., Qiao, Q., Lewington, S., and Di Angelantonio, E. 2013. The age-specific quantitative effects of metabolic risk factors on cardiovascular diseases and diabetes: A pooled analysis. *PLoS One* 8, no. 7: 65174. https://doi.org/10.1371/journal.pone.0065174

Singh, M., Emanuel, N., Kumar, N., Tiwari, M., Tiwari, A, Kumari, P., Singh, S., Taneja, N. K., and Chauhan, K. 2023. Nutritional and Functional Properties of Millets: Processing and Health Benefits. In *Book: Millet Marvels A Sustainable Food Renaissance*: 25–53. New India Publishing Agency-Nipa.

Sinha, R., and Gupta, M. 2020. Cervical cancer screening in India: Current status and future directions. *Indian Journal of Cancer* 57, no. 2: 110–115.

Sinha, R., Rothman, N., Salmon, C. P., Knize, M. G., Brown, E. D., Swanson, C. A., Rhodes, D., Rossi, S., Felton, J. S., and Levander, O. A. 1998. Heterocyclic amine content in beef cooked by different methods to varying degrees of doneness and gravy made from meat drippings. *Food and Chemical Toxicology* 36, no. 4: 279–287. https://doi.org/10.1016/s0278-6915(97)00162-2. PMID: 9651044.

Siroha, A. K., Sandhu, K. S., and Kaur, M. 2016. Physicochemical, functional and antioxidant properties of flour from pearl millet varieties grown in India. *Journal of Food Measurement and Characterization* 10: 311–318. https://doi.org/10.1007/s11694-016-9308-1

Smith, C. J., Perfetti, T. A., and Rumple, M. A. 2016. Biomarkers of tobacco-specific nitrosamine exposure in humans. *Cancer Epidemiology, Biomarkers & Prevention* 25, no. 3: 448–453.

Srivastava, R. K., Bansal, S., and Tomar, R. S. 2020. Development and nutritional evaluation of millet-based ready-to-eat snack. *Indian Journal of Nutrition* 7, no. 1: 206–211.

Straif, K., Benbrahim-Tallaa, L., Baan, R., Grosse, Y., Secretan, B., El Ghissassi, F., and Cogliano, V. 2009. A review of human carcinogens—Part C: Metals, arsenic, dusts, and fibres. *The Lancet Oncology* 10, no. 5: 453–454. https://doi.org/10.1016/S1470-2045(09)70134-2

Sudha, V., Radhika, G., Sathya, R. M., Ganesan, A., and Mohan, V. 2018. Replacing white rice with whole grains in the diet of South Indian adults with type 2 diabetes to improve glycemic control: A randomized controlled trial. *Indian Journal of Medical Research* 148, no. 6: 706–713.

Sung, H., Ferlay, J., Siegel, R. L., Laversanne, M., Soerjomataram, I., Jemal, A., and Bray, F. 2021. Global cancer statistics 2020: GLOBOCAN estimates of incidence and mortality worldwide for 36 cancers in 185 countries. *CA: A Cancer Journal for Clinicians* 71, no. 3: 209–249. https://doi.org/10.3322/caac.21660

Taylor, J. R. N. 2004. Overview: Importance of sorghum in Africa. In *Afripro: Workshop on the Proteins of Sorghum and Millets*. Pretoria, South Africa.

Teo, K. K., Ounpuu, S., Hawken, S., Pandey, M. R., Valentin, V., Hunt, D., Diaz, R., Rashed, W., Freeman, R., Jiang, L., and Zhang, X. 2006. Tobacco use and risk of myocardial infarction in 52 countries in the INTERHEART study: A case-control study. *The Lancet* 368, no. 9536: 647–658.

Timmis, A., Vardas, P., Townsend, N., Torbica, A., Katus, H., De Smedt, D., Gale, C. P., Maggioni, A. P., Petersen, S. E., Huculeci, R., and Kazakiewicz, D. 2022. European Society of Cardiology: cardiovascular disease statistics 2021. *European Heart Journal* 43, no. 8: 716–799. https://doi.org/10.1093/eurheartj/ehac064

Toedebusch, R., Belenchia, A., and Pulakat, L. 2018. Diabetic cardiomyopathy: impact of biological sex on disease development and molecular signatures. *Frontiers in Physiology* 9: 453. https://doi.org/10.3389/fphys.2018.00453

Tomar, V., Kaur, A., Kaur, A., and Kumar, A. 2018. Glycemic index of Indian Flat Breads (Rotis) prepared using multigrain flour and whole wheat flour. *Annals of Biology* 34: 143–147.

Tripathi, G., Patel, H., Kumar, J., and Borah, A. 2023. A review on nutritional and health benefits of millets. *International Journal of Plant & Soil Science* 35, no. 19: 1736–1743. https://doi.org/10.9734/IJPSS/2023/v35i193722

UNSCEAR (United Nations Scientific Committee on the Effects of Atomic Radiation). 2000. *Sources and Effects of Ionizing Radiation*. United Nations Publications.

Vaduganathan, M, Mensah, G, Turco, J., Fuster, V., and Roth, G. A. 2022. The global burden of cardiovascular diseases and risk: A compass for future health. *JACC* 80, no. 25: 2361–2371. https://doi.org/10.1016/j.jacc.2022.11.005

Walboomers, J. M. M., Jacobs, M. V., Manos, M. M., Bosch, F. X., Kummer, J. A., Shah, K. V., and Meijer, C. J. L. M. 1999. Human papillomavirus is a necessary cause of invasive cervical cancer worldwide. *Journal of Pathology* 189, no. 1: 12–19.

Wallingford, S. C., Olsen, C. M., Plasmeijer, E., and Green, A. C. 2011. Skin cancer arising in scars: A systematic review. *Dermatologic Surgery* 37, no. 9: 1239–44. https://doi.org/10.1111/j.1524-4725.2011.02060.x

WCRF/AICR. 2018. *Diet, Nutrition, Physical Activity and Cancer: A Global Perspective*. Continuous Update Project Expert Report. https://www.wcrf.org/dietandcancer

WHO. 2019. *WHO Report on Cancer: Setting Priorities, Investing Wisely and Providing Care for All*. World Health Organization. https://www.who.int/publications-detail-redirect/9789240001299

WHO. 2021. *Healthy Diet*. World Health Organization. https://www.who.int/news-room/fact-sheets/detail/healthy-diet

WHO. 2021a. *Cardiovascular Diseases (CVDs)*. World Health Organization.

WHO. 2021b. *Obesity and Overweight*. https://www.who.int/news-room/fact-sheets/detail/obesity-and-overweight

WHO. 2023. *Diabetes*. https://www.who.int/news-room/fact-sheets/detail/diabetes. Accessed, March 6, 2024.

WHO/ICO. 2007. Information Centre on HPV and Cervical Cancer (HPV Information Centre). Summary Report on HPV and Cervical Cancer Statistics in India 2007. [Last Assessed on 2008 May 1].

WHO/UNEP. 2013. *State of the Science of Endocrine Disrupting Chemicals – 2012*. World Health Organization and United Nations Environment Programme. https://www.who.int/publications/i/item/9789241505031

Wild, C. P., and Gong, Y. Y. 2010. Mycotoxins and human disease: A largely ignored global health issue. *Carcinogenesis* 31, no. 1: 71–82. https://doi.org/10.1093/carcin/bgp264

Wilkins, E., Wilson, L., Wickramasinghe, K., Bhatnagar, P., Leal, J., Luengo-Fernandez, R., Burns, R., Rayner, M., and Townsend, N. 2017. *European Cardiovascular Disease Statistics 2017*. European Heart Network, Brussels.

Xiao, J., Li, Y., Niu, L., Chen, R., Tang, J., Tong, Z., and Xiao, C. 2023. Effect of adding fermented proso millet bran dietary fiber on micro-structural, physicochemical, and digestive properties of gluten-free proso millet-based dough and cake. *Foods* 12, no. 15: 2964. https://doi.org/10.3390/foods12152964

Yager, J. D., and Davidson, N. E. 2006. Estrogen carcinogenesis in breast cancer. *The New England Journal of Medicine* 354, no. 3: 270–282. https://doi.org/10.1056/NEJMra050776

Zhang, L., La, X., Tian, J., Li, H., Li, A., Liu, Y., Wu, C., and Li, Z., 2021. The phytochemical vitexin and syringic acid derived from foxtail fillet bran inhibit breast cancer cells proliferation via GRP78/SREBP-1/SCD1 signaling axis. *Journal of Functional Foods* 85: 104620.

Zhang, L. Z., and Liu, R. H. 2015. Phenolic and carotenoid profiles and antiproliferative activity of foxtail millet. *Food Chemistry* 1, no. 174: 495–501. https://doi.org/10.1016/j.foodchem.2014.09.089

Zheng, W., and Lee, SA. 2009. Well-done meat intake, heterocyclic amine exposure, and cancer risk. *Nutrition and Cancer* 61, no. 4: 437–446. https://doi.org/10.1080/01635580802710741

Zhou, C., Gao, L., Flaws, J. A., and Lichtensteiger, W. 2014. Endocrine-disrupting chemicals and the risk of hormone-related cancers. *Frontiers in Public Health* 2, no. 14. https://doi.org/10.3389/fpubh.2014.00014

Zhu, D., Zhao, G., and Wang, X., 2021. Association of smoking and smoking cessation with overall and cause-specific mortality. *American Journal of Preventive Medicine* 60, no. 4: 504–512.

Zodpey, S., and Subramanian, S. 2018. Epidemiology of cardiovascular diseases and cancer in India: The changing trend. *Indian Journal of Public Health* 62, no. 6: 532–536.

11 Millets for Celiac Disease

T. Tamilselvan[1] *and M. Badhani*[2]

[1] Flour Milling Baking and Confectionery Technology Department, CSIR-Central Food Technological Research Institute, Mysore, Karnataka, India

[2] Department of Food and Nutrition, College of Community Science, Govind Ballabh Pant University of Agriculture and Technology (GBPUAT), Pantnagar, Uttarakhand, India

11.1 INTRODUCTION TO GLUTEN-RELATED DISORDERS

Gluten, the main storage protein found in wheat (*Triticum aestivum*), is primarily present in endosperm and makes up 75–80% of total wheat proteins. Gluten proteins are also found in cereals such as rye (*Secale cereale*) and barley (*Hordeum vulgare*), which are species belonging to the *Poaceae* family. It constitutes two different protein components, gliadins and glutenins. Its unique rheological and viscoelastic properties contribute to the elasticity, expandability, gas retention, and compactness required to produce leavened bread and other baked products (Belton 1999). Most baked products like pizza crusts, burger buns, wheat bread, multi-grain bread, doughs, salad rolls, and pasta are prepared by adding gluten. Gluten is also frequently used as a binding and extending agent in processed foods to improve texture, flavor, and moisture retention. Due to its use in processing, packaging, or as part of ingredients, gluten can be present in several daily-use products.

Due to its ubiquitous nature, ingestion of gluten can trigger symptoms in genetically susceptible individuals. Globally, about 8.4% of the population is suffering from disorders related to gluten consumption. GRDs are defined as adverse reactions to gluten that are mediated by the immune system. Celiac disease (CD), dermatitis herpetiformis (DH), gluten ataxia (GA) as autoimmune, wheat allergy as allergic, and non-celiac gluten sensitivity (NCGS) as non-autoimmune-allergic diseases are the five main categories of GRDs (Figure 11.1). Each GRD occurs following specific pathophysiological responses to gluten, and recent advances have been made in unravelling each of these disorders' pathogenic pathways. GRDs present with typical and atypical manifestations. A long-life adherence to a strict gluten-free diet (GFD) is the only effective GRD treatment, warranting good health in most patients. However, a growing trend in the consumption of gluten-free products or following a GFD is observed among the general population, based on the unfounded belief that avoiding gluten can enhance well-being or that gluten is harmful to everyone (Reilly 2016). Several studies indicate that a significant portion of the general population is interested in reducing or avoiding gluten in their diets (Wu et al 2015; Cabrera-Chávez et al 2017). It underlines the demand for a next-level understanding of the processes of gluten-related diseases. This may assist in the clarification of risk factors, symptoms, and genetic factors that predispose to adverse reactions to gluten in some people.

11.2 CELIAC DISEASE

CD is an immune reaction to gluten that causes inflammatory damage to the small intestine in genetically predisposed individuals due to an inappropriate T cell response. It has a worldwide prevalence of approximately 0.6%–1% (Fasano and Catassi 2012). Gluten is a digestion-resistant protein consumed significantly and contains various non-digestible immunogenic peptides. It may end up in a gluten tolerance failure, wherein the immune system gets activated during intestinal infections. Gluten contains gliadin, a complex protein high in proline and glutamine, which are not

DOI: 10.1201/9781003686668-11

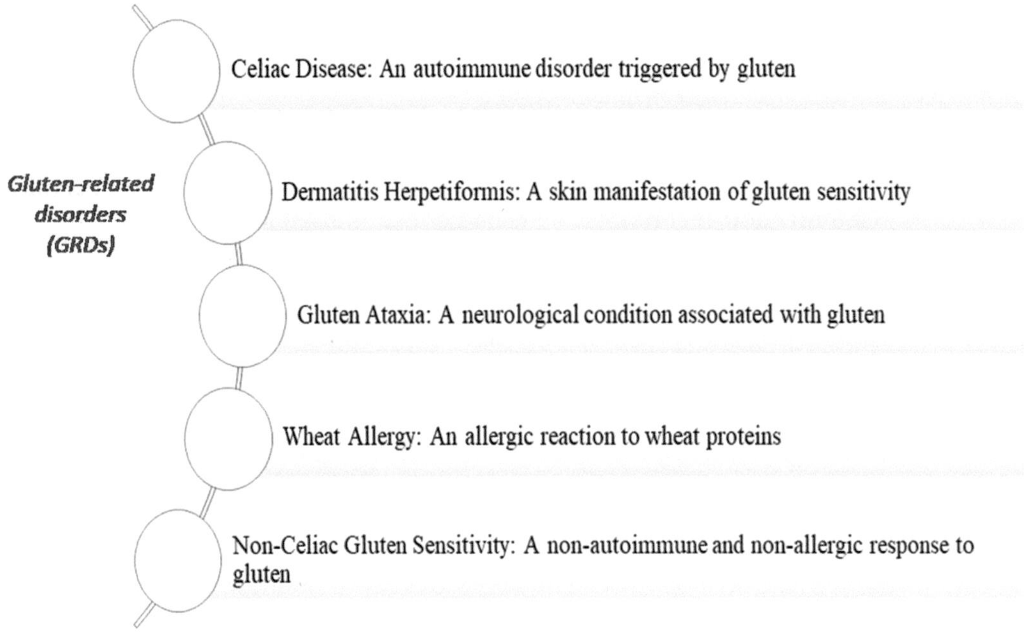

FIGURE 11.1 Types of gluten-related disorders and their responses.

completely digested by intestinal enzymes. The partial digestion results in peptides that may raise gut permeability and provoke immune responses resembling those caused by pathogenic microorganisms (Lammers et al 2011).

CD is an autoimmune disorder with particular genetic factors such as human leukocyte antigen (HLA)-DQ2 and -DQ8, the auto-antigen tissue transglutaminase (tTG), and the environmental trigger gluten. Besides genetic predisposition and gluten exposure-altered intestinal barrier, a pro-inflammatory immune response to gluten, a malfunction of adaptive immune response, and an imbalanced gut microbiome are the most significant factors that play a considerable role in CD development. Poddighe and Abdukhakimova (2021) reported that CD is still underdiagnosed in developing countries and that children are more severely affected. Moreover, CD misdiagnosis has become a prominent problem worldwide. To improve the diagnostic accuracy and avoid complications that can be fatal, such as small bowel carcinoma and lymphoma, an evidence-based approach is necessary. These complications are typically the result of unrecognized CD, whereas wrong prescriptions of a lifelong GFD may cause unnecessary expenses and adversely affect patients' quality of life. Furthermore, CD patients on a GFD must have regular follow-up visits.

11.2.1 Mechanism of Action

It involves a complex interaction between gluten peptides, genetic factors, and immune responses. Key processes include activating both adaptive and innate immune systems, which leads to intestinal damage (Figure 11.2). The following sections detail the mechanisms.

1. *Gluten Peptide Recognition*
   - Gluten peptides, particularly those deamidated by tissue transglutaminase (tTG), are presented by HLA-DQ2 and HLA-DQ8 molecules, activating CD4+ T lymphocytes.
   - Immunodominant peptides, such as A-gliadin P31-43, can trigger innate immune responses without HLA recognition (Falcigno et al 2020).

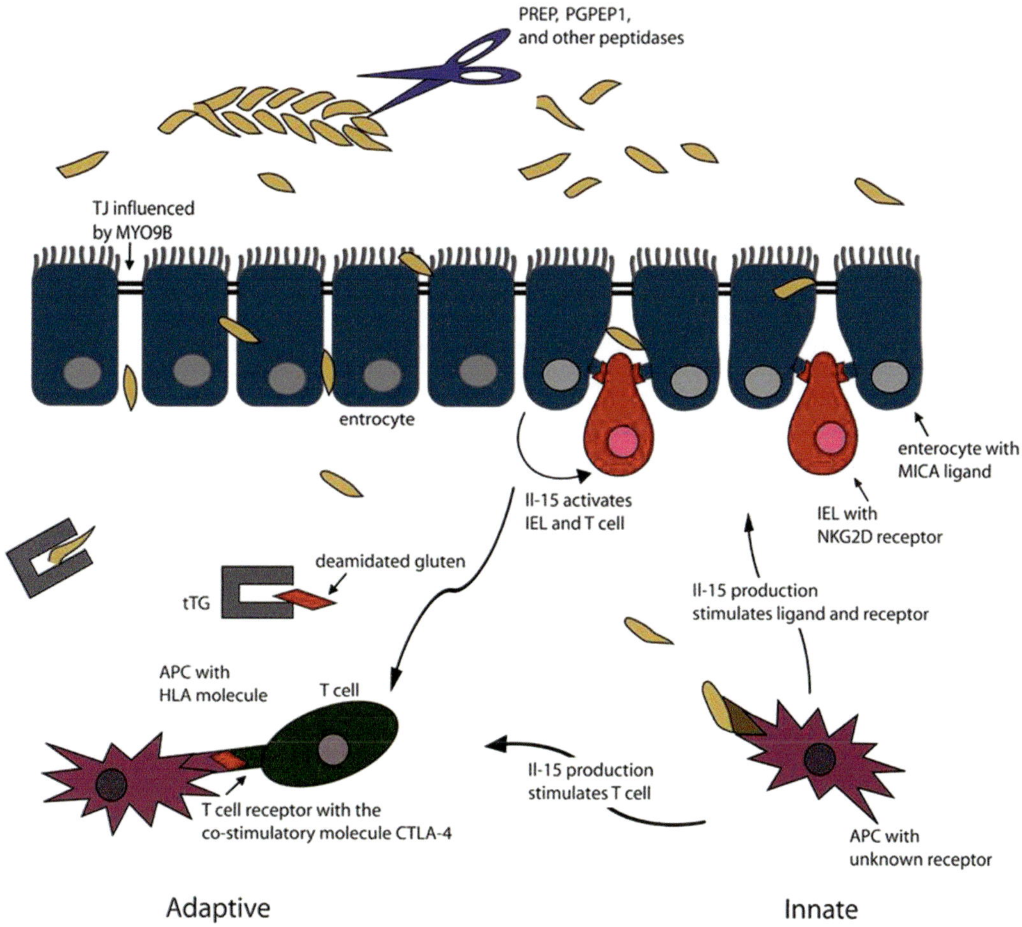

FIGURE 11.2 Mechanism of action in celiac disease. (Image reproduced from Monsuur and Wijmenga (2006).)

2. *Immune Response Activation*
   - The adaptive immune response is characterized by the production of pro-inflammatory cytokines, notably interferons gamma (IFNγ), which contribute to epithelial damage.
   - Cytotoxic CD8+ intraepithelial lymphocytes (IELs) are activated, exacerbating intestinal injury through the JAK/STAT signaling pathway (Levescot et al 2022).
3. *Role of Tissue Transglutaminase (tTG)*
   - tTG modifies gluten peptides, enhancing their binding to HLA-DQ2/DQ8, thus amplifying T cell activation.
   - Increased tTG expression in the gut is linked to the pathogenesis of CD, facilitating gluten's prolonged presence in the mucosa (Dieterich et al 2003).

11.2.2 Signs and Symptoms

CD can present in intestinal and extraintestinal forms. The intestinal form typically shows symptoms like diarrhea, loss of appetite, and abdominal distention, mainly in children under three years of age. In older children and adults, symptoms might include bloating, constipation, and weight loss, while severe malabsorption with chronic diarrhea is rare. Extraintestinal symptoms, such as

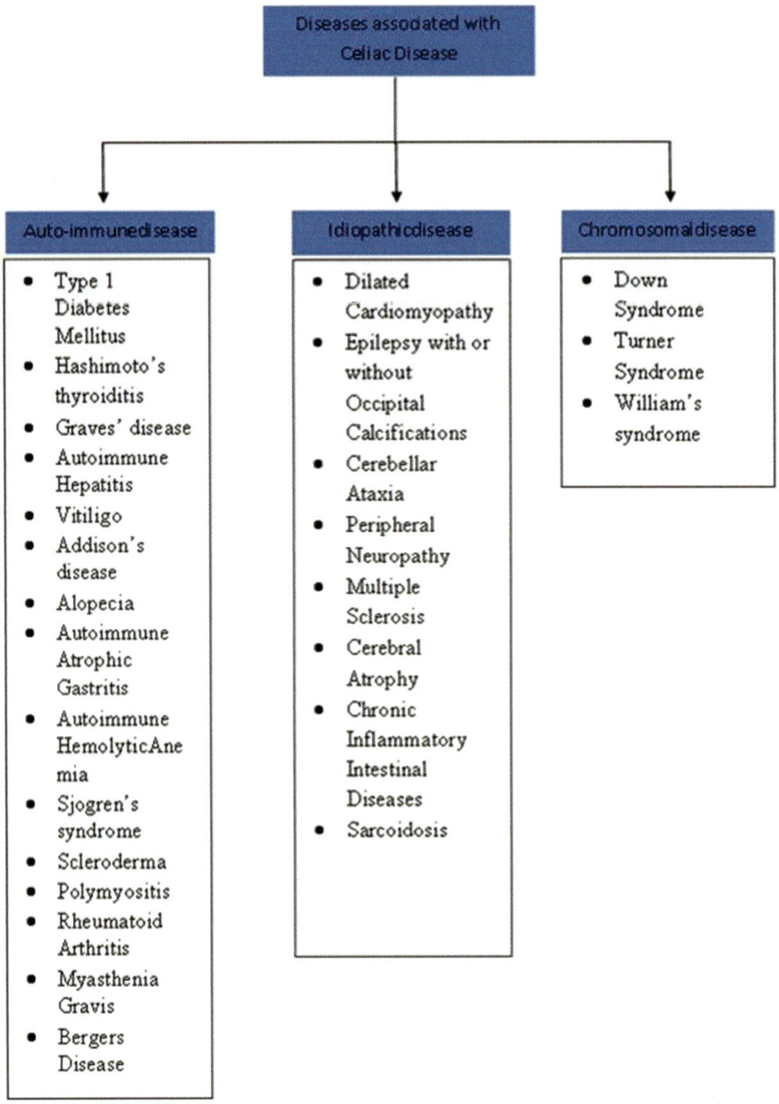

FIGURE 11.3 Categories of diseases associated with celiac disease.

iron deficiency anemia and growth retardation in children, may also occur. Neurological symptoms like headaches, anxiety, and depression can be present, along with reproductive issues such as late menarche and infertility (Figure 11.3). Many of these symptoms can improve with a strict GFD, although some, including fatigue and neurological problems, may persist in certain patients (Saccone et al 2016).

11.2.3 Diet and New Treatments

The sole effective treatment for CD is a lifelong strict GFD. This diet not only resolves symptoms but also results in negative autoantibody tests and the regeneration of intestinal villi, offering some degree of protection against related complications. Adhering to a GFD may deteriorate one's quality of life, cause psychological issues, and increase the worry of unintentional gluten exposure. Furthermore, these individuals might become deficient in certain vitamins and minerals, develop metabolic syndrome, have an increased risk of cardiovascular problems, and suffer from severe constipation. Such problems can be overcome by informing patients about the dangers of the GFD and supplying them with nutritional advice from a professional dietitian. Many individuals with CD feel that the GFD significantly diminishes their quality of life, with approximately 40% expressing dissatisfaction and seeking alternative treatment options (Aziz et al 2011).

Most of the clinical trials are in early phases, with only a few having advanced to later stages. Among these are the trials of larazotide acetate and gluten-specific proteases from a bacterial mixture (ALV003) (Murray et al 2017) that have caught most attention. Acting as a zonulin antagonist, larazotide acetate blocks the disassembly of tight junctions. By doing this, the amount of gluten that can cross a permeable intestinal mucosal barrier is reduced (Leffler et al 2015). Larazotide has been shown to help alleviate gluten-related symptoms, but it does not completely repair the epithelial barrier or stop gluten from entering the mucosal lining. The proteases in ALV003 are gluten-specific and fragment the gluten they encounter in the stomach in a small portion before it reaches the duodenum. The method has been successful in the digestion of small amounts of gluten; thus, it can be used in the case of cross-contamination, while at the same time, it does not offer any protection to patients so as to avoid the negative effects of large doses of gluten. However, a recent phase 2 study by Murray et al (2017) revealed that ALV003 was not associated with histological or symptom score improvements in 494 patients with CD who had moderate to severe symptoms as compared to placebo. Moreover, IL-15 monoclonal antibodies (AMG 714) are being tested in phase 2 studies in gluten challenge and refractory CD (RCD) type II patients. However, more safety studies are required before a license can be granted. At last, Nexvax2 vaccination is another hypothetical therapeutic intervention aimed at the CD desensitization to gliadin peptides. Though substantial side effects like abdominal pain and vomiting were reported, the trial proceeded successfully through phase 1. If further data reveal effectiveness, vaccines might be able to provide a permanent solution to CD (Anderson and Jabri 2013). Although a strict GFD is still the mainstay of treatment, recent studies are looking into vaccine development and alternative therapies to provide better patient outcomes. The subsequent paragraphs present the present trends in vaccine research and different treatment options for CD.

11.2.4 Alternative Therapeutic Approaches

- *Enzymatic Treatments*: Strategies include enzymatic degradation of gluten and transglutaminase inhibitors to prevent gluten peptide modification.
- *Immune Modulation*: Innovative therapies focus on modulating the immune response and enhancing intestinal permeability to reduce symptoms.
- *Nanoparticle Therapies*: These aim to recalibrate the immune response, potentially offering a more flexible treatment approach compared to strict dietary restrictions.

Despite the advancements in vaccine and therapeutic options, the reliance on a GFD remains a significant burden for many patients. Continued research is essential to develop effective treatments that can alleviate this challenge.

11.2.5 Diagnosis

CD is generally more frequent in females, where a female-to-male ratio of 2:1 to 3:1 has been reported (Fasano and Catassi 2012). The disease can be initiated at any time in life, with an occurrence peak shortly after weaning and again in the second or third decades of life. Diagnosis is difficult because of the different symptoms the patients show. A study demonstrated that a late CD diagnosis, especially after the age of 50, together with non-compliance to a strict GFD, may result in higher death rates than in the general population. In addition to being rare and accounting for only about 1% of patients with CD, the complications that accompany CD are hyposplenism, intestinal lymphoma, small bowel adenocarcinoma, and ulcerative jejunitis. These complications should be thought of in all those patients who, despite following a GFD, have unexplained persistence or aggravation of symptoms such as diarrhea, intestinal sub-occlusion, abdominal pain, weight loss, fever, and severe fatigue. Complications are more probable to be present in the elderly and DQ2 homozygous patients who are not strictly adhering to a GFD.

11.3 OTHER GLUTEN DISORDERS

11.3.1 Dermatitis Herpetiformis

DH is a chronic and systemic autoimmune disease related to gluten hypersensitivity, characterized by intense itching and a burning sensation. The lesions are polymorphic and predominantly affect the extensor surfaces, such as elbows and knees, as well as the buttocks and scalp, often in a symmetrical manner. Similar to CD, the etiopathogenesis of DH involves interactions between genetic, environmental, and immunological variables. It is considered an autoimmune disease, since pathognomonic granular immunoglobulin A (IgA) response in the dermis, directed against epidermal transglutaminase (TG3), and circulating autoantibodies against tissue transglutaminase (tTG) and TG3 exist in DH. Moreover, the predisposing genetic background, more specifically HLA-DQ2 or -DQ8 haplotypes, is a necessity for the development of the disease (Vale et al 2019). Currently approximately 13% of patients with CD have DH. It is typically diagnosed during adulthood, and the incidence of DH is highest in females and males aged 50–69 years.

11.3.1.1 Signs and Symptoms

An itchy rash on the elbows, extensor areas of the wrists, knees, and buttocks, especially the sacral areas, characterizes the clinical presentation of DH. Itching is noticeable and is correlated with general sleep disruption. Small blisters, papules, and erythema make up the polymorphic rash, but due to scratching and itching, erosions, post-inflammatory hyperpigmentation, and scaling frequently take center stage in the clinical picture. Direct immunofluorescence (DIF) of IgA granular accumulation in the skin papillae and along the cutaneous epidermal junction is used to make the diagnosis (Rybak-d'Obyrn and Placek 2022). Neutrophilic microabscesses in the dermal papillae are histological findings in DH lesions in skin biopsies, yet it does not mention DH specifically. DIF continues to be the main method for diagnoses.

11.3.1.2 Diagnosis

Anti-tissue transglutaminase (Anti-tTG) along with other autoantibodies can help with illness diagnosis and monitoring, although anti-epidermal transglutaminase (TG3) antibody has recently been demonstrated to be an important serological diagnostic.

11.3.1.3 Management

The essential treatment for DH is a strict, lifelong GFD. Adherence to a GFD leads to healing of the small bowel mucosa and alleviation of the clinical symptoms, but total clearance of the DH rash may take several months or even a couple of years. Therefore, at the beginning of GFD, treatment individuals with widespread, active rash need additional treatment with dapsone. Dapsone is a sulfone drug with potent antimicrobial and anti-inflammatory properties, which relieve the DH rash and itch effectively but does not affect the enteropathy (Salmi and Hervonen 2020). In rare cases of DH, the rash continues despite long-lasting, strict, adherence to a GFD. However, some reports suggest that a proportion of patients with DH following a GFD could later reintroduce gluten to their diet without developing symptoms or signs of DH (Paek et al 2011). The gluten challenge studies have also investigated the possible redevelopment of gluten tolerance in DH. The first gluten-challenge study reported 11 out of 12 (92%) patients with DH relapsed with rash and 7 (64%) of these also with villous atrophy (Leonard et al 1983). Recently, a 12-month gluten-challenge study was performed on 19 long-term GFD-treated DH patients in Finland (Mansikka et al 2019). In this study, 18 (95%) of the patients relapsed in a mean of 6 months; 15 (79%) developed DH rash, 12 of whom also showed small bowel villous atrophy, and 3 patients showed the progression of small bowel mucosal villous atrophy without skin symptoms or cutaneous IgA deposits. At present, it seems that the development of gluten tolerance in DH is rare or even non-existent, and lifelong strict adherence to a GFD is still justified in all patients with DH. New alternative medicines such as colchicine, methotrexate, heparin, cyclosporin, mycophenolate, tetracycline, nicotinamide, azathioprine, and rituximab have been shown to be effective in treating DH, according to a recent case report (Nguyen and Kim 2021).

11.3.2 Gluten Ataxia

GA is a neurological disorder associated with gluten sensitivity, particularly in individuals with CD. It is characterized by progressive cerebellar ataxia, which can lead to significant impairment in coordination and balance. The underlying mechanisms involve autoimmune responses, where specific antibodies target neural tissues, leading to cerebellar degeneration and inflammation. The symptoms often develop insidiously and may include a range of neurological deficits. Following are the key signs and symptoms associated with GA.

11.3.2.1 Key Symptoms of Gluten Ataxia

- *Gait Ataxia*: Patients typically exhibit uncoordinated walking patterns, often described as a wide-based gait (Ortega and Branson 2023).
- *Neurological Deficits*: GA accounts for approximately 15% of all ataxias and 40% of idiopathic sporadic ataxias. Symptoms may include dysarthria (slurred speech), nystagmus (involuntary eye movement), and decreased proprioception (Casella et al 2017). Neuropathological findings include loss of Purkinje cells, cerebellar atrophy, and inflammatory infiltrates, indicating an immune-mediated pathogenesis (Rouvroye et al 2020). MRI studies show cerebellar atrophy in up to 60% of patients, highlighting the structural impact of gluten on the nervous system (Hernández-Lahoz et al 2014).
- *Sensory Changes*: Many patients report sensory disturbances, such as numbness or tingling in the extremities (Krishnaprasad et al 2023).
- *Cognitive Function*: While cognitive impairment is not common, some patients may experience emotional disturbances.

In patients with GA, who also show major neurological symptoms, only 10% of them have gastrointestinal symptoms; thus, the diagnosis can be quite difficult. It emphasizes the significance of identifying neurological symptoms when there are no usual gastrointestinal symptoms. In contrast, there are some patients in whom the gut symptoms precede the neurological symptoms so that they are misdiagnosed, or their treatment is delayed. This point raises the necessity for detailed examinations of those who are thought to be gluten-sensitive, irrespective of whether they have gastrointestinal symptoms or not (Ciacci 2022).

11.3.2.2 Autoimmune Mechanisms

GA is an autoimmune response that occurs when the consumption of gluten leads to the production of antibodies that mistakenly attack neuronal proteins, mainly those in the cerebellum, causing the loss of coordination symptoms (ataxia). GA is mainly related to the presence of anti-gliadin antibodies (AGAs) and antibodies against tissue transglutaminase 6 (tTG6), which bind to neuronal tissues (Hernández-Lahoz et al 2014). The phenomenon of cross-reactivity occurs when antibodies against gluten also recognize glutamic acid decarboxylase-65 (GAD-65), a protein in the cerebellum, thus aggravating the neurological symptoms. Neuropathological examinations show cerebellar microglial activation and lymphocytic infiltration, which is an indication of an immune-mediated mechanism (Floare et al 2024).

11.3.2.3 Diagnosis and Management

Early diagnosis and treatment are important. Patients with neurological symptoms often start treatment later than those with gastrointestinal symptoms (Ortega and Branson 2023). A strict GFD has been shown to improve symptoms for many patients. However, some may need further dietary changes to manage reactions to other proteins. Research shows that sticking to a strict GFD can lead to significant clinical improvements and stabilization of symptoms in patients with GA, even if they do not have gastrointestinal symptoms (Krishnaprasad et al 2023). Patients with GA usually stabilize or improve by strictly following a GFD, no matter if they have enteropathy or not.

11.3.3 Non-Celiac Gluten Sensitivity

NCGS is a condition characterized by symptoms similar to CD but without the associated autoimmune response or intestinal damage. It is a complex and often debated condition due to the lack of specific biomarkers and the potential influence of psychological factors. The mechanisms underlying NCGS are multifaceted, involving various components of wheat and the body's immune response.

11.3.3.1 Mechanisms of Action

- *Immune Activation*: NCGS may involve immune responses to gluten and other wheat components, such as amylase–trypsin inhibitors (ATIs) and fermentable carbohydrates like fructans.
- *Intestinal Barrier Dysfunction*: Evidence suggests compromised intestinal barrier integrity, leading to increased permeability and immune activation.
- *Cytokine Release*: Certain cytokines and biomarkers, including zonulin and antigliadin antibodies, have been implicated in the pathophysiology of NCGS (Shiha et al 2024).

The consuming of gluten can greatly impact symptom severity, showing the important role of the gut–brain axis in NCGS. Recent studies have pointed out the effect of nocebo, where negative beliefs about gluten consumption worsen symptoms. This suggests that NCGS may not be a separate clinical disorder, but rather a mix of conditions with similar symptoms (Mennini et al 2024). Patients often find relief from symptoms when they avoid gluten, but symptoms can return when gluten is reintroduced. The clinical presentation of NCGS varies, with common symptoms discussed below.

11.3.3.2 Gastrointestinal Symptoms

- *Abdominal Pain*: Frequently reported, often resembling irritable bowel syndrome (Catassi et al 2023).
- *Bloating and Dyspepsia*: Many patients experience discomfort and digestive issues after gluten consumption.
- *Nausea*: This symptom can also manifest alongside other gastrointestinal complaints.

Despite these symptoms, the pathophysiology of NCGS remains poorly understood, and no definitive biomarkers exist for diagnosis (Shiha et al 2024). Conversely, some researchers argue that symptoms attributed to NCGS may also arise from other dietary components, such as FODMAPs or non-gluten proteins in wheat, complicating the understanding of this condition.

11.3.3.3 Diagnosis and Treatment

NCGS is a condition that is identified through exclusion; after CD and wheat allergy have been ruled out, NCGS is considered (Kamilova et al 2023). The management of NCGS mainly revolves around dietary changes, especially the use of gluten-restricted diets or GFDs. In NCGS, a GFD is generally advised, but a GRD might be adequate for symptom relief, and it is important that nutritional assessments are carried out regularly to ensure that no deficiencies result from restrictive diets. Intestinal barrier dysfunction and inflammation, which are gluten's toxic effects, may be alleviated by dietary polyphenols. However, much more work is needed to fully understand the mechanisms and to develop better ways of diagnosis and treatment of NCGS. Although diet therapy works well for many NCGS patients, the absence of well-defined diagnostic criteria and the unknown nature of the pathophysiology of the condition make the issue of treatment more difficult.

11.3.4 Wheat Allergy

Wheat allergy is mainly an IgE-mediated allergic reaction that targets certain protein components of wheat, mainly gluten and its fractions, which can have a major impact on the physical health and overall quality of life of the affected individuals. Among children, it is a considerable problem and is basically a condition whose symptoms extend from dermatological manifestations to difficulties in breathing. Therefore, correct diagnosis is key to the right treatment that most of the time is allergen avoidance. Its pathophysiology comprises the process where the subject becomes sensitive to these proteins and thus experiences different allergic symptoms in the subsequent contact with them.

11.3.4.1 IgE Sensitization and Allergens

- Wheat proteins, especially gliadins and glutenins, are the main allergens, with omega-5 gliadin identified as a significant trigger for allergic reactions (Obtułowicz et al 2015).
- Hydrolyzed wheat proteins can also induce allergies due to the formation of neo-allergens through deamidation, which alters the protein structure and enhances IgE binding (Tranquet et al 2018).

11.3.4.2 Role of Amylase/Trypsin Inhibitors (ATIs)

- ATIs, constituting 2–4% of wheat proteins, have been implicated in IgE-mediated reactions and may trigger innate immune responses, contributing to wheat-related disorders.

While the IgE-mediated mechanism is well-documented, some individuals may have non-IgE-mediated reactions to wheat. This highlights the complexity of wheat allergies and the need for more research into these other pathways.

11.3.4.3 Key Symptoms of Wheat Allergy

- *Skin Reactions*: Urticaria (hives) and angioedema are common, presenting as itchy, swollen areas on the skin.
- *Respiratory Issues*: Symptoms may include asthma, rhinitis, and, in severe cases, anaphylaxis, which is a life-threatening reaction (Zheng et al 2024).
- *Gastrointestinal Distress*: Symptoms can also include abdominal pain, nausea, vomiting, and diarrhea, although these are more the characteristic of non-IgE-mediated responses.

11.3.4.4 Dietary Management Strategies

- The cornerstone for managing wheat allergy is the elimination of gluten from the diet to prevent allergic reactions and gastrointestinal symptoms.
- Regular consultations with dietitians are essential to ensure balanced nutrition and to address potential deficiencies associated with GFD.
- Continuous assessment of adherence to the GFD and monitoring for complications such as metabolic syndrome and nutritional deficiencies are crucial.

11.3.4.5 Diagnostic Approaches

Skin prick tests (SPT), specific IgE testing, and oral food challenge (OFC) are the main methods to check for a wheat allergy. While the current diagnostic landscape for wheat allergy is improving, distinguishing wheat allergy from NCGS remains difficult, complicating clinical management (Kamilova et al 2023). Further research is essential to refine diagnostic tools and treatment options. More studies are needed to improve diagnostic tools and therapies.

11.4 MILLETS AS GLUTEN-FREE ALTERNATIVES

Millets are gaining popularity as a nutritious, gluten-free alternative to traditional grains, such as wheat, making them particularly beneficial for individuals with coeliac disease or gluten sensitivity. Millets' high nutritional profile, combined with their ability to adapt to a variety of environmental conditions, makes them a viable option for improving food security and health. They can help to build a sustainable agriculture by ensuring food security, nutritional security, disease prevention, and economic security. They are classified as major or minor based on their grain size and cultivation area. Major millets include sorghum (*Sorghum bicolor*), pearl millet (*Pennisetum glaucum*), and finger millet (*Eleusine coracana*), whereas minor millets include foxtail millet (*Setaria italica*), barnyard millet (*Echinochloa frumentacae*), kodo millet (*Paspalum scrobiculatum*), little millet (*Panicum sumatrense*), and proso millet (*Panicum miliaceum*). Each type has its own unique features and nutritional benefits. Many major and minor millets are grown around the world, but their consumer acceptability is lower.

While grains such as buckwheat and amaranth are nutrient-dense, millets provide an intriguing blend of vital nutrients, dietary fiber, and antioxidants that are at the root of their health-promoting properties. Millets have a strong antioxidant capacity, which is very effective in fighting oxidative stress, the most common problem in gluten-sensitive individuals. They are rich in essential minerals such as calcium, magnesium, and potassium, often surpassing other gluten-free grains in mineral density (Pandey et al 2024). Regular consumption of millets has been linked to positive health outcomes, including improved blood sugar control, reduced risk of cardiovascular diseases, and management of obesity. These benefits are particularly important in combating lifestyle-related health issues.

Millets are naturally gluten-free and versatile, which can be used in various food applications, including bakery products like bread, biscuits, and cookies. As discussed above, millets can be an alternative nutrient-rich source for individuals with gluten-related disorders that are required to maintain appropriate body function without gluten consumption. Also, millets are low glycemic in nature due to the slower digestibility of carbohydrate and their delayed absorption helps in the reduction of blood glucose spike during digestion in diabetic people when consumed. Millets are rich in phytonutrients such as phenolics, flavonoids, dietary fiber, and phytosterols, which help in reducing the risk of various degenerative diseases (Figure 11.4). It potentially offers various health beneficial properties such as anti-inflammatory, antioxidative, anti-ulcerative, anticarcinogenic, anti-cholesterol, antimicrobial, hypoglycemic, and prebiotic (Sharma et al 2021).

11.4.1 Market Potential of Millets

According to the Food and Agriculture Organization (FAO), India is the largest producer and consumer of millets worldwide. India's contribution is about 38.4% of global production. Among the Indian states, Rajasthan is the largest producer followed by Uttar Pradesh, Karnataka, Tamil Nadu, and Maharashtra. In the year 2024, millets were cultivated in an area of 12.19 million hectares with a production of 15.38 million metric tons. During the same period, Indian millets were exported to countries such as UAE, Saudi Arabia, Nepal, and USA, to a volume of 1.46 lakh metric tons and amount of 70.89 million USD (APEDA 2023). The millet market size is expected to significantly

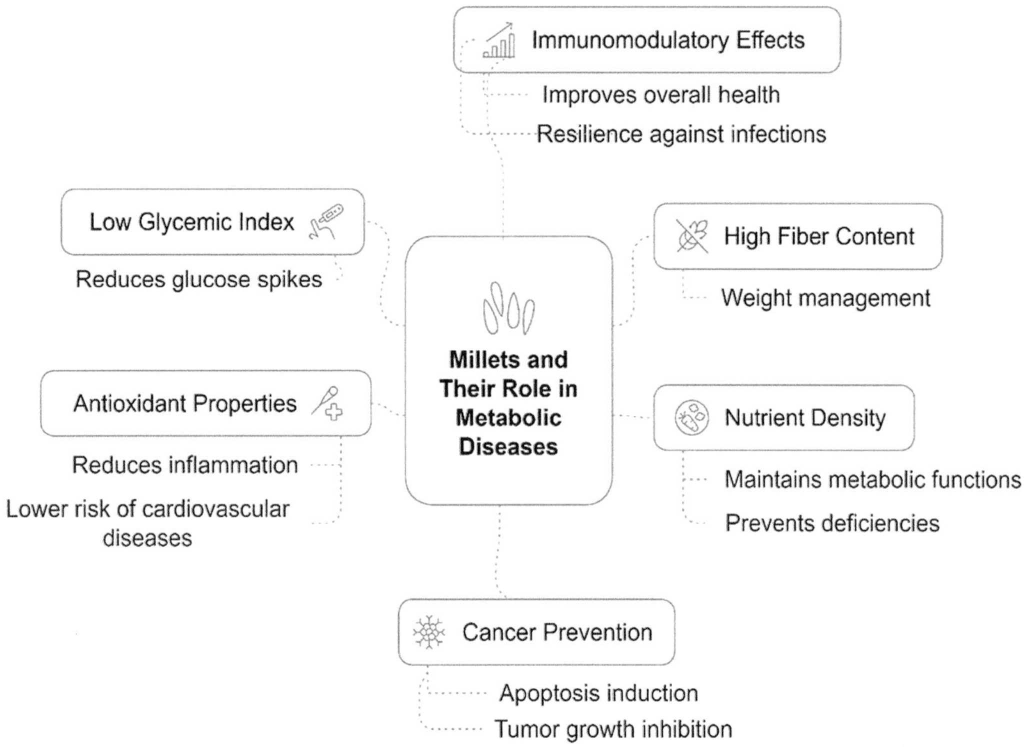

FIGURE 11.4 Health benefits of millets.

expand due to the intersection of environment challenges, health-focused consumer base, and government initiatives. In 2024, the global millet market size was valued at 15.3 billion USD and expected to reach 234 billion USD by 2034 with a CAGR of 4.4% (Global Market Insights 2025). The shifting perception of consumers towards nutritional benefits and clean-label products makes millets stand at the right spot in this trend.

11.4.2 Challenges Associated with Millet Utilization

- However, they are often less accepted by consumers compared to traditional crops, primarily due to taste and texture issues.
- Despite its nutritional benefits, millet products face challenges in consumer acceptability. They are generally considered less palatable than wheat products. To improve this, blending millet flour with wheat flour is a common practice, which helps enhance the taste and texture of the final products.
- Compared to major cereals such as rice and wheat, the techno-functional properties of millet flours were lower and it affected its usage commercially. Processing methods such as starch and protein modifications using thermal and non-thermal treatments may positively influence its functionality, nutritional and bioactive composition.
- Another major reason for poor consumer acceptability response is due to the lack of advanced processing technologies for the production across different categories such as ready to eat, ready to cook, ready to drink compared to other major cereals.
- Reduced shelf life of millets due to rancidity, which affects the storage duration and sensory parameters, is another factor that influences its wider acceptability. Higher fat content and lipase activity also contribute to the poor shelf life of millet flours.

- Although millets exist from ancient times, palatability in terms of taste and flavor reduces their consumption and their chance of becoming a mainstream grain.
- Antinutritional factors, such as tannins, phytic acids, protease inhibitors present in higher amounts in bran and hull, interfere with the nutrient absorption and bioavailability. To remove these factors, primary processing of millets needs to be done with higher efficiency, and reduced cost which is still in growing phase.
- Due to the absence of gluten, the development of fermented gluten-free products such as bread, buns, pizza bases with millets are difficult. Various technologies and compositional approaches can be used to overcome the challenge, but the cost of final product will be higher.
- Other non-fermented gluten-free bakery products such as biscuits, cookies, crackers, pasta, vermicelli, noodles can be prepared easily with the addition of suitable additives.
- In developing countries, crop improvement strategies are mostly focused on other major cereals. This causes the millets to fall behind and slows down farmers' adaptability.
- Lack of efficient primary processing technologies to dehull and polish the minor millets is another challenge. This is due to its smaller size, variation among millets and within its varieties leads to difficulty in designing a common equipment similar to rice and wheat.

More research related to addressing the above-mentioned challenges related to millets is required to improve their consumption and export to other countries, ultimately increasing the farmers' income.

11.5 UTILIZATION OF MILLETS IN GLUTEN-FREE FOODS

In recent times, due to the higher incidence of gluten-related disorders and intake by normal individuals as a healthier option led to significant momentum in the millet-based gluten-free food products (Figure 11.5). Millet is explored extensively in food categories such as bakery products, instant

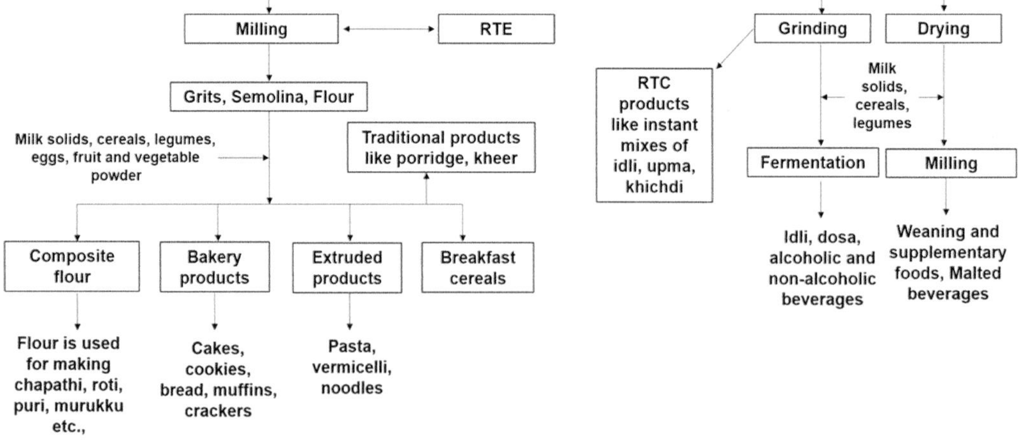

FIGURE 11.5 Schematic diagram for developing millet-based composite foods. (Adapted and modified from Kumar et al (2018).)

mixes and beverages. The processed food market is expanding globally due to changing economic status, increased per capital income, fast pacing life, higher standard of living, and advancements in technology (Aggarwal and Sharma 2020).

11.5.1 Bakery Products

Among the food processing sectors, bakery is one of the largest sectors with huge number of organized and unorganized players. Due to its lower cost, bakery products were widely consumed. The formation of gluten network is an essential for the development of bakery products. The substitution or complete replacement of gluten will lead to product quality changes drastically. To overcome this challenge, various agents such as enzymes, emulsifiers, hydrocolloids, extruded flours or the use of protein addition and various other technologies were widely studied (Table 11.1). The development of gluten-free breads with millet flours improves the nutritional quality, beneficial for human health as it is widely prepared using lesser-nutrient ingredients such as starch and hydrocolloids. Sarabhai et al (2021) reported the development of complete foxtail millet gluten-free bread with the addition of enzymes such as protease, xylanase, and glucose oxidase, which significantly improved the specific volume, crumb springiness, lowered the hardness, and altered the rheological properties than control. Protease addition at 0.1% increased the batter elasticity and overall sensory acceptability than other enzymes used such as xylanase and glucose oxidase. Lazova-Borisova and Angelov (2020) developed gluten-free breads with millet, rice, and chickpeas to find their suitability for preparation. They found that millet flour was highly suitable with higher polyunsaturated fatty acid and omega 3: omega 6 ratio. Pessanha et al (2021) studied the effect of incorporating extruded pearl millet flour at 50 and 100%. The results showed no reduction in nutritional content, increased antioxidant activity, and higher specific volume at 50% extruded flour substitution. This proved that extrusion has great potential in developing GFBs. de Aguiar et al (2024) developed whole pearl millet-based gluten-free bread with the addition of starch, milk, egg, and hydrocolloids. The developed breads received better sensory acceptability and have improved dietary fiber and protein content compared to rice-based bread and wheat bread. Tamilselvan et al (2022) developed complete proso millet bread using different hydrocolloids such as xanthan gum, guar gum, and hydroxypropyl methyl cellulose (HPMC). The results showed that HPMC at 2% showed drastic improvement in batter rheological properties, loaf volume, color, and overall sensory acceptability.

Saberi et al (2023) developed gluten-free sponge cake with 50% corn flour and the replacement of millet flour (50%) with different concentrations of chia seed flour (from 4 to 16%). The addition of chia flour increased cake hardness, radical scavenging activity, reduced the specific volume, porosity, and crust lightness and redness values. Zhang et al (2024) used extruded pearl millet flour-based cake. The extrusion of flour at lower moisture (14%) and higher temperature (170°C) significantly increased the batter viscoelasticity and cake-specific volume, reduced cake hardness, and bettered the overall quality of the cake. The authors suggested that the use of extruded millet flour is an important alternative to improve whole millet cake quality. Flatbread is widely consumed in Indian diet and important carbohydrate source. Kumar et al (2020) developed gluten-free flatbread using pearl millet flour as the base substituted with extruded finger millet flour at various concentrations (10–30%). This substitution significantly increased the nutritional, dough rheological in terms of extensibility, puffing, textural, and overall sensory properties of the flatbread. In the same way, Kumar et al (2023) substituted extruded finger millet flour for maize-based unleavened flatbread at various concentrations (10–30%). The authors observed a significant improvement in dough viscoelasticity; textural properties and taste were similar to control. From these studies, we can conclude that the substitution of extruded finger millet flour can alter the rheology, techno-functional, and nutritional quality of the flatbreads.

Gluten-free cookies are one of the widely consumed bakery products which are higher in fat and sugar and can be developed easier with the addition of additives compared to fermented bakery

TABLE 11.1
Gluten-Free Bakery Products Developed with Millets

Product	Technology/Ingredient Used	Important Outcomes of the Study	Reference
Little millet bread	Planetary ball milling	• Substitution of ball-milled flour at various concentrations (5–25%) altered the flour functional properties and microstructure. • Ball-milled flour improved the batter viscoelasticity, bread loaf, and specific volume, textural and sensorial properties were highest at 15% substitution level.	Tamilselvan et al (2024)
Rice and Foxtail millet-based bread	Hydrocolloids – HPMC (1 and 2%), pectin (1.5 and 2.5%), and concentrated raisin juice (CRJ) (3 and 4%)	• Bread color increased with the addition of HPMC and pectin. • 1% HPMC showed higher volume. • 1% HPMC and 3% CRJ gave bread with better technological and sensory quality.	Abdollahzadeh et al (2024)
Foxtail millet bread	Sourdough technology	• Four strains of lactic acid bacteria used as starter culture. • Sourdough fermentation increased the bread texture such as hardness, springiness, gumminess, and chewiness.	Li et al (2024)
Sorghum gluten-free bread	Extrusion and germination	• Substitution of 5% germinated millet flour in sorghum bread enhanced crumb softness.	Comettant-Rabanal et al (2021)
Proso millet bread	Extraneous protein and enzymes	• Protein incorporation increased the crumb structure strength, specific volume, and sensory acceptability. • Reduced bread hardness and inherent bitter taste removal from millets. • Transglutaminase showed minimal effect.	Tomić et al (2020)
Sorghum cookies	Malting	• Cookies with malted red sorghum flours have higher protein digestibility and gamma aminobutyric acid content.	Garzón et al (2020)
Multi-cereal and legume cookies	Parboiled rice, kodo millet, sorghum, foxtail millet, green gram, Bengal gram, black gram, cowpea, and soybean	• Multi-cereal mix flour showed reduced water and oil absorption capacity than wheat flour. • Lightness reduced and hardness increased with increasing storage time. • Overall acceptability was good.	Vasanthakumari and Jaganmohan (2018)
Pearl millet cookies	Pearl millet and flaxseed flour	• Flaxseed substitution at 17% can be used to develop better-quality cookies. • Flaxseed increased the hardness and decreased the fracturability.	Bashir et al (2020)
Pearl millet biscuit	Orange peel flour substitution	• 5 and 10% peel addition has acceptable sensory quality. • Peel addition increased the dietary fiber, minerals, and antioxidant content.	Obafaye and Omoba (2018)
Pearl millet biscuit	Fermentation and malting	• Both traditional processing improved the biscuit's nutritional composition and amino acid content. • Malted biscuit was found to be highly acceptable.	Adebiyi et al (2017)

(Continued)

TABLE 11.1 (Continued)
Gluten-Free Bakery Products Developed with Millets

Product	Technology/Ingredient Used	Important Outcomes of the Study	Reference
Finger millet biscuits	Spontaneous fermentation (SF)	• SF decreased ash, fiber, and fat contents, while increasing protein, carbohydrates, energy, mineral, and antioxidant contents of biscuits. • SF affected physical and microstructural properties. • 24 h fermented biscuits showed better sensory properties.	Mudau et al (2022)
Foxtail millet biscuit	Hydrocolloid addition – carboxymethylcellulose (CMC)	• Hardness of CMC-added biscuit was similar to control. • CMC altered the morphology and internal structure. • 0.1% CMC was highly acceptable sensorially.	Reaz et al (2023)
Gluten-free pearl millet crackers	Germinated pearl millet flour (70%), defatted sesame flour (20%), and tigernut flour (10%)	• Nutritional content of the developed cracker was superior than wheat crackers. • Antinutrient was reduced and protein digestibility was improved. • 70:20:10 formulation was highly acceptable.	Akeem et al (2023)
Gluten-free millet muffins	chickpea protein isolate (CPI), microbial transglutaminase (MTG), and xanthan gum (XG)	• Addition of CPI, MTG, and XG altered the batter consistency index and apparent viscosity. • The study showed protein network can be formed in gluten-free muffins by adding CPI and MTG.	Shaabani et al (2018)
Gluten-free rice flour and pearl millet-based muffins	Oyster mushroom powder (OMP)	• Addition of OMP at varying concentration in rice flour pearl millet flour blend increased the protein content significantly. • OMP increased hardness, chewiness, and color of the muffins. • 15% OMP substitution was highly acceptable.	Dhillon et al (2023)

products. Aljobair (2022) optimized gluten-free cookies using complete sorghum, millet flour, and their combinations and compared them with wheat flour cookies. Cookies made with the combination of sorghum: millet flour (25:75) showed better nutritional profile, phenolic content, antioxidant activity, and acceptable sensory quality suitable for celiac population. To increase the health benefits, Selvaraju et al (2024) developed finger and pearl millet flour-based gluten-free cookies with the substitution of microalgae *Chlorella minutissima*. This substitution increased the cookie hardness, protein content by 2%, total phenolic content, better *invitro* carbohydrate digestibility leading to lower glycemic index. The authors suggested these cookies for diabetic population too. Brites et al (2018) aimed to prepare gluten-free cookies similar to wheat cookies in terms of physical and textural characteristics. They achieved this by optimizing the formulation consisting of 7.5% chia seeds, 40% proso millet flour, and 52.5% buckwheat flour. Lestari et al (2017) developed low GI cookie bar using gluten-free ingredients such as foxtail millet flour (15%), kidney bean (30%) and arrowroot flour (15%) with good sensory score. Higher millet flour substitution led to darker color, harder texture, and higher protein content.

Biscuits are one of the important instant snacks consumed globally due to its convenience, taste, and shelf life. Adugna et al (2024) developed gluten-free finger millet biscuit by preparing flour from different processing methods such as fermentation and malting. The processed flour-added biscuits showed higher sensory acceptability, increased proximate and mineral contents, while reducing their antinutritional content compared to native biscuits. Manchanda et al (2024) developed multi-millet biscuit with finger millet, pearl millet, and buckwheat. Compared to refined wheat flour biscuits, these biscuits have higher protein, mineral content, energy density, and sensory acceptability. In contrast, to achieve calorie reduction, Singh and Kumar (2018) prepared composite mix of ger minated foxtail millet (85%) and copra meal (15%), substituted this mix with amaranth (60:40), and developed gluten-free biscuits. The authors achieved drastic reduction in calorie, antinutrients, and acrylamide formation. Di Cairano et al (2021) developed biscuits using buckwheat, millet, sorghum, and legume at varying proportions. Biscuits found to have darker crust, reduced hardness, and low glycemic index than soft wheat flour biscuit. Similarly, Hymavathi et al (2020) developed sorghum biscuits with different variations such as sweet, salt, coconut, and peanut and found all of them to be nutrient-dense and low glycemic. Millets are naturally low glycemic in nature, tapping this potential will help in developing nutrient-rich biscuits for consumers.

11.5.2 Extruded Products

Extrusion technology is widely used to produce value-added products from millets and other grains. The market for extruded snacks market is valued at 63.38 billion dollars in 2024 and is predicted to reach 74.52 billion dollars by 2030 with a growth rate of 4.7% (Grand View Research 2024). Compared to conventional methods, extrusion has various advantages such as continuous processing, multifunctional equipment, and better control over the output. Extrusion is of two types: (1) Cold extrusion uses no heat and minimal shear to extrude the product; (2) hot extrusion is a thermo-mechanical process which involves the use of high heat, high pressure, and high shear rate to extrude the product.

Cold extruded products such as pasta, noodles, and vermicelli were consumed globally. Traditionally, wheat semolina is the major ingredient widely used to develop pasta, whereas the gluten-free pasta developed using non-gluten sources is not available commercially. This might be due to the lack of processing ability. Rudra et al (2020) developed gluten-free pasta using blends of hydrothermally treated barnyard millet and amaranth flour. Pasta developed with 50:50 ratio showed lower cooking loss, higher firmness, least stickiness, and easy digestibility. Manoj Kumar et al (2019) successfully prepared depigmented pearl millet flour-based pasta by using milk proteins (sodium caseinate and whey protein concentrate) along with transglutaminase. Enzyme addition drastically improved the pasta firmness, sensory attributes and drastically reduced the cooking loss. In another study, Pessanha et al (2023) found that the substitution of whole millet precooked flour (50%) prepared by extrusion in raw millet flour helps in the development of gluten-free pasta with better quality parameters such as better texture, higher antioxidant, and antihyperglycemic activity, and nutritional content than raw flour. The sensory evaluators flagged only the cooked texture as poor in the developed product. Gwekwe et al (2024) prepared gluten-free sorghum pasta using sorghum flour, pearl millet flour, and bean flour (20%). The final-developed pasta has higher protein and fiber content, better physical and sensory properties. Similarly, Palavecino et al (2019) developed gluten-free sorghum pasta with better nutritional quality that especially altered the starch hydrolysis rate due to multi-fold increment in slowly digestible starch, lower glycemic index, antioxidant activity, and higher potentially bioaccessible polyphenol contents. Tyl et al (2020) suggested cooking of pasta drastically induced changes in protein solubility and its secondary structure. Also, they found that proso millet can be utilized as a promising ingredient to develop gluten-free pasta. In the same way, Motta Romero et al (2017) evaluated the addition of hydrocolloids on the dough

TABLE 11.2
Gluten-Free Extruded Products Developed with Millets

Product	Technology/Ingredient Used	Important Outcomes of the Study	Reference
Foxtail millet pasta	Tapioca flour addition	• 70% foxtail millet flour and 30% tapioca flour were optimized formulation with better sensory quality. • Higher protein, mineral, fiber, and fat were observed than standard pasta.	Rao et al (2021)
Pearl millet pasta	Amaranth flour substitution (0–50%)	• The higher the pearl millet, the higher the cooking loss. • 60% pearl millet and 40% amaranth flour had better yield similar to conventional pasta. • Cooking loss is within limit and has a good sensory score.	Rathore and Pandey (2023)
Sorghum pasta	Peanut flour substitution	• 90% sorghum and 10% peanut flour were highly acceptable by the panelists. • Peanut substitution significantly affected the functional properties and improved pasta nutritional composition.	Sobowale et al (2019)
Gluten-free rice noodles	Finger millet (FM) substitution (10–30 g/100 g)	• 20% FM substitution was accepted sensorially. • FM substitution increased the antioxidant activity, nutritional and cooking parameters. • Resistant starch content was higher than control.	Chen et al (2021)

rheological properties of proso millet pasta. Xanthan gum at 2% significantly improved the elasticity and the network strength of the developed pasta dough. Proso millet pasta with higher amylose and high molecular weight prolamins showed higher firmness, chewiness with lower cooking loss and stickiness score (Cordelino et al 2019).

Noodles are also widely consumed. It belongs to a fast-growing sector and is popularized due to its convenience, shelf life, cost effectiveness, and easy cooking ability. It is mainly prepared using wheat flour. Functional pasta, developed with multi-millet flour blend (40% proso millet, 30% little millet, and 30% kodo millet) with addition of inulin at various concentrations, was developed by Mubeena and Haripriya (2021). A 20% inulin addition showed better textural and sensory acceptability similar to control and recommended for commercialization by the panelists. Dahal et al (2021) developed corn- and millet-based gluten-free noodles using hydrocolloids in response surface methodology. The optimized formulation consists of 98.77 g corn flour, 60 g millet flour, 50 g egg, 1.5 g of xanthan gum, and 1.47 g of guar gum. Hydrocolloids addition improved the textural properties, water-holding capacity, tensile strength, and stability of the noodles. Limited research work has been done on the development of gluten-free noodles and its evaluation (Table 11.2). This area needs to be explored in detail to tap its market potential globally.

11.5.3 Beverage Products

In recent years, plant-based or non-dairy functional beverages have been growing at international markets, and the consumer trend in their consumption showing positive signs of growth due to new concepts, health concerns, and clean label trend (Table 11.3). In a study by Joseph et al (2025),

TABLE 11.3
Gluten-Free Beverages Developed with Millets

Product	Technology/Ingredient Used	Important Outcomes of the Study	Reference
Millet milk	Coconut milk substitution at various concentrations (40–60%)	• 50:50 substitution was found to have better nutritional profile than other combinations. • Selected combination has better sensory acceptability.	Dhankhar et al (2019)
Millet ready to drink beverage	Sorghum and finger millet was used as base	• Sorghum and finger millet (26:26) was acceptable sensorially. • Antioxidant activity was significantly higher in coconut-flavored beverage, while phenolic content was higher in carrot-flavored beverage.	Bembem and Agrahar-Murugkar (2020)
Millet and sprouted legume-based beverage	Base ingredient contains 5.8% of sorghum and pearl millet each flavored with jaggery, buttermilk, and salt	• Jaggery flavored has higher sensory acceptability. • Buttermilk flavored was having better nutritional composition in terms of protein, calcium, iron, and phosphorous. • Total phenolics, flavonoids, and antioxidants are also higher in buttermilk-flavored one.	Agrahar-Murugkar et al (2020)
Multifunctional prebiotic functional beverage	Barnyard, foxtail, and kodo millet	• D-optimal design found that combination of barnyard (7 g/100 g): foxtail (10 g/100 g): kodo (8 g/100 g). • Fructooligosaccharides was added to improve taste, soluble fiber content, and prebiotic property.	Arya and Shakya (2021)
White finger millet probiotic beverage	Fermented using *Lactobacillus rhamnosus*	• Response surface methodology (RSM) identified a combination of 14% finger millet, 1% microbial inoculum, and 5% sugar received highest acceptability. • This combination has higher viscosity and lighter color than other combinations.	Navyashree et al (2023)

barnyard millet milk-based drink added with *Spirulina* sp., fermented with *Lactobacillus rhamnosus* and *Saccharomyces cerevisiae* suitable for diabetic population, was developed. Bacterial fermented drink showed higher phenolic content and antimicrobial activity. The flavored fermented combination received better sensory scores with a shelf life of five days at 4°C. Vila-Real et al (2022) developed finger millet-based yogurt-like beverage cocultured with *Weissella confusa* and *Lactobacillus plantarum*. Both strains improved the count above 10^8 CFU/ml, improved gamma aminobutyric acid, dextran content, protein digestibility significantly and sensorially acceptable. In the follow-up study, Vila-Real et al (2025) found that the developed beverage has higher antidiabetic activity and phenolic content, which improved with fermentation. Also, they suggested the possibility of consuming fermented finger millet on impacting blood glucose levels and gut microbiota. Udeh et al (2025) explored the effect of fermentation time on functional finger millet malt beverages fermented with *Lactobacillus fermentum*. The higher the fermentation time, the lower the phenolic content. At 24 h fermentation, this developed malt beverage has better phenolic and antioxidant content. An innovative product millet skim beverage was developed by Pan et al (2019), optimizing the processing parameters such as soaking with 0.5 g/100 g sodium bicarbonate solution and 15 min blanching. Srivastava et al (2025) developed novel synbiotic beverage using pearl millet and soy milk fermented with *L. plantarum*. Compared to unfermented beverage, this developed beverage with pearl millet (40%) has strain count greater than 10^8 CFU/ml with higher viability percentage, better sensory acceptability during the 25 days storage duration. Challa et al (2025) developed foxtail millet beverage with *Lactobacillus* culture by fermenting at different incubation periods. About 8 h of incubation were accepted sensorially with a consumer acceptability index of 89%. The authors suggested production of this beverage into larger scale due to its higher nutritional, mineral content, and antioxidants.

11.5.4 Future Perspectives

- Future work should focus on diversifying millet-based products beyond traditional staples (like rotis or porridge) to include pasta, noodles, bread, cookies, breakfast cereals, and snacks tailored for gluten-intolerant populations.
- One major hurdle in the wider acceptance of millet-based gluten-free products is their crumbly texture and earthy flavor. Future research should emphasize on hydrocolloid use, enzymatic treatments, composite blending, and fermentation techniques to enhance mouthfeel, softness, and shelf life.
- There is a lack of standardized protocols for millet-based gluten-free product development and labeling.
- Developing uniform processing standards and validated gluten-testing methods for millet products will build consumer trust and ensure food safety for celiac patients.
- Despite the known nutritional benefits, clinical trials evaluating the therapeutic benefits of millets in celiac patients are limited.
- Future efforts should include longitudinal studies assessing the impact of regular millet consumption on gut health, micronutrient status, and inflammatory markers in celiac individuals.
- Microbiome-based studies to validate the role of millets in restoring gut health post-gluten damage.
- The millet-based gluten-free segment remains underutilized due to limited consumer awareness and product availability.
- A major issue in gluten-free food production is the risk of cross-contamination during cultivation, storage, and processing. Establishing dedicated gluten-free millet value chains and certification systems will enhance food safety and compliance.

11.6 CONCLUSION

CD, a chronic autoimmune disorder triggered by gluten ingestion, presents a significant dietary challenge for affected individuals. The increasing global prevalence of this condition has intensified the demand for safe, nutritious, and gluten-free food alternatives. Millets offer a promising solution due to their naturally gluten-free nature, rich nutrient profile, and adaptability to diverse agro-climatic conditions. Beyond their nutritional advantages, millets possess functional and sensory properties that support the development of a wide array of gluten-free food products. However, challenges such as limited consumer awareness, processing constraints, price and variability in taste and texture still hinder their mainstream acceptance. Scientific validation of millet safety for celiac patients' consumption, coupled with innovations in product development and processing technologies, can pave the way for millets to become a staple in gluten-free dietary regimes. Integrating millets into therapeutic nutrition not only benefits individuals with CD but also supports sustainable agriculture and food security.

REFERENCES

Abdollahzadeh, A., Vazifedoost, M., Didar, Z., Haddadkhodaprast, M. H., & Armin, M. 2024. Comparison of the effect of hydroxyl propyl methyl cellulose, pectin, and concentrated raisin juice on gluten-free bread based on rice and foxtail millet flour. *Food Science & Nutrition*, *12*(1), 439–449. https://doi.org/10.1002/FSN3.3741

Adebiyi, J. A., Obadina, A. O., Adebo, O. A., & Kayitesi, E. 2017. Comparison of nutritional quality and sensory acceptability of biscuits obtained from native, fermented, and malted pearl millet (*Pennisetum glaucum*) flour. *Food Chemistry*, *232*, 210–217. https://doi.org/10.1016/J.FOODCHEM.2017.04.020

Adugna, A. A., Tolesa, G. N., Abera, S., & Deme, G. D. 2024. Effect of grain fermentation and malting time on nutrient and anti nutrient composition of biscuits from Aksum finger millet (*Eleusine coracana*). *Cogent Food and Agriculture*, *10*(1). https://doi.org/10.1080/23311932.2024.2336690

Aggarwal, M., & Sharma, D. 2020. Millet flour for baked food products. *Plant Archives*, *20*, 458–461.

Agrahar-Murugkar, D., Bajpai-Dixit, P., & Kotwaliwale, N. 2020. Rheological, nutritional, functional and sensory properties of millets and sprouted legume based beverages. *Journal of Food Science and Technology*, *57*(5), 1671–1679.

Akeem, S. A., Mustapha, B. O., Ayinla, R. O., Ajibola, O., Johnson, W. O., & Akintayo, O. A. 2023. Physical characteristics, nutritional composition and acceptability of gluten-free crackers produced from germinated pearl millet (*Pennisetum glaucum*), defatted-sesame seed (*Sesamum indicum*) and defatted-tigernut (*Cyperus esculentus*) composite flours. *Discover Food*, *3*(1), 1–17.

Aljobair, M. O. 2022. Physicochemical properties and sensory attributes of cookies prepared from sorghum and millet composite flour. *Food Science and Nutrition*, *10*(10), 3415–3423.

Anderson, R. P., & Jabri, B. 2013. Vaccine against autoimmune disease: Antigen-specific immunotherapy. *Current Opinion in Immunology*, *25*, 410–7.

APEDA. 2023. *Indian Millets*. https://apeda.gov.in/apedawebsite/SubHead_Products/Indian_Millets.htm

Arya, S. S., & Shakya, N. K. 2021. High fiber, low glycaemic index (GI) prebiotic multigrain functional beverage from barnyard, foxtail and kodo millet. *LWT*, *135*, 109991. https://doi.org/10.1016/J.LWT.2020.109991

Aziz, I., Evans, K. E., Papageorgiou, V., & Sanders, D. S. 2011. Are patients with coeliac disease seeking alternative therapies to a gluten-free diet? *Journal of Gastrointestinal and Liver Diseases*, *20*, 27–31.

Bashir, S., Yaseen, M., Sharma, V., Ranjan Purohit, S., Barak, S., & Mudgil, D. 2020. *Rheological and Textural Properties of Gluten Free Cookies Based on Pearl Millet and Flaxseed*. https://doi.org/10.33263/BRIAC105.65656576

Belton, P. 1999. Mini review: On the elasticity of wheat gluten. *Journal of Cereal Science*, *29*(2), 103–7. https://doi.org/10.1006/jcrs.1998.0227

Bembem, K., & Agrahar-Murugkar, D. 2020. Development of millet based ready-to-drink beverage for geriatric population. *Journal of Food Science and Technology*, *57*(9), 3278–3283.

Brites, L. T. G. F., Ortolan, F., da Silva, D. W., Bueno, F. R., Rocha, T. de S., Chang, Y. K., & Steel, C. J. 2018. Gluten-free cookies elaborated with buckwheat flour, millet flour and chia seeds. *Food Science and Technology*, *39*(2), 458–466. https://doi.org/10.1590/FST.30416

Cabrera-Chávez, F., Dezar, G. V., Islas-Zamorano, A. P., Espinoza-Alderete, J. G., Vergara-Jiménez, M. J., Magaña-Ordorica, D., & Ontiveros, N. 2017. Prevalence of self-reported gluten sensitivity and adherence to a gluten-free diet in Argentinian adult population. *Nutrients*, *9*(1), 81. https://doi.org/10.3390/nu9010081

Casella, G., Santilli, I., Di Bella, C., Crisafulli, V., Villanacci, V., et al. 2017. Cerebellar ataxia, celiac disease and non-celiac gluten sensitivity. *Archives of Neuroscience*, *4*(2), e44187. https://doi.org/10.5812/archneurosci.44187.

Catassi, C., Catassi, G., & Naspi, L. 2023. Nonceliac gluten sensitivity. *Current Opinion in Clinical Nutrition and Metabolic Care*, *26*(5), 490–494. https://doi.org/10.1097/MCO.0000000000000925

Challa, M., Kuna, A., Kata, L., & Das, D. 2025. Probiotic foxtail millet beverage formulation and evaluation of nutritional, physicochemical, and sensory parameters. *International Journal of Food Science and Technology*, *60*(1), 28. https://doi.org/10.1093/IJFOOD/VVAE028

Chen, J., Wang, L., Xiao, P., Li, C., Zhou, H., & Liu, D. 2021. Informative title: Incorporation of finger millet affects in vitro starch digestion, nutritional, antioxidative and sensory properties of rice noodles. *LWT*, *151*, 112145. https://doi.org/10.1016/J.LWT.2021.112145

Ciacci, C. 2022. Clinical features of GRDs. *Gluten-Related Disorders*, 107–112. https://doi.org/10.1016/b978-0-12-821846-4.00005-x

Comettant-Rabanal, R., Carvalho, C. W. P., Ascheri, J. L. R., Chávez, D. W. H., & Germani, R. 2021. Extruded whole grain flours and sprout millet as functional ingredients for gluten-free bread. *LWT, 150*, 112042. https://doi.org/10.1016/J.LWT.2021.112042

Cordelino, I. G., Tyl, C., Inamdar, L., Vickers, Z., Marti, A., & Ismail, B. P. 2019. Cooking quality, digestibility, and sensory properties of proso millet pasta as impacted by amylose content and prolamin profile. *LWT, 99*, 1–7. https://doi.org/10.1016/J.LWT.2018.09.035

Dahal, A., Sadiq, M. B., & Anal, A. K. 2021. Improvement of quality of corn and proso millet-based gluten-free noodles with the application of hydrocolloids. *Journal of Food Processing and Preservation*, *45*(2), e15165. https://doi.org/10.1111/JFPP.15165

de Aguiar, E. V., Centeno, A. C. L. S., Garcia dos Santos, F., & Capriles, V. D. 2024. Whole grain pearl millet-based gluten-free bread: A novel alternative with nutrition and sensory appeal. *Applied Food Research*, *4*(2), 100520. https://doi.org/10.1016/J.AFRES.2024.100520

Dhankhar, J., Kundu, P., & Mehla, R. 2019. Preparation and physicochemical evaluation of dairy free alternative based on coconut and millet milk. *International Journal of Pharmacy and Biological Sciences-IJPBS TM, 1*, 9.

Dhillon, G. K., Kour, A., & Salazar, B. M. 2023. Potential of Pleurotus ostreatus as a novel protein source in rice-millet-based gluten-free muffins. *Cogent Food and Agriculture*, *9*(1). https://doi.org/10.1080/23311932.2023.2191888

Di Cairano, M., Condelli, N., Caruso, M. C., Cela, N., Tolve, R., & Galgano, F. 2021. Use of underexploited flours for the reduction of glycaemic index of gluten-free biscuits: Physicochemical and sensory characterization. *Food and Bioprocess Technology*, *14*(8), 1490–1502. https://doi.org/10.1007/S11947-021-02650-X

Dieterich, W., Esslinger, B., & Schuppan, D. 2003. Pathomechanisms in celiac disease. *International Archives of Allergy and Immunology*, *132*(2), 98–108. https://doi.org/10.1159/000073710

Falcigno, L., Calvanese, L., Conte, M., Nanayakkara, M., Barone, M. V., & D'Auria, G. 2020. Structural perspective of gliadin peptides active in celiac disease. *International Journal of Molecular Sciences*, *21*(23), 9301. https://doi.org/10.3390/ijms21239301

Fasano, A., & Catassi, C. 2012. Clinical practice. Celiac disease. *The New England Journal of Medicine*, *367*, 2419–2426. https://doi.org/10.1056/NEJMcp1113994

Floare, M. L., Wharton, S. B., Simpson, J. E., Aeschlimann, D., Hoggard, N., & Hadjivassiliou, M. 2024. Cerebellar degeneration in gluten ataxia is linked to microglial activation. *Brain Communications*, *6*(2), fcae078. https://doi.org/10.1093/braincomms/fcae078

Garzón, A. G., Erben, M., Osella, C. A., & Drago, S. R. 2020. Effects of baking on γ-aminobutyric acid and free phenolic acids from gluten-free cookies made with native and malted whole sorghum flours. *Journal of Food Processing and Preservation*, *44*(8), e14571. https://doi.org/10.1111/JFPP.14571

Global Market Insights. 2025. *Millets Market Size & Share, Growth Forecasts Report 2025–2034*. https://www.gminsights.com/industry-analysis/millets-market

Grand View Research. 2024. *Extruded Snacks Market Size, Share | Industry Report, 2030*. https://www.grandviewresearch.com/industry-analysis/extruded-snacks-market

Gwekwe, B., Nyanga, L. K., Matsungo, T. M., Chidewe, C., Mukanganyama, S., Nyakudya, E., Mtambanengwe, F., Mapfumo, P., & Chopera, P. 2024. Development and sensory properties of extruded sorghum-based gluten-free pasta. *Food and Feed Research*, *1*(1), 1–17.

Hernández-Lahoz, C., Rodrigo-Sáez, L., Vega-Villar, J., Mauri-Capdevila, G., & Mier-Juanes, J. 2014. Familial gluten ataxia. *Movement Disorders: Official Journal of the Movement Disorder Society*, *29*(3), 308–310. https://doi.org/10.1002/mds.25783

Hymavathi, T. V., Robert, P., Thejasri, V., Jyosthna, E., & Wang, H.-Y. 2020. Proximate composition and glycemic index profiling of differently composed nutri-cereal biscuits. *International Research Journal of Pure and Applied Chemistry, IRJPAC*, (1), 39–46. https://doi.org/10.9734/IRJPAC/2020/V21I2130288

Joseph, B., Bhavadharini, M., Nivetha, S., Lavanya, M., Jaganmohan, R., Baskaran, N., & Vignesh, S. 2025. Synbiotic fermented barnyard millet drink: Exploring its nutritional profile, sensory attributes, and bioactive health potentials. *Food Chemistry Advances*, *6*, 100872. https://doi.org/10.1016/J.FOCHA.2024.100872

Kamilova, A. T., Azimova, N. D., & Zakharova, I. N. 2023. Gluten-related disorders: wheat allergy and non-celiac gluten sensitivity. *Pediatrics. Consilium Medicum*, (4), 246–251.

Krishnaprasad, P., Gallati, C., Dhillon, J., & Bakst, B. 2023. S4093 understanding gluten ataxia in a newly diagnosed celiac disease patient: A case report. *The American Journal of Gastroenterology*, *118*(10S), S2596. https://doi.org/10.14309/01.ajg.0000966012.02404.d7

Kumar, A., Tomer, V., Kaur, A., Kumar, V., & Gupta, K. 2018. Millets: A solution to agrarian and nutritional challenges. *Agriculture and Food Security*, *7*(1), 1–15.

Kumar, P., Kaur, C., Rudra, S. G., & Arora, B. 2023. Extruded finger millet improves rheology and quality of composite maize flatbread. *International Journal of Gastronomy and Food Science*, *31*, 100638. https://doi.org/10.1016/J.IJGFS.2022.100638

Kumar, P., Kaur, C., Sethi, S., & Kaur Jambh, H. 2020. Effect of extruded finger millet on dough rheology and functional quality of pearl millet-based unleavened flatbread. *Cereal Chemistry*, *97*(5), 991–998. https://doi.org/10.1002/CCHE.10321

Lammers, K. M., Khandelwal, S., Chaudhry, F., et al. 2011. Identification of a novel immunomodulatory gliadin peptide that causes interleukin-8 release in a chemokine receptor CXCR3-dependent manner only in patients with coeliac disease. *Immunology*, *132*, 432–40.

Lazova-Borisova, I., & Angelov, L. 2020. Fatty acid composition of rice flour millet and chickpeas for the production of gluten free bread. *AgroLife Scientific Journal*, *9*(2). https://agrolifejournal.usamv.ro/index.php/agrolife/article/view/269

Leffler, D. A., Kelly, C. P., Green, P. H., et al. 2015. Larazotide acetate for persistent symptoms of celiac disease despite a gluten-free diet: A randomized controlled trial. *Gastroenterology*, *148*, 1311–9.

Leonard, J., Haffenden, G., Tucker, W., Unsworth, J., Swain, F., McMinn, R., Holborow, J., & Fry, L. 1983. Gluten challenge in dermatitis herpetiformis. *The New England Journal of Medicine*, *308*(14), 816–819. https://doi.org/10.1056/NEJM198304073081406

Lestari, L. A., Huriyati, E., & Marsono, Y. 2017. The development of low glycemic index cookie bars from foxtail millet (*Setaria italica*), arrowroot (*Maranta arundinacea*) flour, and kidney beans (*Phaseolus vulgaris*). *Journal of Food Science and Technology*, *54*(6), 1406–1413.

Levescot, A., Malamut, G., & Cerf-Bensussan, N. 2022. Immunopathogenesis and environmental triggers in coeliac disease. *Gut*, *71*(11), 2337–2349. Advance online publication. https://doi.org/10.1136/gutjnl-2021-326257

Li, S., Zhang, A., Zhao, W., Li, P., Si, X., Liu, J., & Yi, H. 2024. Physicochemical properties of whole grain foxtail millet sourdough and steamed bread quality: Co-fermentation of lactic acid bacteria and yeast in whole grain fermented foods. *Food Bioscience*, *57*, 103581. https://doi.org/10.1016/J.FBIO.2024.103581

Manchanda, M., Rawat, D., Chandra, A., & Saini, R. K. 2024. Development and evaluation of calcium-fortified multi-millet biscuits: A nutritious alternative to refined wheat flour. *Foods*, *13*(11), 1696. https://doi.org/10.3390/FOODS13111696

Manoj Kumar, C. T., Sabikhi, L., Singh, A. K., Raju, P. N., Kumar, R., & Sharma, R. 2019. Effect of incorporation of sodium caseinate, whey protein concentrates and transglutaminase on the properties of depigmented pearl millet-based gluten free pasta. *LWT*, *103*, 19–26. https://doi.org/10.1016/J.LWT.2018.12.071

Mansikka, E., Hervonen, K., Kaukinen, K., Ilus, T., Oksanen, P., Lindfors, K., Laurila, K., Hietikko, M., Taavela, J., Jernman, J., Saavalainen, P., Reunala, T., & Salmi, T. 2019. Gluten challenge induces skin and small bowel relapse in long-term gluten-free diet-treated dermatitis herpetiformis. *The Journal of Investigative Dermatology*, *139*(10), 2108–2114. https://doi.org/10.1016/j.jid.2019.03.1150

Mennini, M., Ferrari, F., Parisi, P., & Di Nardo, G. 2024. Gluten and non-coeliac gluten sensitivity: The nocebo effect and future avenues. *The Lancet. Gastroenterology & Hepatology*, *9*(4), 292–293. https://doi.org/10.1016/S2468-1253(23)00444-2

Monsuur, A. J., & Wijmenga, C. 2006. Understanding the molecular basis of celiac disease: What genetic studies reveal. *Annals of Medicine*, *38*(8), 578–591. https://doi.org/10.1080/07853890600989054

Motta Romero, H., Santra, D., Rose, D., & Zhang, Y. 2017. Dough rheological properties and texture of gluten-free pasta based on proso millet flour. *Journal of Cereal Science*, *74*, 238–243. https://doi.org/10.1016/J.JCS.2017.02.014

Mubeena, S. A., & Haripriya, A. 2021. Optimization and functionality of inulin added minor millet based gluten-free noodles. *The Indian Journal of Nutrition and Dietetics*, 68–78. https://doi.org/10.21048/IJND.2021.58.1.25902

Mudau, M., Mashau, M. E., & Ramashia, S. E. 2022. Nutritional quality, antioxidant, microstructural and sensory properties of spontaneously fermented gluten-free finger millet biscuits. *Foods*, *11*(9), 1265.

Murray, J. A., Kelly, C. P., & Green, P. H. R., et al. 2017. No difference between latiglutenase and placebo in reducing villous atrophy or improving symptoms in patients with symptomatic celiac disease. *Gastroenterology, 152*, 787–98. https://doi.org/10.1053/j.gastro.2016.11.004

Navyashree, N., Buvaneswaran, M., Sunil, C. K., Rawson, A., & Natarajan, V. 2023. Development of white finger millet probiotic beverage using *Lactobacillus rhamnosus* (LGG): Process optimization and study of physicochemical and nutritional properties. *Journal of Food Process Engineering, 46*(10), e14200. https://doi.org/10.1111/JFPE.14200

Nguyen, C. N., & Kim, S. J. 2021. Dermatitis herpetiformis: An update on diagnosis, disease monitoring, and management. *Medicina (Kaunas, Lithuania), 57*(8), 843. https://doi.org/10.3390/medicina57080843

Obafaye, R. O., & Omoba, O. S. 2018. Orange peel flour: A potential source of antioxidant and dietary fiber in pearl-millet biscuit. *Journal of Food Biochemistry, 42*(4), e12523. https://doi.org/10.1111/JFBC.12523

Obtułowicz, K., Waga, J., & Dyga, W. 2015. Gluten–mechanisms of intolerance, symptoms, and treatment possibilities of IgE-related allergy for gluten in the light of actual clinical and immunological studies. Przeglad lekarski, *72*(12), 747–753.

Ortega, D., & Branson, C. 2023. S4000 a rare case of early onset gluten ataxia. *The American Journal of Gastroenterology, 118*(10S), S2542. https://doi.org/10.14309/01.ajg.0000965640.74562.a8

Paek, S. Y., Steinberg, S. M., & Katz, S. I. 2011. Remission in dermatitis herpetiformis: A cohort study. *Archives of Dermatology, 147*(3), 301–305. https://doi.org/10.1001/archdermatol.2010.336

Palavecino, P. M., Ribotta, P. D., León, A. E., & Bustos, M. C. 2019. Gluten-free sorghum pasta: starch digestibility and antioxidant capacity compared with commercial products. *Journal of the Science of Food and Agriculture, 99*(3), 1351–1357. https://doi.org/10.1002/JSFA.9310

Pan, M., Cao, Y., Chi, X., Song, Z., Ai, N., & Sun, B. 2019. Influence of processing conditions on the physicochemical properties of a new-type of nutritional drink—Millet skim milk beverage. *Molecules, 24*(7), 1338. https://doi.org/10.3390/MOLECULES24071338

Pandey, M., Singh, S., Tripathi, R., Mishra, A., Singh, P. K., Tiwari, H., Dwivedi, P., & Kumar, S. 2024. *Millets for Food and Nutrition Security: A Review*. https://doi.org/10.9734/ijpss/2024/v36i24385

Pessanha, K. L. F., de Menezes, J. P., dos Anjos Silva, A., da Silva Ferreira, M. V., Takeiti, C. Y., & Carvalho, C. W. P. 2021. Impact of whole millet extruded flour on the physicochemical properties and antihyperglycemic activity of gluten free bread. *LWT, 147*, 111495. https://doi.org/10.1016/J.LWT.2021.111495

Pessanha, K. L. F., Santos, M. B., de Grandi Castro Freitas-Sá, D., Takeiti, C. Y., & Carvalho, C. W. P. 2023. Impact of whole millet extruded flour on the physicochemical properties and antihyperglycemic activity of gluten free pasta. *Journal of Food Science and Technology, 60*(6), 1738–1748.

Poddighe, D., & Abdukhakimova, D. 2021. Celiac Disease in Asia beyond the Middle East and Indian subcontinent: Epidemiological burden and diagnostic barriers. *World Journal of Gastroenterology, 27*, 2251–2256. https://doi.org/10.3748/wjg.v27.i19.2251

Rao, A., Dhas, A., Dhas, T. A., Esther, M., Sharon, M., Manoharan, A. P., & Nithyalakshmi, V. 2021. Development of fibre enriched ready-to-cook pasta with foxtail millet and tapioca flour. *The Pharma Innovation Journal, 10*(5), 1432–1435.

Rathore, S., & Pandey, A. K. 2023. Effectual study, statistical optimization, and neural network-based predictive model of pearl millet and amaranth flours formulations for gluten-free pasta. *JSFA Reports, 3*(11), 572–581. https://doi.org/10.1002/JSF2.160

Reaz, A. H., Abedin, M. J., Mohammad Abdullah, A. T., Satter, M. A., & Farzana, T. 2023. Physicochemical and structural impact of CMC-hydrocolloids on the development of gluten-free foxtail millet biscuits. *Heliyon, 9*(6). https://doi.org/10.1016/J.HELIYON.2023.E17176

Reilly, N. R. 2016. The gluten-free diet: Recognizing fact, fiction, and fad. *The Journal of Pediatrics, 175*, 206–10.

Rouvroye, M. D., Zis, P., Van Dam, A. M., Rozemuller, A. J. M., Bouma, G., & Hadjivassiliou, M. 2020. The neuropathology of gluten-related neurological disorders: A systematic review. *Nutrients, 12*(3), 822. https://doi.org/10.3390/nu12030822

Rudra, S. G., Anand, V., Kaur, C., Bhooshan, N., & Bhardwaj, R. 2020. Hydrothermal treatment to improve processing characteristics of flour for gluten-free pasta. *Starch/Staerke, 72*(9–10), 1900320. https://doi.org/10.1002/STAR.201900320

Rybak-d'Obyrn, J., & Placek, W. 2022. Etiopathogenesis of dermatitis herpetiformis. *Advances in Dermatology and Allergology, 39*, 1–6. https://doi.org/10.5114/ada.2020.101637

Saberi, A., Zolfaghari, M. S., & Qomi, M. S. M. 2023. Improvement of gluten -free sponge cake with a combination of chia seed flour and millet flour. *Journal of Nutrition and Food Safety*, *9*(4), 663–671. https://jnfs.ssu.ac.ir/article-1-784-en.pdf

Saccone, G., Berghella, V., Sarno, L., et al. 2016. Celiac disease and obstetric complications: A systematic review and metanalysis. *American Journal of Obstetrics and Gynecology*, *214*, 225–34. https://doi.org/10.1016/j.ajog.2015.09.080

Salmi, T., & Hervonen, K. 2020. Current concepts of dermatitis herpetiformis. *Acta dermato-venereologica*, *100*(5), adv00056. https://doi.org/10.2340/00015555-3401

Sarabhai, S., Tamilselvan, T., & Prabhasankar, P. 2021. Role of enzymes for improvement in gluten-free foxtail millet bread: It's effect on quality, textural, rheological and pasting properties. *LWT*, *137*, 110365. https://doi.org/10.1016/J.LWT.2020.110365

Selvaraju, K., Mathur, M., SSM, S., Sahu, J. K., Hariprasad, P., & Malik, A. 2024. Deciphering the effect of *Chlorella minutissima* incorporation in gluten-free millet cookies: Physical and functional properties. *Algal Research*, *82*, 103683. https://doi.org/10.1016/J.ALGAL.2024.103683

Shaabani, S., Yarmand, M. S., Kiani, H., & Emam-Djomeh, Z. 2018. The effect of chickpea protein isolate in combination with transglutaminase and xanthan on the physical and rheological characteristics of gluten free muffins and batter based on millet flour. *LWT*, *90*, 362–372. https://doi.org/10.1016/J.LWT.2017.12.023

Sharma, R., Sharma, S., Dar, B. N., & Singh, B. 2021. Millets as potential nutri-cereals: A review of nutrient composition, phytochemical profile and techno-functionality. *International Journal of Food Science & Technology*, *56*(8), 3703–3718. https://doi.org/10.1111/IJFS.15044

Shiha, M. G., Raju, S. A., Penny, H. A., & Sanders, D. S. 2024. Non-coeliac gluten sensitivity: from Salerno to Rome. *The Lancet. Gastroenterology & Hepatology*, *9*(2), 94–95. https://doi.org/10.1016/S2468-1253(23)00358-8

Singh, A., & Kumar, P. 2018. Gluten free approach in fat and sugar amended biscuits: A healthy concern for obese and diabetic individuals. *Journal of Food Processing and Preservation*, *42*(3), e13546. https://doi.org/10.1111/JFPP.13546

Sobowale, S. S., Adebo, O. A., & Mulaba-Bafubiandi, A. F. 2019. Production of extrudate pasta from optimal sorghum–peanut flour blend and influence of composite flours on some quality characteristics and sorption isotherms. *Transactions of the Royal Society of South Africa*, *74*(3), 268–275. https://doi.org/10.1080/0035919X.2019.1639563

Srivastava, U., Singh, A., Ahmed, M., Iqbal, U., & Saini, P. 2025. Functional and physicochemical characterization of a novel pearl millet—Soy milk-based synbiotic beverage. *Food Safety and Health*, *3*(1), 115–127. https://doi.org/10.1002/FSH3.12076

Tamilselvan, T., Saravanan, M., & Prabhasankar, P. 2024. Influence of mechanical activation of starch using planetary ball milling on the development of little millet gluten free bread. *Innovative Food Science & Emerging Technologies*, *98*, 103860. https://doi.org/10.1016/J.IFSET.2024.103860

Tamilselvan, T., Sharma, S., Thomas, P. E., Goyal, K., & Prabhasankar, P. 2022. Role of hydrocolloids in improving the rheology, quality characteristics, and microstructure of gluten-free proso millet bread. *International Journal of Food Science & Technology*, *57*(11), 7156–7166. https://doi.org/10.1111/IJFS.16058

Tomić, J., Torbica, A., & Belović, M. 2020. Effect of non-gluten proteins and transglutaminase on dough rheological properties and quality of bread based on millet (*Panicum miliaceum*) flour. *LWT*, *118*, 108852. https://doi.org/10.1016/J.LWT.2019.108852

Tranquet, O., Larré, C., & Denery-Papini, S. 2018. Allergic reactions to hydrolysed wheat proteins: clinical aspects and molecular structures of the allergens involved. *Critical Reviews in Food Science and Nutrition*, *60*(1), 147–156. https://doi.org/10.1080/10408398.2018.1516622

Tyl, C., Marti, A., & Ismail, B. P. 2020. Changes in protein structural characteristics upon processing of gluten-free millet pasta. *Food Chemistry*, *327*, 127052. https://doi.org/10.1016/J.FOODCHEM.2020.127052

Udeh, H. O., Duodu, K. G., & Jideani, A. I. O. 2025. Effect of fermentation time on the physicochemical properties and phenolic composition of malted finger millet beverages. *Food Science and Nutrition*, *13*(3), e4659. https://doi.org/10.1002/FSN3.4659

Vale, E.C., Dimatos, O.C., Porro, A.M., & Santi, C.G. 2019. Consensus on the treatment of autoimmune bullous dermatoses: dermatitis herpetiformis and linear IgA bullous dermatosis – Brazilian Society of Dermatology. *Anais Brasileiros de Dermatologia*, *94*, 48–55. https://doi.org/10.1590/abd1806-4841.2019940208

Vasanthakumari, P., & Jaganmohan, R. 2018. Process development and formulation of multi-cereal and legume cookies. *Journal of Food Processing and Preservation*, *42*(12), e13824. https://doi.org/10.1111/JFPP.13824

Vila-Real, C., Costa, C., Pimenta-Martins, A., Mbugua, S., Hagrétou, S. L., Katina, K., Maina, N. H., Pinto, E., & Gomes, A. M. P. 2025. Novel fermented plant-based functional beverage: Biological potential and impact on the human gut microbiota. *Foods*, *14*(3), 433. https://doi.org/10.3390/FOODS14030433

Vila-Real, C., Pimenta-Martins, A., Mbugua, S., Hagrétou, S. L., Katina, K., Maina, N. H., Pinto, E., & Gomes, A. M. P. 2022. Novel synbiotic fermented finger millet-based yoghurt-like beverage: Nutritional, physicochemical, and sensory characterization. *Journal of Functional Foods*, *99*, 105324. https://doi.org/10.1016/J.JFF.2022.105324

Wu, J. H., Neal, B., Trevena, H., Crino, M., Stuart-Smith, W., Faulkner-Hogg, K., Yu Louie, J. C., & Dunford, E. 2015. Are gluten-free foods healthier than non-gluten-free foods? An evaluation of supermarket products in Australia. *British Journal of Nutrition*, *114*(3), 448–54. https://doi.org/10.1017/S0007114515002056

Zhang, X., Wu, Z., Wang, J., Bian, N., Zhao, P., Sun, N., & Chen, J. 2024. Insight into elevated quality of whole millet (*Pennisetum glaucum*) cake through the process of extrusion. *Journal of Cereal Science*, *118*, 103931. https://doi.org/10.1016/J.JCS.2024.103931

Zheng, W., Wai, C. Y. Y., Sit, J. K. C., Cheng, N. S., Leung, C. W. M., & Leung, T. F. 2024. Routinely used and emerging diagnostic and immunotherapeutic approaches for wheat allergy. *Biomedicines*, *12*(7), 1549. https://doi.org/10.3390/biomedicines12071549

12 Millet-Based Food Options
A Review of Commercially Available Products

Shivli Srivastava[1] *and Shefali Srivastava*[2]
[1] Nestle Development Center, Manesar (Gurugram), Haryana, India
[2] Symbiosis Institute of International Business, Symbiosis International (Deemed University), Pune, Maharashtra, India

12.1 INTRODUCTION

Millets contribute 10% to the country's food grains supporting especially 12 million people who belong to vulnerable groups either rural or urban. India is the biggest producer (11,849,190 tonnes) of millets in the world whereas the second producer is Niger (3,656,958 tonnes) [Food and Agricultural Organization of the United Nations (FAO) 2024].

Over the past few years, the market for millets in India has achieved remarkable expansion. Area under millet cultivation increased from 12.29 million ha in 2013–14 to 15.48 million ha in 2021–22, according to government data [Press Information Bureau (PIB) 2023].

The estimated millet yield in India has more than doubled since 1966, and India's average yield in millet farming in 2021–22 is 1208 kg/ha. This significant upsurge in millet production and yield has not only strengthened the supply chain but has also opened doors for a wide variety of millet-based products in the market.

Several reports emphasize the increasing demand for healthy foods globally, mainly due to the increase in lifestyle diseases such as diabetes, obesity, cardiovascular diseases and cancers. India too witnessed a similar trend. Present-day consumers have a greater concern about food ingredients, safety and quality. The consumers believe that food companies should be responsible for keeping people healthy and should also address societal nutrition issues. Commercialization of the millet products is the best way for increasing consumption of various millets as the present-day consumer demands convenience foods for numerous reasons.

Despite the growing recognition of millets for their nutritional and environmental benefits, there are various challenges which hamper their widespread acceptance and commercialization in global markets. All of which jointly limit the potential of millets as a staple food and commercial commodity. The millet supply chains pose significant challenges, particularly for small-scale farmers, including women and young entrepreneurs as they struggle to integrate into formal value chains (Aayog et al 2023).

12.2 MILLET-BASED PACKAGED FOOD MARKET – SCOPE AND OVERVIEW

Shifting consumer preference towards healthier and more sustainable food options has encouraged many food entrepreneurs in India to have millet startups. These wonder grains have made a strong comeback in recent years. Millet-based food products come in various categories, catering to diverse consumer preferences. These include pearled grains, flour, snacks, breakfast cereals and ready-to-cook and ready-to-eat meals and beverages.

India and China, in particular, lead in both production and consumption, with local brands innovating to meet evolving consumer needs. Meanwhile, North America and Europe are witnessing a surge in interest, driven by a growing affinity for superfoods and a focus on sustainable agriculture.

DOI: 10.1201/9781003686668-12

The millet market is estimated to expand at a compound annual growth rate (CAGR) of 4.60%, increasing from $11.02 billion in 2023 to $13.80 billion by 2028. The millet packaged food sector was valued at $39.5 million in 2022 and is expected to project a CAGR of 10.2% from 2023 to 2029, potentially reaching nearly $78.5 million. The chief component within this market is millet-based snacks, followed by millet-based breakfast cereals and millet-based breads (Shah & Tripathy 2023).

The market for packaged food made from millet in India was valued at US$37.7 million in 2022. It is projected to expand at a CAGR of 9.2% from 2022 to 2032. By the end of 2032, the Indian millet-based packaged food market is forecast to reach US$91.1 million. Notably, the millet-based packaged food market is expected to hit US$85.91 million by 2030 (Transparency Market Research 2025).

The demand for millet products varies significantly across various regions of India. Southern states like Karnataka, Tamil Nadu and Andhra Pradesh have historical depth and continuity of millet consumption culture. This part accounts for a significant portion of the millet market. However, millet food products are also gaining popularity in other regions, which include the northern and western states. The number of millet entrepreneurs in India has concurrently experienced a remarkable upsurge.

In India there were approximately 1000 millet-product startups in 2023, as reported by the Indian Council of Agriculture Research. These entrepreneurs have swiftly noticed the potential of millet as a sustainable and healthy food source and therefore promptly diversified their product portfolios accordingly. Furthermore, many entrepreneurs in India have plans to expand the production, consumption and exports of millet-based products.

E-commerce platforms are instrumental in leading market expansion, providing consumers with easy access to a variety of millet-based food products. The convenience of online shopping, together with dynamic marketing push and eco-friendly packaging options, enhances product visibility and consumer engagement. This move towards digital retail has become a bedrock of the market's expanding reach and acceptance.

The India millet-based packaged food market is fragmented. There are large numbers of small-scale manufacturers. Large players hold a minimum share of the market. Most of the millet-based processed food companies are focusing on comprehensive research and development activities. They are striving to expand their product portfolios and create innovative millet-based packaged food. The millet-based packaged food market is highly competitive, with both large and small players present. Some of the market's key players include the following: Tata Consumer Soulfull Pvt. Ltd., Kellogg's, Natureland Organics, Early Foods, Patanjali Ayurved Ltd., General Mills Inc, Bambino Agro Industries, Bliss Tree India, Coastal Foods, Early Foods, FirmRoots Private Limited, ITC Limited, Marico, Moon Foods, Naturally Yours, Num Num, OGMO Foods, Priya Foods, Quaker Oats Company, Slurrp Farm, Sri Lakshmi Foods, Swiss Bake Ingredients Pvt. Ltd., Tropolite, Truefarm Foods, Urban Millets Pvt. Ltd. and Urban Monk Private Limited.

12.3 MILLET-BASED FOOD PRODUCTS AVAILABLE IN MARKET

To gain a competitive advantage in the market, the companies are focusing on product innovation, expanding distribution channels and strategic partnerships and collaborations. The literature reveals that the Indian market for millet food products could be segmented on the basis of occupation (public/private), food preference (vegetarian/non-vegetarian), income group, age group, family size, education, gender, patients of lifestyle disorders, diabetes and celiac diseases etc. (Lalita & Radhika 2014). On the other hand, consumer preferences of millet products in India are determined by product-related factors, price, health and nutrition benefits, promotional efforts and awareness (Krishnasamy et al 2025). In fact, consumer choices regarding millets are influenced by a combination of demographic, social, psychological and cultural influences (Sulthana 2014). Factors like age, gender and education significantly impact these preferences. An increased awareness of the nutritional advantages of millets correlates with higher consumption rates. There is a positive relationship between age and the consumption of millets, largely due to traditional dietary habits and heightened health awareness. Older individuals, raised on a diet that included millets, tend to be more knowledgeable about their taste and health advantages, which include aiding digestion and supplying fibre, minerals and antioxidants. In addition, cultural importance, such as the consumption of millets during festivals, affects buying behaviour (Negi & Sahu 2024).

Variety of millet-based food products are available in the market which for convenience and easy access purposes have been categorized as below. The sales are also affected by the choice of sales channels such as, modern trade, specialty stores, convenience stores, online retail, other sales channel etc. To collect the information about millet food products, a search on the e-commerce website, Amazon (www.amazon.in), was done using the keywords related to millet-based food items such as "millet namkeen", "baked millet products", "millet-based beverages", "millet-based snacks", "millet flour", "millet grains" etc. were used.

12.3.1 Breakfast Items

A wide range of different types of millet food products are available in the market, viz., ragi bites choco fills, millet dalia, multigrain millet oatmeal, millet muesli, millet flakes, jowar flakes, masala millet containing bajra and barley flakes. The Table 12.1 lists the major millet food products available in the market as retrieved from the website of Amazon, a leading e-commerce platform. Maggi instant noodles with millets can be eaten during breakfast, lunch/dinner. Besides millet bread, millet pancake mix and millet hakka noodles are available in the market and can serve as healthy breakfast items.

Ingredients of various products reveal that different millets have been used in the products such as finger millet, sorghum, kodo millet and foxtail millet. Tata Soulfull ragi bites chocofills contain 34.1% millet (ragi). Vasani G mix millet dalia contains pearl millet along with wheat, rice and green gram.

Ragi flakes along with jowar flakes with rolled oats, wheat and barley flakes are included in the multigrain millet oatmeal. Tata soulfull millet muesli contains 13% ragi flakes with rolled oats, rice flakes, corn flakes and other ingredients. Health Sutra millet flakes contain only ragi/bajra flakes. Likewise, True Elements jowar flakes contain only jowar flakes. A variety of flakes viz., bajra flakes, barley flakes, potato flakes and other ingredients have been added in Nestle a$^+$ Masala millet. Britannia millet bread contains 21% of millets. Sprouted jowar has been used in The Naturik Co. waffle and pineapple mix. Slurrp Farm hakka noodles contain foxtail millet flour with wheat flour and other ingredients. Hence, a variety of millet-based food items which are either ready to eat or can be easily prepared are available for breakfast.

12.3.2 Lunch/Dinner Items

In Indian diet, staple grains generally wheat and rice are eaten. Wheat flour is used for making chapati. Rice is consumed in boiled form. Various flours available in the market include Ashirvaad Nature's Superfoods gluten-free flour containing sorghum flour and finger millet flour along with other ingredients. This can be used as a substitute for wheat flour for making chapati and other preparations such as paratha, puri etc. Pearl millet grains as well as unpolished millet grains of browntop, foxtail, kodo, barnyard and little millet are available in the market which can be used as a substitute of rice for making various dishes such as khichdi, pulav etc. to be consumed during lunch/dinner. The Table 12.2 lists the commercially available lunch/dinner items as retrieved from the Amazon website. Besides ready-to-cook multi-millet khichdi containing kodo, proso, little, barnyard and foxtail millets along with other ingredients are available in the market. One such product is from Fresco Farm. Millet dosa/idli mixes, which are ready to cook, are also available in the market which can be conveniently used.

TABLE 12.1
Breakfast Items

Product Name	Ingredients	Method of Preparation	Occasion of Consumption	Product Claims	Price*
Tata Soulfull Ragi Bites Choco Fills	Ragi (34.1%), chocolate cream filling (32%) (sugar, interesterified vegetable fat, cocoa powder (2.8%), milk solids, emulsifier (INS (322(i)), rice, refined sugar, Bengal gram dal (1.8%), cocoa powder, iodized salt, nature-identical flavouring substance, stabilizer (INS 170(i)), natural colour (INS 150d), edible vegetable oil (palmolein), antioxidant (INS 320), emulsifier (INS 322(i))	Just add the cereal to your bowl. Pour some milk of your choice. Best served with cold milk.	Breakfast	No Maida Ragi calcium Dal protein	Rs. 384/kg
VGBNP Vasani G (Mix Millet Dalia)	Skinned green gram (moong dal), white sesame (til), pearl millet dalia (bajra dalia), wheat dalia (gehu dalia) rice (chaval), carom seed (ajwain)	Not given on pack.	Breakfast	No chemical Premium quality Rich fibre	Rs. 199.50/kg
Multigrain Millet Oatmeal	Multigrain blend 96% (rolled oats, wheat flakes, barley flakes, ragi flakes, jowar flakes), flax seeds, chia seeds This product contains 10% millets	1. Boil 90 ml water/milk in a pan, then remove from heat. 2. Add 45 g of millet multigrain oats to the boiled water/milk and stir well. 3. Cover with a lid and let it sit for 4–5 minutes. Millet multigrain oats are now ready. Sweet preparation – add sweetener of choice, fresh fruits and nuts. Savoury preparation – mix in sauteed veggies before serving.	Breakfast	1.2× more plant protein, 1.5× fibre, no added sugar (as compared to ordinary oats)	Rs. 89/500 g

(Continued)

TABLE 12.1 *(Continued)*
Breakfast Items

Product Name	Ingredients	Method of Preparation	Occasion of Consumption	Product Claims	Price*
Tata Soulfull 0% Added Sugar Millet Muesli	Rolled oats (37%), rice flakes (19%), ragi flakes (13%), corn flakes (9%), flax seeds (8%), black raisins (4%), almonds (3%), rice bran oil, pumpkin seeds (2%), chia seeds (2%), antioxidant (INS 320). CONTAINS ADDED NATURAL FLAVOURING SUBSTANCE (ROSEMARY)	READY TO EAT: Just add it to your bowl, pour some milk and enjoy!	Breakfast	Made with 97% whole grains, fruit, nuts and seeds, our millet muesli is high in fibre and rich in protein. 0% added sugar.	Rs. 477.14/kg
Health Sutra Millets Flakes Combo – Ragi Flakes and Bajra Flakes	Ragi/bajra flakes	Ready to eat: Take flakes in a bowl, pour hot milk/cold milk/buttermilk.	Breakfast	Calcium-rich, high-fibre, low-fat Complex carbs, protein-rich, mineral-rich	Rs. 440/kg
True Elements Jowar Flakes	Jowar flakes	Jowar flakes can be consumed with warm/cold milk for a healthy breakfast. Fruits or nuts may be added as toppings for extra crunch and taste. They can also be consumed as a snack.	Breakfast/ snacking	Strengthens immune system, maintains heart health, promotes bone health	Rs. 444.44/kg

Nestlé a⁺ Masala Millet	Pearled bajra flakes (42%), pearled barley flakes (23%), potato flakes (potato, margarine, iodized salt, turmeric), soyabean oil, dehydrated vegetables (5.5%), [carrot (2.5%), green beans (1.5%), peas (1.5%)], iodized salt, potassium chloride, sugar, mixed spices (1.8%), (turmeric, cumin, coriander (0.3%), aniseed, black pepper (0.2%), red chilli (0.1%), fenugreek, ginger, cardamom (0.02%), clove (0.02%), nutmeg (0.02%)), green chilli, flavour enhancers (627, 631), natural flavouring substances and acidity regulator (330). Contains barley, milk, soy	Add sachet contents to 200 ml (1 cup) water in a pan and bring it to a boil while stirring. Cook for 2 minutes on a low to medium flame. Mix well. Allow it to stand for a minute. Enjoy hot!	Breakfast/ snacking	High in fibre: Nestlé a⁺ Masala Millets are high in fibre. - 30% lower in calories: Contains 30% lower calories. - Goodness of bajra: Bajra is a climate-smart crop and requires less water to cultivate. - No Added Preservatives: It contains no added preservatives.	Rs. 50/100 g
Britannia Millet Bread	Wheat flour (atta), water, millets 21% (softgrain millet, bajra millet, kodo millet, jowar millet, ragi flour), yeast, rolled oats, wheat bran, gluten, sugar, iodized salt, refined palmolein, broken wheat, preservative (282), emulsifier (472e), acidity regulator (260) and flour treatment agent (510)	Ready to consume.	Breakfast	Goodness of millets – ragi, jowar, bajra 0% maida added Source of fibre	Rs. 50/300 g

(Continued)

TABLE 12.1 *(Continued)*
Breakfast Items

Product Name	Ingredients	Method of Preparation	Occasion of Consumption	Product Claims	Price*
THE NATURIK CO. Waffle and Pancake Mix	Sprouted jowar, sprouted masoor flour, oats, jaggery powder, chocolate powder, vanilla powder, banana powder, baking powder	Mix ½ cup of milk to 1 cup of mix. Stir well to remove any lumps. Pour a spoonful of batter and cook on both sides till it becomes golden brown. Serve with honey syrup, dry fruits and nuts.	Breakfast	No preservatives 100% vegan Gluten-free ingredients High-protein High-fibre	Rs. 179/150 g
Slurrp Farm No Maida Hakka Noodles, Not Fried, No MSG, Classic Millet and Mild Millet Noodles	Noodles Super grain blend (whole wheat flour, foxtail millet flour), cluster bean powder (natural gum, iodized salt, antioxidant (rosemary extract) INS 392, food additives – none Spice mix Spices (coriander, chilli, onion, garlic, cumin, turmeric, black pepper)	Cook the noodles in 1 L boiling water for 4 minutes. Drain the hot water and rinse the noodles with cold water.	Breakfast/ snacking between meals/tea time	No maida and not fried, zero junk	Approximately Rs. 60/100 g

*[a] Price may vary with pack size and discount offer.

TABLE 12.2
Lunch/Dinner Items

Product Name	Ingredients	Method of Preparation	Occasion of Consumption	Product Claims	Price*
Fresco Farm Fresco's Diabetics Wellness Pack (Foxtail Millet Khichdi, Finger Millet Dosa, Multi Millet Idli)	Multi-millet idli – kodo, proso (cheena), little (kutki), barnyard (sanwa), foxtail (kangani) and sorghum millets (jowar), urad dal, salt, citric acid and baking soda sachet Multi-millet khichdi – kodo, proso, little, barnyard and foxtail millets, moong dal, salt, masala sachet and rice bran oil Finger millet dosa – finger millet (ragi), urad daal, salt, fenugreek powder and citric acid	Ready to cook	Lunch/dinner	100% chemical and preservative-free, NO JUNK GUARANTEED. Weight control, gluten free, diabetic-friendly, low GI, rich in protein	Rs. 60.40/100 g
MAGGI Nutri-licious Masala Oats Instant Noodles With Millet (260), Magic	Flour blend (oat flour (34.5%), resultant wheat flour (resultant atta), sorghum flour (5.3%), ragi flour (3%), palm oil, wheat gluten, iodized salt, humectants (451(i) and 452(i))	Step 1: Break the oats noodle cake into two parts. Step 2: Add noodles and masala tastemaker to 240 ml (approx. 1¼ cups) of boiling water. Step 3: Cook for 4 minutes while stirring occasionally in an open pan; don't drain the remaining water. Step 4: Hold for 2 minutes, and it's ready.	Breakfast/ lunch or dinner	Delight your taste buds with the all-new recipe where 20 spices and herbs meet the goodness of oats and millet. Each serving (74.5 g) of MAGGI oats noodles with millet is a source of fibre and protein.	Rs. 0.47/g

(Continued)

TABLE 12.2 ***(Continued)***
Lunch/Dinner Items

Product Name	Ingredients	Method of Preparation	Occasion of Consumption	Product Claims	Price*
Aashirvaad Nature's Superfoods Gluten-Free Flour	Jowar flour, flaked rice flour, starch, ragi flour, dehydrated potato, milk solids, thickener (INS 415) psyllium husk powder, emulsifier (INS 471) and iodized salt.	Pour boiling water into flour, knead the dough until it becomes non-sticky, let the dough rest for about 20 minutes, cook the roti on both sides on the flame and let it puff up.	Lunch/dinner	Naturally gluten free, rich in dietary fibre, source of protein	Price approximately Rs. 237/kg
The Millet Company 1 kg (500 g × 2) Unpolished Millet Combo Pack of 5, Browntop, Foxtail, Kodo, Barnyard, and Little Millet (Total 5 kg), Natural Farm Grown, High Fibre Millets	Browntop, foxtail, kodo, barnyard and little millet	Not given on pack	Lunch/dinner	Unpolished grains, preserving nature's goodness	Rs. 1515/5 kg (303.05/kg)

*[a] Price may vary with pack size and discount offer.

12.3.3 Items for Snacking between Meals/Beverages/Tea Time

The table 12.3 lists the commercially available items for snacking between meals/beverages/tea time items as retrieved from the Amazon website. True Elements millet chikki contains 27% millets in combination of jowar, ragi and bajra and is claimed to contain two times more fibre, 16% less fat and clean labelled. Gleevita chocolate moon and star millet crunchies for kids contain a higher percentage of millets i.e. 50% in combination of jowar, bajra and ragi. Several types of millet biscuits/cookies are available in the market. One such type is Me and Millet cookies with different millets claimed to be clean label. Artinci eggless, sugar-free chocolate cake is diabetic-friendly, high-protein, low-calorie for weight loss. The cake is low GI. It contains blend of erythritol, fructooligosaccharides and stevia as sweetening agents. It does not contain dextrose or maltodextrin, maida and hydrogenated fat.

A variety of millet drinks are available which are processed in different ways. Millet drinks serve as excellent alternative to sugary or carbonated beverages and are suitable for all age groups. Being rich in minerals, vitamins and fibre, they improve digestion and give a feeling of fullness. In addition, millet drinks are good for weight management, boosting immunity and heart health. Bliss Body sugar-free millet fermented drink is diabetic-friendly, good for gut health, rich in antioxidants with other benefits. Sweet Karam Coffee health mix contains 56% millets viz., little, foxtail, kodo, barnyard, pearl, finger and sorghum. This is rich in fibre, calcium with no added sugars and preservatives. Eats instant sprouted and roasted ragi malt with natural cocoa powder mix is high in calcium and easy to digest. This product does not contain artificial additives. Another malted millet drink is Millet House Premium instant malt nutrition health drink which contains Sridhanya millets viz., foxtail, kodo, little, barnyard and browntop. Better Bet Vegan original Millet $^{+}$Oats drink contains sprouted millets. This is high in calcium with no lactose and added sugar.

It is general practice to consume namkeen with tea. Millet Namkeen Desi Masala contains ragi and jowar. The namkeen is roasted and low glycaemic index. Millet and jowar puffs are made using a baking technique. Puffs are blend of jowar, foxtail millet, corn and rice. Millet Kurmura contain jowar, bajra and ragi. The product is claimed to be healthy as it is roasted not fried. It has no palm oil and no MSG. Roasty Tasty Millet Munch chatpata main ingredient is sorghum flakes. It is roasted whole grain product.

12.4 CONSUMER ACCEPTANCE OF MILLET-BASED FOOD PRODUCTS

Millets serve as a viable, nutritious and healthy alternative to wheat in food production. However, products derived from millets often face challenges in consumer acceptance due to sensory quality. Comparatively lower viscoelastic properties owing to lack of gluten in millets particularly in bakery formulations result in decreased acceptability. Products formulated from millets have some drawbacks related to taste, texture and anti-nutrient factors. Compared to wheat, millet products are the least acceptable. So, to improve its acceptability, products are prepared by blending millet flour with wheat flour. Furthermore, millet-based products typically exhibit a harder texture, increased weight and a less porous structure. Moreover, the less desirable taste and flavour profile of millets constrains their application in product formulations. Additionally, some millets contain a high concentration of anti-nutrient, which can hinder the absorption of essential nutrient, posing a significant concern for consumption. Proper cooking methods are crucial to mitigate these issues. Pearl millet contains goitrogens, compounds that can disrupt thyroid function by hindering iodine uptake, particularly in excessive quantities (Siroha & Punia Bangar 2024). Finally, accessibility and cooking challenges further hinder millet adoption in global markets. Unlike major cereals wheat and rice, millets are not widely available in supermarkets, which limits their accessibility for consumers (Alekhya & Raj Shravanthi 2019). Additionally, certain millet varieties require prolonged cooking times or specific preparation methods such as fermentation or pounding. These labour-intensive processes may discourage urban consumers who prefer convenient, ready-to-cook food options (Aayog et al 2023).

TABLE 12.3
Items for Snacking between Meals/Beverages/Tea Time

Product Name	Ingredients	Method of Preparation	Occasion of Consumption	Product Claims	Price[a]
True Elements Millet Chikki with Jaggery – Made with Peanuts, Millets and Raw Honey	Peanuts (32%), millets (27%), jowar (10%), ragi (10%), bajra (7%), raw honey (15%), jaggery powder (15%), oats flour (6%), amaranth puff (5%), rosemary extract	Ready to Consume	Snacking between meals	2× more fibre 27% millets 16% less fat No added preservatives and colours, made with jaggery and raw honey	Rs. 78.75/100 g
Gleevita Chocolate Moon and Star Millet Crunchies For Kids	Millets (50% – jowar, ragi, bajra), jaggery (30%), corn (10%), cocoa powder (4%), sunflower oil (3%), unrefined sugar (2.5%), chocolate flavour (0.4%), vanilla powder (0.1%)	Ready to Consume	Snacking between meals	Goodness of millets and jaggery	Rs. 73.70/100 g
Me and Millets Combo Ragi Twist, Bajra Bites and Jowar Delight Cookies, Millets Biscuits, Millets Cookies	Ragi flour (33%), jaggery, oats flour, butter, milk solids, almond flour, coconut powder, raising agent [(Ins 500(Ii)], cardamom powder, jowar flour (33%),	Ready to Consume	Snacking between meals/tea time	No artificial flavours, colours and preservatives No maida and no refined flours, No Palm Oil.	Rs. 95.67/count

Artinci Eggless Sugar Free Chocolate Cake (150 g) - Diabetic Friendly and High Protein, Healthy Low-Calorie Cake with Millets, Healthy snack for Weightloss, as seen on Shark Tank India	House low-carb flour (whole wheat, foxtail millet, soy, coconut, oat flours), low GI sweetener (blend of erythritol, fructooligosaccharides, stevia), butter, cocoa powder, milk solids, prebiotic fibre, whey protein concentrate, natural and nature-identical flavours (vanilla and chocolate extracts), baking powder, baking soda, wheat protein	Ready to consume	Snacking/tea time	N dextrose or maltodextrin or other sneaky high-GI ingredients, No hydrogenated fats, no maida	Rs. 199/150 g
Bliss Body Sugar-Free Millet Fermented Drink I Diabetic Friendly I Gut Care-Best for bloating, constipation II Mango Flavour 100% Natural, No Artificial Sweeteners and Refreshing Taste Healthy for Body	Foxtail millet, water, plant-based stevia glycosides, alphonso mango fruit powder, E202, E211	Ready to consume	Breakfast/ snacking between meals/tea time	Fermented millet beverage, rich in authentic fruit powder, rich in polyphenols, flavonoids and antioxidants	Approximately Rs. 50/200 ml as on 19 October 2025
Sweet Karam Coffee Millet Health Mix (Kanji Maavu) – 500g I 100% Natural Millet Drink Powder I Rich in Fiber and Calcium I No Refined Sugar I Perfect for Kids and Adults I Pack of 2 (250 g Each)	Millets [56% (little, foxtail, kodo, barnyard, pearl, finger, sorghum)], chickpeas, moong dal, horse gram, black urad dal, peanuts, wheat, rice [7% (Mapillai, samba, kavuni)], soya beans, almonds, cashews, barley, sago and cardamom	Boil for 3 minutes and consume	Breakfast/ snacking between meals/tea time	Source of dietary fibre, no added sugar, no added preservatives	Approximately Rs. 89.80/100 g

(Continued)

TABLE 12.3 *(Continued)*
Items for Snacking between Meals/Beverages/Tea Time

Product Name	Ingredients	Method of Preparation	Occasion of Consumption	Product Claims	Price[a]
Eat5 Instant Sprouted and Roasted Ragi Malt with Natural Cocoa Powder I (15 g × 25 Sachet) I Nutritious and Delicious Instant Drink Mix I High in Calcium and Iron I 100% Natural, No Preservatives I Vegan and Gluten-Free	Sprouted and roasted ragi flour, jaggery powder, cocoa powder and gaur gum	Add ragi malt content to warm milk or water. Stir continuously to prevent lumps from forming. Keep stirring until the ragi malt blends smoothly into the liquid (optional). You can add sweeteners like jaggery powder or honey to taste	Breakfast/snacking between meals/tea time	100% natural ingredients, natural energy for active kids, easy-to-digest sprouted ragi, no artificial additives, jaggery instead of refined sugar	Approximately Rs. 52.80/100 g
Millet House Premium Instant Malt Nutrition Health Drink I Siridhanya Millets Cereals Dry Fruits Pulses Organic Health Mix Drink I Meal Supplement Instant Drink for IT, Officials, Students (250 g)	Siridhanya millets (foxtail, kodo, little, barnyard, browntop), cereals and pulses (proso millet, bajra, ragi, green gram, horse gram, black-eyed peas, chickpeas, maize, jowar, toor seeds, peas), dry fruits and nuts (almond, pista, dates, cashew, groundnut, dry grapes), seeds (fenugreek, flax, watermelon, pumpkin, sunflower), sabudana, cardamom, dry ginger	Take 250 ml of hot milk. Add a tablespoon (10–15 g) of instant malt powder. Add sweetener (jaggery etc.) as per requirement and stir	Breakfast/snacking between meals/tea time	Wheat-free, soya-free, white rice-free, no added sugar, no preservatives, no artificial colours	Approximately Rs. 99.60/100 g

Better Bet Vegan Original Millets+ Oats Drink 1.44 L (8 × 180 ML) I Plant Based I No Added Sugar I Lactose Free I No Added Preservatives I No Cholesterol I No Trans Fat	Water, 10% millets and oats blend sprouted sorghum (jowar), oats, sprouted finger millets (ragi), amaranth (rajgir), sunflower oil, stabilizer – INS 170(I), acidity regulator – INS 340(ii), nature flavours substances, emulsifiers – INS 322(I), salt, citrus fibre, stabilizer – INS 418, vitamins (B2, B12, D2)	Use it like milk	Breakfast/ snacking between meals/tea time	Made with sprouted millets, high in calcium, 0% dairy, 0% lactose, 0% added sugar, 100% cruelty-free, no artificial preservatives	Approximately Rs. 23.54/100 ml
Mille Not Fried Jowar Puffs Combo – Magic Masala and Chatpata Treat, Naturally Gluten Free, No Preservatives, Healthy Ready to Eat Millet Snacks	Puff: Supergrain blend (jowar, foxtail millet, corn, rice), rice bran oil Seasoning: Vegetables and spices (onion, garlic, tomato, chilli, amchur, tamarind), salt, natural and nature-identical flavours, raw sugar, acidity regulators (INS 330, INS 296, INS 334), potassium chloride – salt substitute (INS 508), rosemary extract – antioxidant (INS 392)	Ready to consume	Snacking between meals/tea time	Baked not fried, no preservatives, naturally gluten free	Approximately Rs. 55.71/100 g
Eat Anytime Premium Creamy and Onion Millet Kurmura I Healthy Snacking Alternative I Made with Nutritious Millet I High In Fiber I Gluten Free I Healthy Snacks for Adults and Kids	Jowar crisps, bajra crisps, ragi crisps, rice bran oil, signature cream and onion seasoning: milk solids, processed cheese powder, real cream powder, dehydrated triple onion blend (green, white and regular), garlic powder, dried herbs, acidifying agents INS 330, INS 296, flavour enhancers INS 627, INS 631, anticaking agents INS 170(i)	Ready to eat	Snacking between meals/tea time	Source of protein, roasted not fried, healthy namkeen, no palm oil, no MSG	Approximately Rs. 155/100 g

(Continued)

TABLE 12.3 *(Continued)*
Items for Snacking between Meals/Beverages/Tea Time

Product Name	Ingredients	Method of Preparation	Occasion of Consumption	Product Claims	Price[a]
Millet Namkeen - Desi Masala	Peanuts, ragi sev (ragi, rice), chana, jowar crisps (jowar, rice), ragi crisps (ragi, rice), rice crisps, sunflower oil, seasoning chilli powder, sugar, jeera, amchoor, sonth, rai, hing, acidity regulator (citric acid), iodized salt	Ready to consume	Snacking between meals/tea time	No palm oil, roasted not fried, low glycaemic index, no transfat	Approximately Rs. 65/100 g
Slurrp Farm No Maida Hakka Noodles, Not Fried, No MSG, Classic Millet and Mild Millet Noodles	Noodles Super grain blend (whole wheat flour, foxtail millet flour), cluster bean powder (natural gum, iodized salt, antioxidant (rosemary extract) INS 392, food additives – none Spice Mix Spices (coriander, chilli, onion, garlic, cumin, turmeric, black pepper)	Cook the noodles in 1 L boiling water for 4 minutes. Drain the hot water and rinse the noodles with cold water	Breakfast/ snacking between meals/tea time	No maida and not fried, zero junk	Approximately Rs. 60/100 g
Eat Anytime Premium Creamy and Onion Millet Kurmura I Healthy Snacking Alternative I Made with Nutritious Millet I High In Fiber I Gluten-Free I Healthy Snacks for Adults and Kids	Jowar crisps, bajra crisps, ragi crisps, rice bran oil, signature cream and onion seasoning: milk solids, processed cheese powder, real cream powder, dehydrated triple onion blend (green, white and regular), garlic powder, dried herbs, acidifying agents INS 330, INS 296, flavour enhancers INS 627, INS 631, anticaking agents INS 170(i)	Ready to eat	Snacking between meals/tea time	Source of protein, roasted not fried, healthy namkeen, no palm oil, no MSG	Approximately Rs. 155/100 g

Roasty Tasty Millet Munch Chatpata 200g – Gluten-Free Healthy Snacks | Ideal for Weight Management | Cholesterol-Free Millet Namkeen	Sorghum flakes, peanuts, Bengal gram, edible vegetable oil, rice bran oil (antioxidant INS 307b), rice puff, sugar, seasoning mix [iodized salt, sugar, spices and condiments (red chilli), coriander, dried mango powder (amchur), garlic, onion, cumin, ginger, black pepper, turmeric, fenugreek], milk solids, hydrolyzed vegetable protein (soy), yeast extract powder, acidity regulator [citric acid (INS/E 330), lemon juice powder, anticaking agent, silicon dioxide (INS/E 551)], flavour enhancer INS/E 635 tamarind powder (tamarind pulp, maltodextrin), red chilli, salt, curry leaves	Ready to consume	Snacking between meals/tea time	100% roasted, whole grain snack	Approximately Rs. 62/100 g

[a] Price may vary with pack size and discount offer.

Despite these limitations, millets are treasure house of nutrients as they are rich in dietary fibre, antioxidants and essential nutrients specially minerals and vitamins. Therapeutic roles of millets in various non-communicable diseases have been well established. They can be a valuable addition to a balanced diet, especially for those seeking alternative grains or gluten-free options (Muskan et al 2025). Pearl millet and finger millet are commonly utilized in food product formulations owing to their favourable taste and flavour profiles (Siroha & Punia Bangar 2024).

12.5 CONCLUSION

Consumer perception plays a vital role in the market expansion of millets. However, challenges such as lack of awareness of millets health benefits, confusion in terminology and competition with major cereal grains limit adoption of these super foods. Addressing these obstacles requires targeted interventions which include improved infrastructure, support for innovations through research and development, consumer education for millets health benefits and enhanced market integration strategies. Moreover, the burgeoning interest in gluten-free diets and functional foods presents an opportunity for the commercialization of millet-based food products, specially, in urban and health-conscious markets. In addition, policy initiatives, such as government-backed subsidies and international collaborations, can further spur millet production and market growth. Advancements in processing technologies, efficient value chains and sustainable agricultural practices will play a pivotal role in establishing millets as a viable alternative to major cereals like wheat and rice. By nurturing ingenuity, policy support and consumer engagement, millets can transition from underutilized grains to mainstream staple crops.

REFERENCES

Aayog, N., Sen, R. K., Meena, H. K., & Shekhar, V. (2023). *Promoting millets in diets: Best practices across states/UTs of India*. National Institution for Transforming India: NITI Aayog, New Delhi, India.

Alekhya, P., & Raj Shravanthi, A. (2019). Buying behaviour of consumers towards millet based food products in Hyderabad district of Telangana, India. *International Journal of Current Microbiology and Applied Sciences*, *8*(10), 223–236. https://doi.org/10.20546/ijcmas.2019.810.023

FAO (Food and Agricultural Organization of the United Nations). (2022). *The statistical division*. http://www.fao.org/faostat/en/#data/QC (Accessed 10 February 2024).

Krishnasamy, J. R., Parthasarathy, K., & Nawaz, N. (2025). Analyzing the factors influencing consumer purchasing decisions for millet foods. In S. Kot, B. Khalid, & A. ul Haque (Eds.), *New challenges of the global economy for business management*. EEEU 2024. *Springer Proceedings in Business and Economics*. Springer, Singapore. https://doi.org/10.1007/978-981-96-4116-1_83

Lalita, A., & Radhika, P. (2014). *Consumer perception and market segmentation of millet products: A case study of Utukur Krishi Vigyan Kendra in YSR district of Andhra Pradesh*. PG Thesis.

Muskan, F., Redhu, M., Redhu, S., & Rahimi, M. M. (2025). Millets in the global market: A critical review of challenges and opportunities. *Food Production, Processing and Nutrition*, *7*, 37. https://doi.org/10.1186/s43014-025-00316-1

Negi, N., & Sahu, G. K. (2024). Understanding millet consumption in India: A comprehensive review of consumption patterns, influencing factors and consumer preferences. *MPJSS*, *151*.

PIB (Press Information Bureau). (2023). *International year of millets: India leading the way*. https://static.pib.gov.in/WriteReadData/specificdocs/documents/2023/mar/doc2023318173501.pdf (Accessed 6 September 2025).

Shah, P., & Tripathy, N. (2023). *From fields to plates: Millets startups transforming India's food market*. https://www.policycircle.org/opinion/millets-consumption-in-india/ (Accessed 6 September 2025).

Siroha, A. K., & Punia Bangar, S. (2024). Millet-based food products: An overview. *Current Food Science and Technology Reports*, *2*(2), 213–220. https://link.springer.com/article/10.1007/s43555-024-00031-x

Sulthana, C. P. (2014). *Consumer acceptability and demand for health foods: A study of millet-based ANGRAU foods in metro Hyderabad.* Unpublished MBA project report, Agricultural University Rajendranagar, School of Agribusiness Management, College of Agriculture, India. https://krishikosh.egranth.ac.in/server/api/core/bitstreams/643d7f0b-cafd-424f-bde9-65ff7d8a383f/content

Transparency Market Research. (2025). *India millet-based packaged food market (2022–2032) – Industry analysis, share, size, growth, trends & forecast.* Retrieved from https://www.transparencymarket-research.com/india-millet-based-packaged-food-market.html

13 Millet Magic
Healthy Recipes for Every Day

Tarvinder Jeet Kaur
Professor and Chairperson, Department of Home Science,
Kurukshetra University, Kurukshetra, Haryana

13.1 INTRODUCTION

Millets are making their comeback as nutritional champions in India's mission towards sustainable diets and holistic health. India proudly took the global lead with the United Nations declaring 2023 as 'International Year of Millets', branding millets as '*Shree Anna*' – The Revered Food. Through policy frameworks like National Millet Mission, POSHAN Abhiyaan and the Mid-Day Meal Program, these nutri-cereals are now transitioning from marginal to mainstream. Millets adapts well to India's soils, climate and culinary traditions, carrying with them not just forgotten flavours but formidable therapeutic potential. Moreover, millets grow in arid zones, need little water, thrive without the need of pesticides and replenish soil fertility. Their reintroduction doesn't just promise resilient farms but healthier plates and sustainable food sovereignty.

But what makes these ancient grains therapeutically relevant today?

We live in an age of climate change, global warming and ever-increasing lifestyle diseases such as obesity, cardiovascular diseases, cancer and diabetes mellitus (type 2); millets may just be the quiet revolution our food systems need. Major millets (sorghum, finger millet, pearl millet) and minor millets (proso, kodo, barnyard, foxtail, little) are getting renewed attention due to their rich nutritional profile and health-promoting characteristics. By switching refined wheat and highly polished rice with millet variations, Indian diets can accomplish better gut health and improved micronutrient intake along with steadier glucose level. For diabetics, millets offer meals that nourish without causing blood sugar spikes. For growing girls, these nutri-cereals provide calcium and iron-rich alternatives without fortification. For vulnerable population, millets supply much needed calcium and biologically available protein along with essential amino acids. For one and all, millets deliver digestible starch, support gut health by improving good gut bacteria, hence reducing gastrointestinal inflammation.

Millets – the nutri-cereals – provide a distinctive nourishing matrix: slowly digestible complex carbohydrates, resistant starch and low-to-moderate glycaemic indices along with notable micronutrients concentrations especially calcium, iron, magnesium, phosphorus and polyphenols. Finger millet, for instance, rich in calcium and phosphorus adds to strengthening bones and teeth, a blessing for populations prone to osteomalacia, osteoporosis and bone demineralization. Barnyard millet, kodo millet and pearl millet being rich in phenolic compounds, flavonoids and iron reduce oxidative stress hence lower the risk of chronic diseases like cancer, premature ageing, Alzheimer and anaemia. Millet's resistant starch supports satiety and glucose regulation, making them ideal for obesity, overweight and diabetes management. Being naturally gluten-free, millets are perfect for persons having coeliac disease, gluten sensitivity and irritable bowel syndrome.

Scientific research further authenticates traditional wisdom. Sowunmi et al (2024) reported significantly reduced postprandial glycaemic spikes among type 2 diabetics with fermented finger millets–based preparations. Chandrasekara and Shahidi (2011) observed that millet's antioxidant aid in preventing LDL oxidation, indicating strong cardioprotective benefits. The role of millet in improving gut microbiota and systemic health is further supported by mounting evidence. The ability of millet in enriching gut microbiota, improving intestinal health, immunological balance, nutrient

 DOI: 10.1201/9781003686668-13

absorption and better mental health was highlighted by Saleh et al (2013) and Jacob et al (2024). The gut–brain axis interface mediated by dietary fibre and polyphenols through millet intake may also have a role in mental health regulation (Balkrishna et al 2024).

For more than 7,000 years, millets, one of the oldest grains ever cultivated, have been a staple of traditional diets across continents (Tripathi & Vyas 2023). These hardy grains have nurtured generations and influenced regional cuisines from Africa and Asia to Europe and America. Teff serves as the foundation for Ethiopia's famous injera flatbread. Fonio used in porridges and couscous-style dishes is prized in West Africa for its light texture and swift cooking. Proso millet has long been used in fermented drinks and porridges in Eastern Europe, and since Neolithic times, it has been used in steamed foods and congees in China. India's varied culinary traditions centred around these hardy grains are exemplified by regional staples like Karnataka's finger millet *mudde*, Rajasthani *rotis,* Maharashtra's *bhakris* and millet khichdi (Jha 2024).

Today, as the world confronts environmental damage and rising health problems, millets emerge as one promising option. Naturally gluten-free, high in prebiotic fibre and low on glycaemic index, millets provide satiety, support gut health and help to regulate blood sugar and cholesterol (Kumar et al 2024; Wale 2024). Furthermore, millets' capability to flourish in arid, nutrient-poor soils with minimal water and inputs makes them a climate-resilient crop, perfect for sustainable farming in the face of worldwide climate change.

Millet repossession is not merely a new food trend; it is a renewal of ancestral wisdom supported by modern nutrition science. Including millets into routine meals is a practical way to respond worldwide challenges related to poor nutrition, chronic disease prevention and sustainable agriculture (Thakur et al 2025). Millets, while traditionally a staple in various cuisines, are now finding their way into unconventional dishes such as ready-to-cook mixes, extruded food products and baked food products, showcasing their versatility and nutritional value beyond familiar recipes (Bisht 2022). Whether in the form of breads, porridges, flatbreads, fermented foods or healthy beverages, millets are slowly finding their way back on to plates around the world (Chaudhuri 2025; Muskan et al 2025).

Millet-based recipes' development take along a diverse portfolio of recipes formulated with both ethnic adaptability and therapeutic efficiency in mind. Recipes such as ***malai kofta*** **curry, finger millet *moong* salad, sorghum *kadi,*** kodo **millet curd rice, sorghum** ***gattae curry,*** **foxtail beetroot *dosa*, little millet vegetable** pulao, ***thalipeeth*, sorghum choco pancakes, pearl millet veggie** khichdi, **sorghum tacos and finger millet** ***masala lassi*** showcase the nutritional cum therapeutic potential of millet-based diets rich in resistant starch, dietary fibre, calcium, iron, magnesium and antioxidants favourable to glycaemic moderation, digestive health and cardiovascular support. Accompanying them are nutrient-dense, healthier indulgences developed with natural sweeteners like desi khand and coconut jaggery, contributing lower glycaemic effect than refined sugars. These include kodo ***kheer*** **bliss, foxtail turmeric** ***halwa*****, choco finger millet brownie, finger millet banana bread, finger millet chocolate shake** and **finger millet *halwa*** crafted to deliver mindful indulgence without compromising metabolic balance. By combining health benefits with familiar and delicious ingredients, this recipe collection shows how millet-based foods can be part of routine meals. It inspires individuals to eat in ways that support long-lasting well-being by combining traditional knowledge with modern nutrition science.

13.2 MILLET-BASED HEALTHY RECIPES

Millets, owing to their cultural significance, nutritional prospective and adaptability have appeared as significant components in the formulation of therapeutic and functional recipes. This chapter offers a carefully curated collection of millet-based recipes that exhibit the culinary adaptability and versatility of nutri-cereals, including pearl millet, finger millet, foxtail millet, sorghum, little millet and kodo millet. These recipes have been considerately selected and adapted to suit varied dietary preferences, meal patterns and seasonal contexts.

The collection contains both traditional preparations and contemporary variations, spanning across starters, snacks, beverages, main courses and desserts. Each recipe reflects the diverse culinary potential of millets to be incorporated into balanced diets through familiar aromas and formats, thereby simplifying their acceptance and long-lasting sustainability in daily meal planning. The objective is not only to preserve traditional culinary knowledge but also to explore possibilities for innovation that align with modern lifestyle goals and well-being. Explore, experiment and enjoy the rich tapestry of aromas, textures and taste that these time-honoured grains have to offer.

List of Millet Recipes:

A. Sorghum *Malai Kofta* Curry
B. Kodo *Kheer* Bliss
C. Finger millet *Halwa*
D. Foxtail Turmeric *Halwa*
E. Finger millet Choco Brownie
F. Finger millet Choco Shake
G. Finger millet Choco Banana Bread
H. Finger millet *Moong* Protein Salad
I. Kodo Millet Curd Rice
J. Foxtail Beetroot *Dosa*
K. Sorghum Kadi
L. Sorghum *Thalipeeth*
M. Sorghum Gattae Curry
N. Little Millet Vegetable *Pulao*
O. Pearl millet Veggie *Khichdi*
P. Sorghum Tacos
Q. Finger millet Spiced Lassi
R. Sorghum Choco Pancakes

13.2.1 Preparation Techniques

For improved culinary functionality, sensory qualities and best nutritional benefits, understanding of apposite preparation techniques is must. This chapter summaries the key methods for the processing such as soaking, germination, fermentation and roasting along with cooking different types of millets. These preparation techniques influence not just the appearance, flavour, texture, taste and overall acceptability of millet-based preparations but also enhance digestibility and bioavailability of nutrients. With a strong overview of preparation methods, this chapter supports both the scientific and practical aspects of millet incorporation to daily diets.

A.) SORGHUM *MALAI KOFTA* CURRY

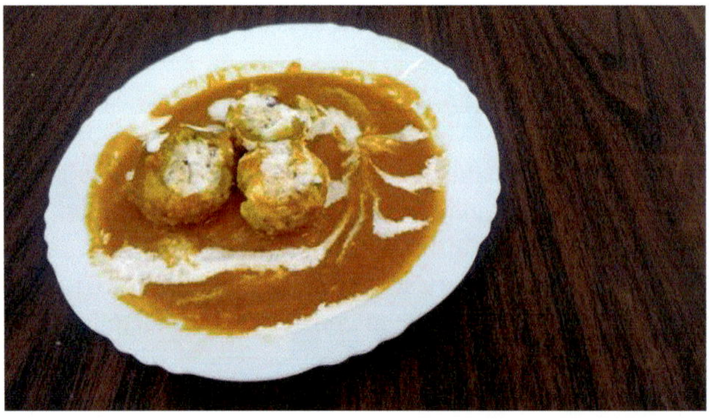

INGREDIENTS

For *kofta*

- Germinated sorghum flour – 100 g
- Red chilli powder to taste
- Turmeric – 2.5 g
- *Carom seeds* – 2.5 g
- *Kasoori methi* – 2 g
- Oil – 20 ml
- Curd – 20 ml
- Cumin seeds – 2.5 g
- Warm water – 30 ml
- Salt to taste

For filling

- *Paneer – 50 g*
- *Khoa – 15 g*
- Cashew – 5 g
- Almond – 5 g
- Black pepper to taste
- Salt to taste

For curry/gravy

- Ginger – 10 g
- Garlic – 5 g
- Onion – 60 g
- Tomato – 150 g
- Cream – 30 g
- Curd – 20 ml
- *Kasoori methi – 2.5 g*
- Mustard oil – 10 ml
- Cumin seeds – 5 g
- Turmeric powder – 5 g
- Red chilli powder – 2 g

METHOD

Prepare dough for *kofta*:

- In a mixing bowl, add germinated sorghum flour, spices, curd and oil and knead a soft dough with warm water.
- Set it aside for 5–10 minutes.

For filling:

- In another bowl, prepare filling for *kofta* by mixing grated *paneer*, *khoa*, chopped dry fruits, black pepper and salt.
- Mix well to form a smooth dough and make small balls from it.

Prepare and cook *kofta*:

- Divide the sorghum dough into equal parts. Roll each part into small circles.
- Take a filling ball, place it in the centre of dough circles and roll it to make *koftas.*
- Heat a steamer, add some water and place a tray on it.
- Place the *kofta* on it and steam it for 6–8 minutes till cooked or in *appe* pan cook till golden brown.

Prepare the curry/gravy:

- Heat oil in a pan, add cumin seeds and let them splutter.
- Add ginger and garlic and sauté until fragrant.

- Sauté chopped onions until golden. Add tomato puree, turmeric powder, red chili powder and cook until oil separates.
- Add cream and *kasoori methi* and cook for another 2–3 minutes, by adding water to adjust consistency like curry/gravy.
- Add millet *koftas* to the curry/gravy and simmer for another 2–3 minutes.

Garnish and serve:

- Garnish with cream and serve hot.

Cooking time: 45 minutes
Mentioned ingredients makes 9 *koftas* (wt. per *kofta*: 25–30 g)
Gravy weight: 300 g **Total weight: 570 g**
Total serve: 3 **Per serve: 190 g**

B.) KODO *KHEER* BLISS

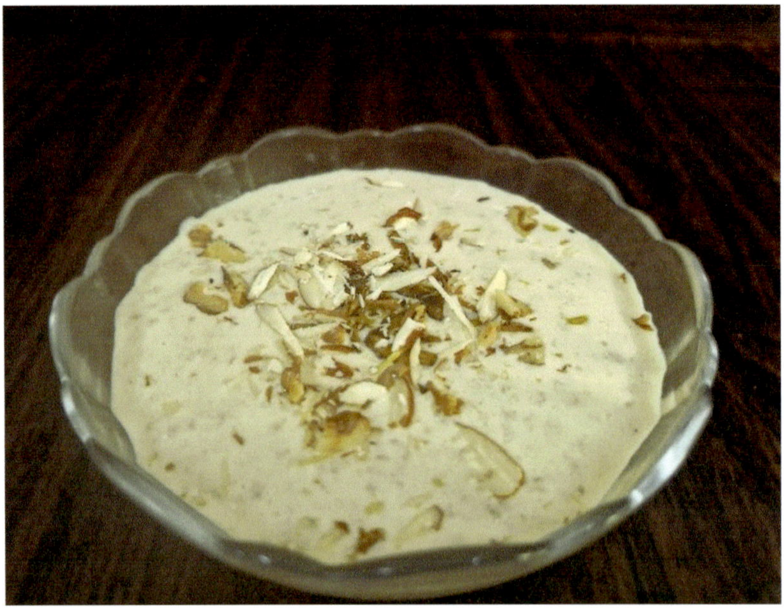

INGREDIENTS

- Kodo millet – 60 g
- Milk – 300 ml
- Coconut jaggery – 10 g
- Cardamom powder – 5 g
- Almonds – 10 g

PRE-PREPARATION

- Wash the kodo millet thoroughly under running water.
- Soak it in clean water for 5–6 hours or overnight.
- Drain the soaked water and wash kodo millet under water.

METHOD

Cook the millet:

- In a pressure cooker, add soaked kodo millet followed by water.
- After 1 whistle, simmer/cook kodo millet for 5–6 minutes.

Prepare kheer:

- In a pan, bring the milk to boil over medium heat.
- Once the milk boils, reduce the heat and add pressure-cooked kodo millet.
- Mix and cook on low flame for 10–12 minutes.
- Stir occasionally to prevent it from sticking to the bottom.

Add coconut jaggery and flavour:

- Add coconut jaggery and cardamom powder.
- Cook for another 5–6 minutes on low flame or till desired consistency.

Garnish and serve:

- Garnish with chopped cashews.
- Serve hot/chilled.

Cooking time: 25 minutes **Total cooked weight: 250 g**
Total serve: 2 **Per serve: 125 g**

C.) FINGER MILLET *HALWA*

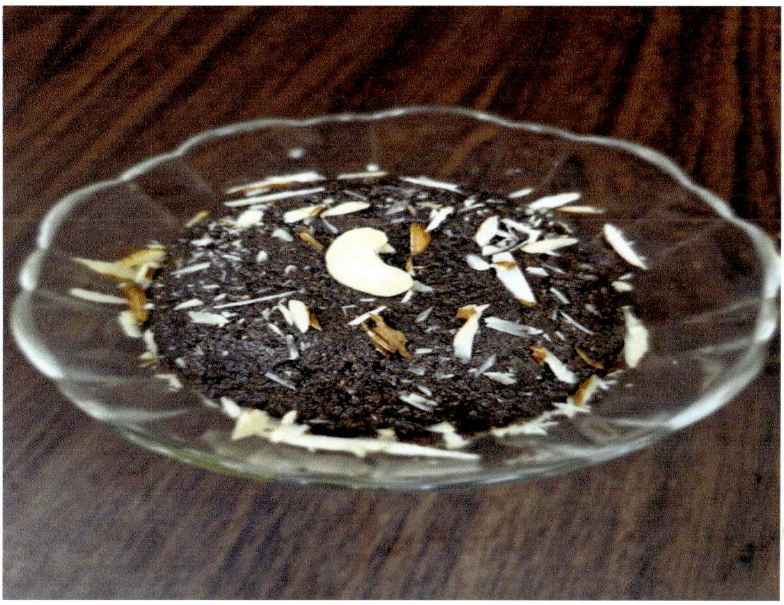

INGREDIENTS

- Germinated finger millet flour – 70 g
- *Desi ghee* – 50 g
- Desi khand – 70 g
- Water – 250 ml
- Cashews – 10 g
- Almond – 10 g

METHOD

Prepare desi khand **syrup:**

- In a heated pan add water and desi khand and give a quick boil until desi khand dissolves properly.

Roast the germinated finger millet flour:

- Melt *ghee* in a heavy bottom pan on medium heat.

- Add the germinated finger millet flour to it and roast it on low flame, stirring continuously to prevent burning.
- Roast it until it turns aromatic and *ghee* separates.

Add desi khand **syrup:**

- Reduce the heat and carefully pour the prepared desi khand syrup into the roasted flour.
- Stir continuously to prevent lumps from forming until it thickens and leaves the sides of the pan.

Garnish and serve:

- Garnish with chopped almonds and cashews.
- Serve hot.

Cooking time: 20–25 minutes **Total cooked weight: 450 g**
Total Serve: 4 **Per serve: 110–115 g**

D.) FOXTAIL TURMERIC *HALWA*

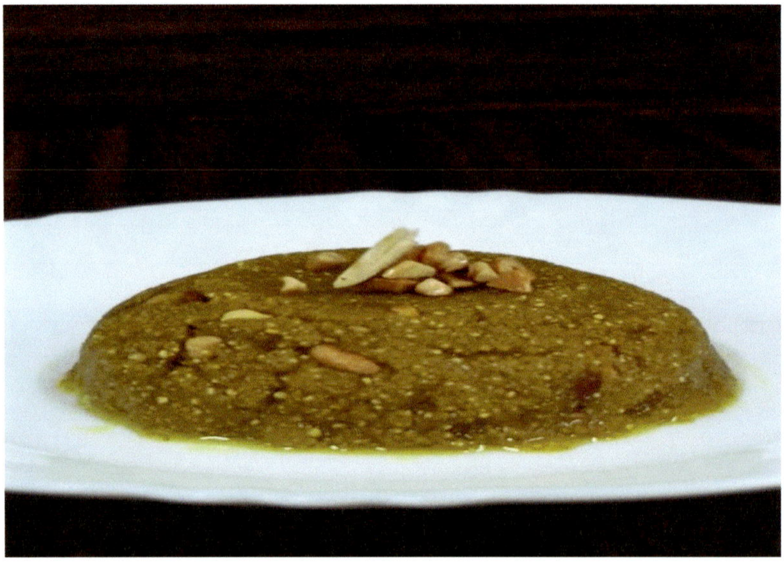

INGREDIENTS

- Foxtail flour – 25 g
- Desi khand – 25 g
- *Ghee* – 15 g
- Cashew – 10 g
- Turmeric powder – 5 g
- Water – 100 ml

METHOD

Prepare desi khand **syrup:**

- Heat water in a pan and add desi khand and turmeric powder to it.
- Bring it to a boil or until desi khand dissolves properly.

Roast the flour:

- In a heated heavy bottomed pan, melt *ghee* and add foxtail millet flour.
- Roast it on low flame until it turns aromatic or golden.
- Stir continuously to prevent burning.

Prepare *halwa*:

- When foxtail flour turns aromatic, add the prepared *desi* khand syrup to it carefully.
- Stir it well to avoid lumps formation.
- Cook it until the mixture thickens smoothly.

Garnish and serve:

- Garnish with cashews and serve hot.

Cooking time: 25 minutes **Total cooked weight: 170 g**
Total serve: 3 **Per serve: 55–60 g (1 small bowl)**

E.) FINGER MILLET CHOCO BROWNIE

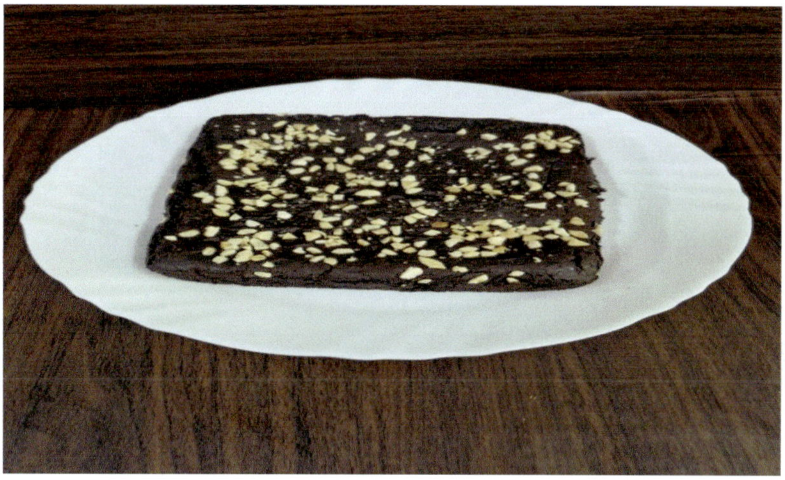

INGREDIENTS

- Olive oil/melted *desi ghee* – 44 g
- Germinated finger millet flour – 115 g
- Cacao powder – 23 g
- Desi khand – 79 g
- Milk – 115 ml
- Vanilla essence – 5 ml
- Dark chocolate compound – 100 g
- Baking powder – 5 g
- Baking soda – 2.5 g
- Cashew – 10 g

METHOD

Pre-preparation:

- Preheat oven to 180°C for 10 minutes beforehand.
- Grease a loaf pan or line it with parchment paper.
- In a double boiler or microwave oven, melt dark chocolate compound.

Beat desi khand **and *ghee*:**

- In a large mixing bowl, add olive oil/*desi ghee*.
- Add desi khand and vanilla essence and mix well with the help of beater.

Assemble all the ingredients:

- Place a sieve over the bowl, add germinated finger millet flour, cacao powder, baking powder and baking soda to it.

- Sift and add to the oil/*ghee* and *desi khand* mixture.
- Add melted chocolate to the above mixture followed by milk.
- Mix all well.

Bake:
- Pour the batter into the prepared cake tin and smooth the top with a spatula.
- Sprinkle chopped cashew/nuts of your choice.
- Bake it in a preheated oven for 25 minutes at 180°C or until a toothpick inserted into centre comes out clean.

Serve:
- Serve hot.

Cooking time: 35 minutes	**Total Weight: 480 g**
Total serve: 10	**Per serve: 48 g**

F.) FINGER MILLET CHOCO SHAKE

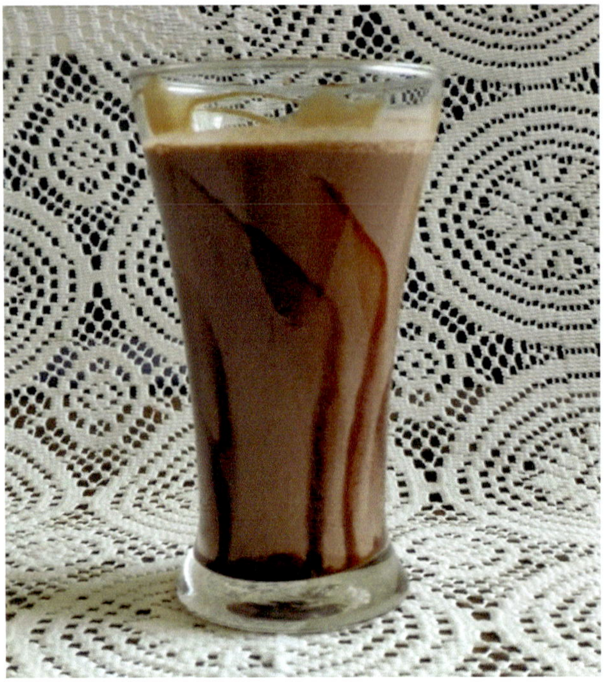

INGREDIENTS
- Germinated finger millet flour – 20 g
- Cacao powder – 7 g
- Water – 150 ml
- *Desi khand* – 15 g
- Milk – 250 ml
- Hershey's chocolate syrup* for garnish (optional)

*Nutritional information not included in the final nutritive value

METHOD:
Prepare germinated finger millet base:
- In a saucepan, mix germinated finger millet flour with water to form a lump-free paste.

- Heat the mixture on low flame, stir continuously, until it thickens.
- Set it aside to cool.

Blending the shake:

- In a blender, combine cooled finger millet base, milk, cocoa powder and desi khand.
- Blend until smooth and creamy.
- Add ice cubes (optional) and blend again for a chilled shake.

Serve:

- Spread Hershey's syrup on glass top edges (optional).
- Pour chocolate finger millet shake into glass.
- Serve chilled.

Cooking time: 15 minutes **Total weight: 400 ml**
Total serve: 2 **Per serve: 1 medium glass (200 ml)**

G.) FINGER MILLET CHOCO BANANA BREAD

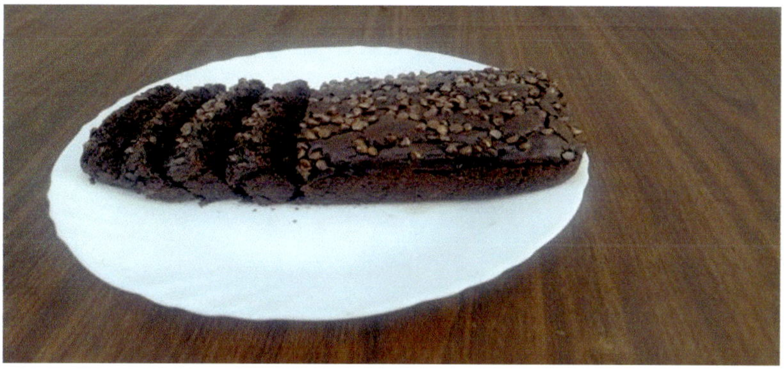

INGREDIENTS

- Germinated finger millet flour – 100 g
- Cacao powder – 35 g
- Desi khand – 100 g
- Milk – 100 ml
- Olive oil – 80 ml
- Flax seeds – 20 g
- Baking powder – 5 g
- Baking soda – 2.5 g
- Ripe banana – 2 (200 g)
- Chocolate chips 10 g
- Ghee 25 g

METHOD

Pre-preparation:

- Preheat oven to 180°C for 10 minutes beforehand.
- Grease a loaf pan or line it with parchment paper.

Make the batter:

- In a blender jar, add germinated finger millet flour, cacao powder, desi khand, milk, olive oil, flax seeds, baking powder, *ghee*, baking soda, banana and milk.
- Blend it well to mix all ingredients evenly.

Bake:

- Pour the batter into the prepared loaf pan and smooth the top with a spatula.
- Sprinkle choco chips or nuts of your choice (optional).
- Bake for 40 minutes at 180°C or until a toothpick inserted into centre comes out clean.

Cool and serve:

- Remove the bread from the oven and let it cool in the pan for 10 minutes.
- Transfer it to a tray, and cut it into slices.

Cooking time: 40 minutes **Total cooked weight: 680 g**
Total serve: 10 **Per serve: 68 g**

H.) FINGER MILLET MOONG PROTEIN SALAD

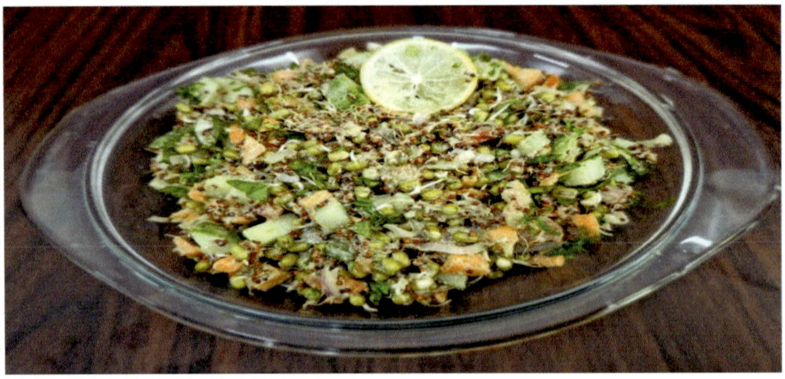

INGREDIENTS

- Germinated finger millet grains – 100 g
- Germinated moong – 100 g
- Onion – 30 g
- Tomato – 50 g
- Carrot – 30 g
- Cucumber – 30 g
- Black pepper – 2 g
- Coriander leaves – 2.5 g
- Salt – as per taste

FOR DRESSING

- Cottage cheese – 10 g
- Green chili – 5 g
- Cashew – 10 g
- Mint leaves – 5 g
- Coriander leaves – 2.5 g
- Ginger – 5 g
- Salt – as per taste

PRE-PREPARATION

- **Sprouting finger millet:** Rinse the finger millet and soak it for 8–12 hours. After soaking, drain the water (to eliminate anti-nutrients) and place the finger millet in a clean muslin cloth for 1–2 days with sprinkling water to maintain moisture.

- **Sprouting whole moong:** Wash and soak the moong for 8–12 hours in water. After soaking, drain and leave it to sprout for 1–2 days in a damp muslin cloth.

METHOD

Cooking sprouted finger millet and moong:

- Bring water to boil in a steamer and add sprouted finger millet and moong separately on steamer plate for 10 minutes. Ensure that the sprouts are soft and tender before adding/using them to salad.

Chop the vegetables:

- Finely chop the vegetables mentioned in the ingredients (onion, tomato, cucumber, and carrot).

Salad dressing:

- Prepare salad dressing by blending cottage cheese, ginger, green chili, cashew, mint, coriander and salt to taste in a blender jar.
- Adjust the consistency with adding water.

Assembling the salad:

- In a large mixing bowl, add steamed sprouted finger millet, steamed moong sprouts, chopped vegetables, black pepper and salt.
- Pour the dressing over the salad and toss every asafoetida together gently until all the ingredients are coated well.

Serve:

- Serve the salad by garnish asafoetida with fresh coriander leaves.

Cooking time: 15 minutes **Total cooked weight: 410 g**
Total serve: 6 **Per serve: 65–70 g**

I.) KODO MILLET CURD RICE

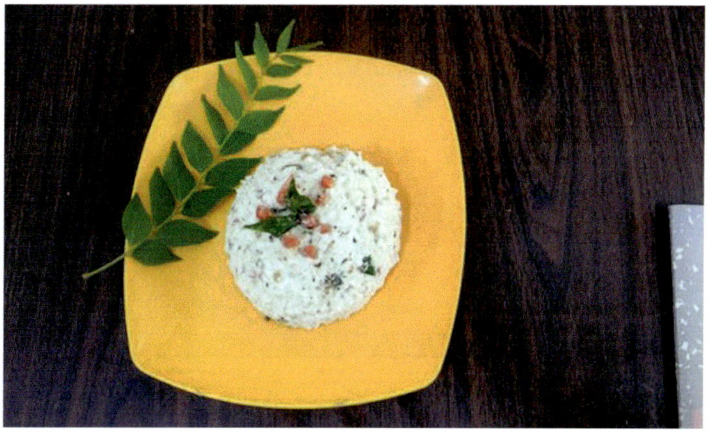

INGREDIENTS

- Kodo millet – 50 g
- Curd – 100 g
- Chana dal – 10 g
- Curry leaves – 5 g
- Mustard seed – 5 g
- Mustard oil – 5 ml
- Salt to taste

PRE-PREPARATION

Soak the millet:

- Wash kodo millet thoroughly and soak it overnight.
- Wash and soak chana dal for 4–6 hours.

METHOD

Cook the kodo millet:

- Rinse the soaked kodo millet under running water to remove anti-nutrients.
- In a pressure cook, add soaked kodo millet, water and salt to taste.
- Cook the millet until soft but not mushy (cook for 2 whistles).
- Once cooked, let it cool at room temperature.

Add curd to millet:

- In a large mixing bowl, add the cooked millet.
- Whisk curd for smooth consistency.
- Add this curd to the millet bowl and mix well.

Tempering:

- Heat oil in a pan, add mustard seeds and let them splutter.
- Add soaked and washed chana dal and roast it for a minute.
- Add curry leaves.
- Pour the tempering over the curd millet mixture and mix gently.
- Serve.

Cooking time: 25 minutes **Total Cooked weight: 420 g**
Total serve: 2 **Per serve: 210 g**

J.) FOXTAIL BEETROOT *DOSA*

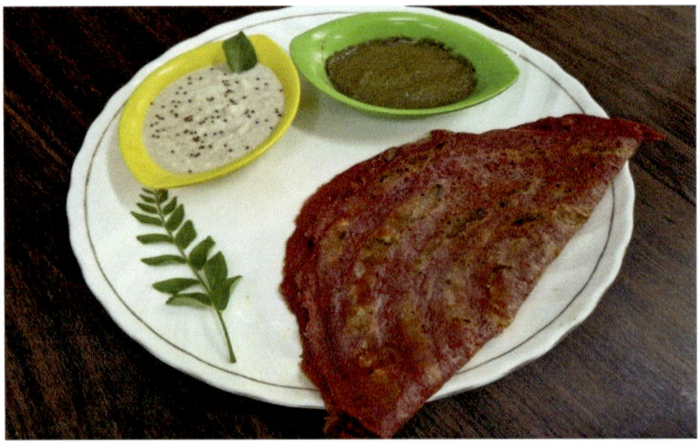

INGREDIENTS

For batter:

- Foxtail millet – 50 g
- *Urad dal* – 50 g
- Beetroot – 25 g

For filling:

- Onion – 20 g
- Capsicum – 30 g
- Carrot – 50 g
- Green chilli – 5 g
- Coriander leaves – 5 g
- Black pepper – 2 g

- Salt to taste
- Oil/*ghee* – 10 ml

PRE-PREPARATION

Soak millet and *urad dal*:

- Wash and soak foxtail millet and *urad dal* separately for 6–8 hours or overnight.

Prepare the batter:

- After soaking, drain the millet and *urad dal* and rinse under water.
- Grind *urad dal* and foxtail millet together with minimal water.
- Pour it into a large bowl and let it ferment for 8–12 hours in a warm place.
- The batter should rise and become light and fluffy.

METHOD

Prepare the beetroot puree:

- Cut beetroot into small pieces.
- Steam beet root and blend it into a smooth puree in a blender jar.

Mix the batter and beetroot puree:

- In a bowl, add beetroot puree to fermented batter.
- Add salt to taste and mix gently.

Prepare filling:

- Finely chop onion, carrot, capsicum, green chillies and coriander.
- Add black pepper and salt to the chopped vegetables.

Make *dosas*:

- Heat a *dosa* pan, lightly grease it with oil or *ghee.*
- Pour a ladleful of the batter on the pan and spread it in a circular motion to form a thin *dosa.*
- Drizzle a few drops of oil or *ghee* around the edges of *dosa.*
- Place a spoonful filling on it and fold it.
- Cook until *dosa* turns golden or crispy.

Serve:

- Serve hot with *chutney* or *sambar.*

Cooking time: 20 minutes **Total cooked weight: 390 g**
Total serve: 2 **Per serve: 2 *dosa* (90–100 g each)**

K.) SORGHUM *KADI*

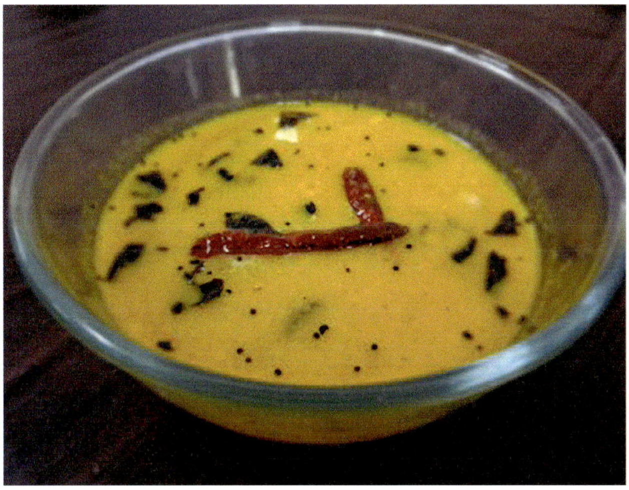

INGREDIENTS

For *kadi*:

- Germinated sorghum flour – 40 g
- Curd – 150 g
- Water – 400 ml
- Salt – to taste
- Red chilli powder – to taste
- Onion – 70 g
- Garlic – 5 g
- Turmeric – 2.5–5 g
- Fenugreek seeds – 5 g
- Ginger – 5 g
- Coriander leaves – 5 g
- Mustard oil – 5 ml

For tadka/tempering:

- Mustard oil/ghee – 5 ml
- Mustard seeds – 5 g
- Dry red chilli – 2
- Curry leaves – 5
- Cumin seeds – 5 g
- Asafoetida – 1 pinch
- Ginger – 5 g

METHOD

Prepare the *kadi* mixture:

- In a large mixing bowl, whisk curd until smooth.
- Add germinated sorghum flour, turmeric powder, chilli powder and salt.
- Add water, mix and make a lump-free batter. Set aside.

Cook the *kadi*:

- In a heated pan, add *ghee*/oil and fenugreek seeds followed by ginger and garlic. Sauté it for a minute on low flame.
- Add onion and fry until it turns golden.
- Pour the *kadi* mixture in it and cook on medium heat, continuously stirring to avoid lumps.
- Once it comes to a boil, reduce the heat and simmer it for 10–15 minutes.

Prepare the *tadka*/tempering:

- Heat oil/*ghee* in a pan, add mustard seeds, cumin, curry leaves and asafoetida. Sauté it for a few seconds.
- Add dry red chilli and off the flame.
- Pour this *tadka* on the prepared *kadi* and mix well.

Garnish and serve:

- Garnish with fresh coriander leaves.
- Serve hot with rice or *roti*.

Cooking time: 40 minutes **Total cooked weight: 560 g**
Total serve: 4 **Per serve: 1 big bowl (140 g)**

L.) SORGHUM *THALIPEETH*

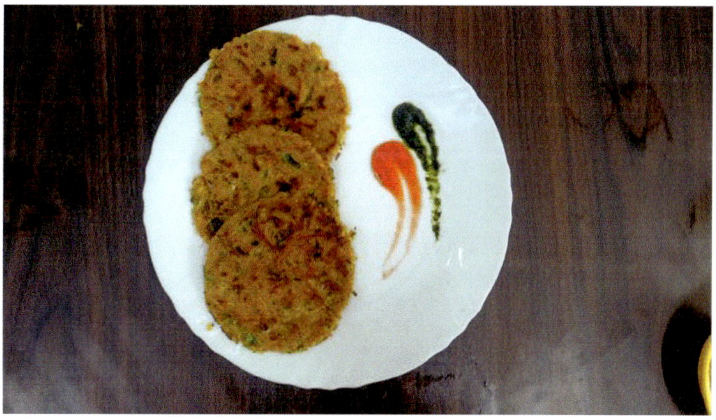

INGREDIENTS

- Germinated Sorghum flour – 100 g
- Onion – 20 g
- Carrot – 30 g
- Capsicum – 30 g
- Green chilli – 5 g
- Coriander leaves – 5 g
- Ginger – 5 g
- Oil – 5 ml
- Water – 70 ml
- Turmeric – 2.5 g
- Salt – as per taste

METHOD

Chop the vegetables:

- Finely chop onion, carrot, capsicum, green chilli and coriander leaves.
- Grate the ginger.

Prepare the dough:

- In a large mixing bowl, add germinated sorghum flour, chopped vegetables, grated ginger, turmeric and salt to taste.
- Add water gradually and knead into a soft dough.
- Cover the dough with a cloth and let it rest for 10 minutes.

Shaping and cooking *thalipeeth*:

- Divide the dough into equal-sized ball.
- On a clean surface, place a ball of dough between two parchment/plastic sheets.
- Gently flatten it with your fingers into a thin disc.
- Make two to three small holes in the centre of the disc (this helps the thalipeeth cook evenly).
- On a lightly greased-heated tawa, transfer *thalipeeth.*
- Cook on medium heat from both sides until golden brown spots appear.

Serve:

- Serve hot with curd/chutney/pickle.

Cooking time: 30 minutes **Cooked weight: 120 g** **Total *Thalipeeth*: 8**
Total serve: 4 **Per serve: 2 *Thalipeeth* (15 g each)**

M.) Sorghum *Gattae* Curry

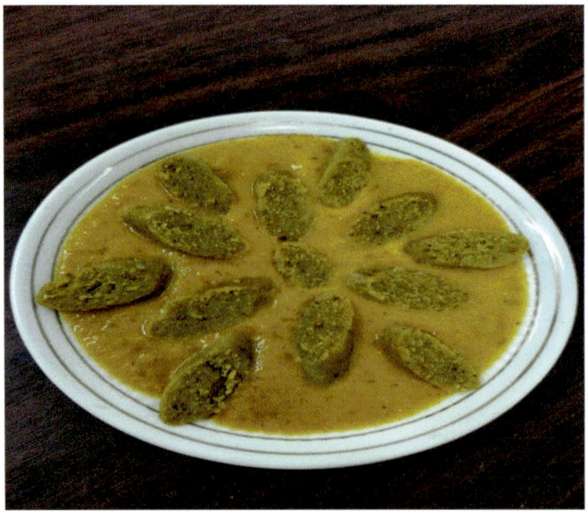

INGREDIENTS

For *gattae*:

- Germinated sorghum flour – 100 g
- Cumin powder – 5 g
- Carom seeds – 2.5 g
- Black pepper – to taste (2 g)
- Turmeric powder – 2.5 g
- Salt – to taste
- Oil – 15 ml

For curry/gravy

- Onion – 50 g
- Tomato – 100 g
- Green chilli – 5 g
- Garlic – 10 g
- Ginger – 10 g
- Salt – to taste
- Red chilli powder – 2.5 g
- Turmeric powder – 2.5 g
- Cashew – 20 g
- Cumin seeds – 5 g
- Asafoetida – 1 pinch
- *Kasoori methi* – 3 g
- Coriander leaves – 5 g
- Oil/*ghee* – 5 ml

METHOD

Prepare sorghum *gattae*:

- In a bowl, mix germinated sorghum flour, carom seeds, cumin powder, black pepper, turmeric powder and salt.
- Add oil and mix well together.
- Gradually add water and knead into a smooth dough.
- Divide the dough into equal portion and roll them into cylindrical logs.
- Boil water in a large pot. Place a sieve or steam tray in it and add the logs. Steam it for 6–8 minutes or until cooked.

- Remove the cooked sorghum *gattae*, let them cool slightly and cut into small oblique pieces.

Prepare the curry/gravy:

- Heat oil in a pan, add cumin seeds and asafoetida. Sauté the onion until golden, then add the ginger–garlic paste and cook.
- Add chopped tomatoes and cashews. Cook it for 2–3 minutes until it becomes soft.
- Cool it at room temperature and blend it to make puree.
- In another heated pan, cook the puree while adding spices and water to adjust consistency.

Assemble curry and *gattae:*

- Add the sliced sorghum *gattae* to the simmering gravy. Let them cook for 5–7 minutes to absorb the flavours.

Garnish and serve:

- Sprinkle *kasoori methi* and coriander leaves to garnish.
- Serve hot with chapatti/parantha/naan.

Cooking time: 35 minutes
***Gattae* weight: 200 g**
Total serve: 3
Total cooked weight: 500 g
Curry/gravy weight: 300 g
Per serve: 1 big bowl (160–170 g)

N.) LITTLE MILLET VEGETABLE PULAO

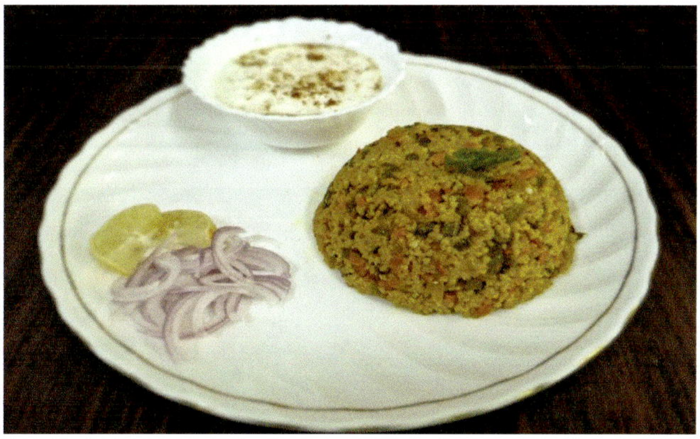

INGREDIENTS

- Little millet – 100 g
- Onion – 50 g
- Tomato – 50 g
- Capsicum – 20 g
- Beans – 20 g
- Green chilli – 5 g
- Ginger – 5 g
- Garlic – 5 g
- Coriander leaves – 10 g
- Cumin – 5 g
- Asafoetida – 1 pinch
- Turmeric powder – 2.5 g
- Bay leaf – 1
- Cloves – 4
- Mustard oil/*ghee* – 5 ml
- Salt – to taste

PRE-PREPARATION

Soak the little millet:

- Rinse little millet thoroughly and soak in clean water for 5–6 hours.
- Drain the soaked water and rinse under water.

METHOD

Chop the vegetables:

- Finely chop onion, tomato, capsicum, beans, green chillies and coriander.
- Crush ginger and garlic.

Preparing the base:

- Heat mustard oil/ghee in a pan, add cumin, asafoetida, bay leaf and cloves. Sauté until aromatic.
- Add chopped onion and cook until golden brown.
- Stir in the ginger–garlic paste and sauté until the raw smell disappears.
- Add chopped tomato, green chili, and vegetables (mentioned in the ingredients) and cook for 1–2 minutes.

Add little millet:

- Add soaked and washed little millet into the vegetable pot with water.
- Reduce the heat and cook for 20–25 minutes or until softens.

Garnish and serve:

- Garnish with coriander leaves and serve hot.

Cooking time: 35 minutes **Cooked weight: 420 g**
Total serve: 2 **Per serve: 210 g**

O.) PEARL MILLET VEGGIE *KHICHDI*

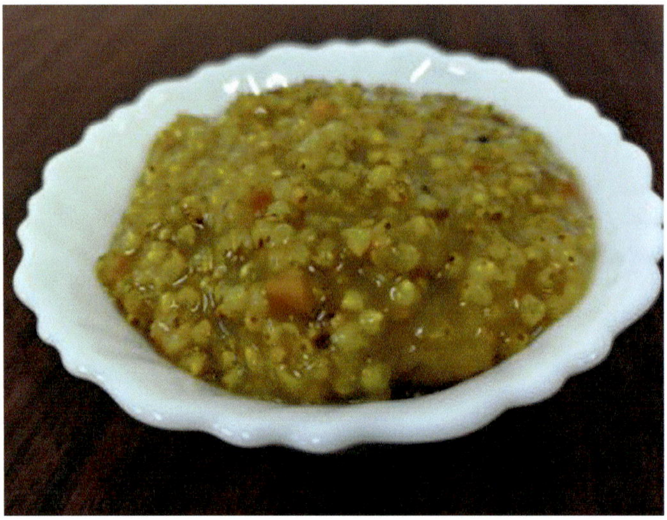

INGREDIENTS

- Germinated pearl millet – 100 g
- Onion – 25 g
- Carrot – 20 g
- Capsicum – 20 g
- Tomato – 30 g
- Garlic – 5 g
- Ginger – 10 g

- Green chillies – 5 g
- Coriander leaves – 5 g
- Turmeric – 2.5 g
- Cumin seeds – 2.5 g
- *Ghee* – 20 ml
- Salt – to taste

PRE-PREPARATION

Soak the pearl millet grains:

- Rinse pearl millet under running water and soak for 6–8 hours or overnight.
- After soaking, drain the soaked water and wash pearl millet under water.

METHOD

Prepare and cook the pearl millet:

- Coarsely grind soaked pearl millet grains in a blender or using mortar and pestle.
- In a pressure cooker, add soaked pearl millet grains, turmeric powder, salt and water and pressure-cook it for three to four whistle on medium flame.

Chop and cook the vegetables:

- Finely chop the vegetables mentioned in the ingredient.
- Heat a pan, add *ghee* and cumin seeds and let them splutter.
- Sauté ginger and garlic for a minute followed by chopped onion, tomato, carrot, capsicum and green chilli.
- Sauté it for 5–6 minutes until vegetables soften.

Assemble pearl millet and vegetables:

- In the pressure-cooked pearl millet, add cooked vegetables and cook for another 4–5 minutes or until smooth consistency (like khichdi).

Garnish and serve:

- Garnish with fresh coriander and serve hot with yogurt or pickle.

Cooking time: 35 minutes **Total cooked weight: 480 g**
Total serve: 2 **Per serve: 240 g**

P.) SORGHUM TACOS

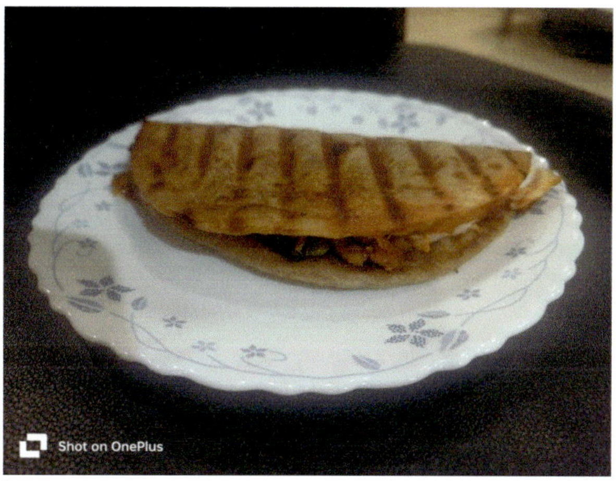

INGREDIENTS

For tacos:

- Germinated sorghum flour – 100 g

- Salt – to taste
- Turmeric – 2.5 g
- Oil/*ghee* – 5 ml

For filling:

- *Paneer* – 50 g
- Capsicum – 20 g
- Carrot – 20 g
- Onion – 30 g
- Green chili – 5 g
- Black pepper – to taste
- Pizza sauce – 10 ml (to taste)
- Salt – to taste

METHOD

Prepare the filling:

- Finely chop capsicum, carrot, onion, green chilli and grate *paneer.*
- In a large mixing bowl, add chopped vegetables, grated paneer, pizza sauce, black pepper and salt.
- Toss it well and ensure all ingredients mix well together.

Make sorghum tacos:

- In a bowl, add sorghum flour, turmeric and salt.
- Add water gradually to make a thick pouring batter.
- In a heated non-stick pan, drizzle oil, pour a spoonful of batter and spread evenly to make medium-sized tacos.
- Cook it from both sides.
- Add a spoon of filling on half of taco.
- Fold it and grill it in griller, until crisp.

Serve:

- Sorghum tacos are ready, serve them with sauce or *chutney.*

Cooking time: 25 minutes
Total serve: 4 medium
Total weight: 290 g
Per serve: 1 medium (70–75 g)

Q.) FINGER MILLET SPICED *LASSI*

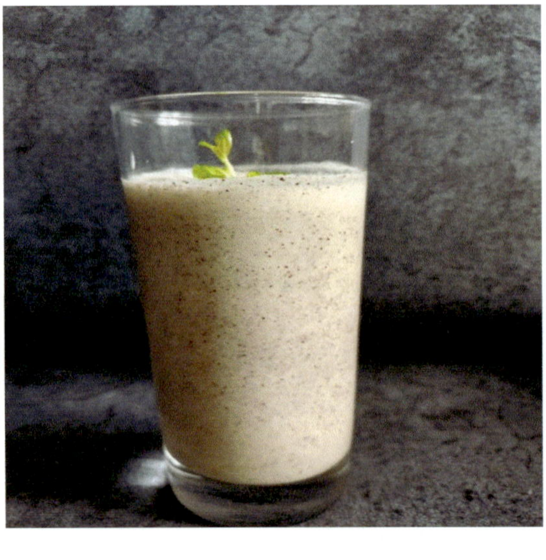

INGREDIENTS

- Germinated finger millet flour – 30 g
- Curd – 250 g
- Water – 500 ml
- *Ghee* – 5 g
- Mustard seeds – 7 g
- Cumin seeds – 7 g
- Asafoetida – 5 g
- Fresh coriander leaves – 30 g
- Curry leaves – 5 g
- Salt – to taste

METHOD

Dry-roast germinated finger millet flour:

- Heat a heavy bottomed pan and dry-roast germinated finger millet flour on low flame.
- Stir continuously until it turns aromatic.
- Transfer it into a bowl and cool it at room temperature.

Make the slurry:

- In a pan add water, bring it to boil.
- Add roasted finger millet flour while continuously stirring to avoid lumps.
- Cook it until it thickens and let it cool.

Add curd:

- When it cools down, add curd and salt and whisk properly.

Prepare the tempering:

- In a heated *tadka* pan, add *ghee*, asafoetida, cumin seeds, mustard seeds and curry leaves. Let them splutter.
- Add this *tadka/masala/tempering* to finger millet *lassi*.

Serve:

- Finger millet *masala lassi* is ready to serve.

Cooking time: 15 minutes **Total weight: 850 ml**
Total Serve: 3 **Per serve: 1 big glass (280 ml)**

R.) SORGHUM CHOCO PANCAKE

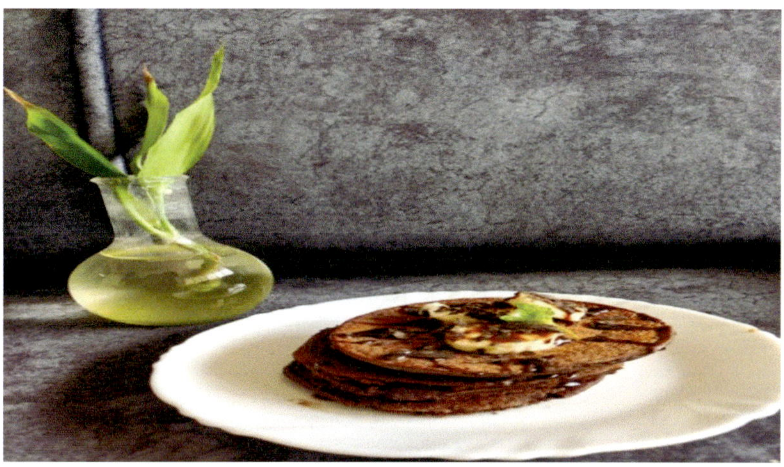

INGREDIENTS

- Germinated sorghum flour – 100 g
- *Desi khand* – 25 g
- Milk – 30 ml
- Cacao powder – 15 g
- Baking powder – 2 g
- *Ghee* – 5 g (for cooking)

METHOD

Prepare the batter:

- In a large mixing bowl, sift together the germinated sorghum flour, baking powder, *desi khand* and cacao powder.
- Mix it well and add water/milk gradually, whisk until combined.
- The batter should be thick but pourable.

Cook the pancakes:

- Heat a non-stick or cast-iron pan and lightly grease it with *ghee*.
- Pour a spoonful batter onto pan and gently spread the batter evenly into a circle using back of the spoon.
- Cook until bubbles on the surface and edges look set.
- Flip and cook the other side until golden brown.

Serve:

- Serve warm with choice of syrup* (choco/honey/maple) and fruit* (optional).
  *Nutritional information not included in the final nutritive value.

Cooking time: 15 minutes
Mentioned ingredients makes 6 pancakes
Weight per pancake: 30 g **Total cooked weight: 180 g**
Total serve: 3 **Per serve: 2 pancakes (60 g)**

13.2.2 Nutritional Composition

This chapter aims to help readers better understand the nutritional value of millets and their relevance in everyday diets. By emphasizing the main nutrients present in varied millets, it offers hands-on insights into how these nutri-cereals can support overall health and well-being. Whether you are selecting millets for their health potential or exploring them as substitutes to commonly consumed cereals, this chapter delivers a sensible understanding of their nutritional potential and how they can add to a more balanced and nourishing diet.

The nutritional data discussed in this chapter is primarily derived from the dietary guidelines for Indians published by NIN (ICMR – NIN, India 2024) and is further supported by recent peer-reviewed studies exploring the impact of processing techniques such as germination on the nutritional quality of millets. Research findings has shown that on germination, pearl millet (*Pennisetum glaucum*), sorghum (*Sorghum bicolor*) and finger millet (*Eleusine coracana*) demonstrated improved nutrients bioavailability while reduced anti-nutritional factors (Sharma et al 2023). Furthermore, germinated moong grain (*Vigna radiata*) and other millets also reported improved antioxidant activities and notable functional attributes (Sharma et al 2023).

A.) Nutritive Value (Sorghum *Malai Kofta* Curry)

Nutrients	Per Serve
Energy (Kcal)	334
Protein (g)	9.08
Fat (g)	20.32
Total carbohydrates (g)	30.14
Dietary fibre (g)	5.65
Iron (mg)	2.24
Calcium (mg)	158.78

B.) Nutritive Value (Kodo *Kheer* Bliss)

Nutrients	Per Serve
Energy (Kcal)	249
Protein (g)	9.13
Fat (g)	9.18
Total carbohydrates (g)	34.90
Dietary fibre (g)	2.71
Iron (mg)	3
Calcium (mg)	172

C.) Nutritive Value (Finger Millet *Halwa*)

Nutrients	Per Serve
Energy (Kcal)	259
Protein (g)	2.60
Fat (g)	15.40
Total carbohydrates (g)	30.60
Dietary fibre (g)	2.75
Iron (mg)	1.12
Calcium (mg)	62.52

D.) Nutritive Value (Foxtail Turmeric *Halwa*)

Nutrients	Per Serve
Energy (Kcal)	126
Protein (g)	1.65
Fat (g)	6.84
Total carbohydrates (g)	15.09
Dietary fibre (g)	1.08
Iron (mg)	0.43
Calcium (mg)	3.71

E.) Nutritive Value (Finger millet Choco Brownie)

Nutrients	Per Serve
Energy (Kcal)	184
Protein (g)	2.21
Fat (g)	9.08
Total carbohydrates (g)	23.19
Dietary fibre (g)	1.92
Iron (mg)	1.11
Calcium (mg)	57.82

F.) Nutritive Value (Finger millet Choco Shake)

Nutrients	Per Serve
Energy (Kcal)	172
Protein (g)	6.05
Fat (g)	14.45
Total carbohydrates (g)	14.45
Dietary fibre (g)	1.93
Iron (mg)	1.52
Calcium (mg)	190.22

G.) Nutritive Value (Finger millet Choco Banana Bread)

Nutrients	Per Serve
Energy (Kcal)	232
Protein (g)	2.72
Fat (g)	13.22
Total carbohydrates (g)	24.83
Dietary fibre (g)	2.93
Iron (mg)	1.59
Calcium (mg)	61.36

H.) Nutritive Value (Finger millet *Moong* Protein Salad)

Nutrients	Per Serve
Energy (Kcal)	137
Protein (g)	7
Fat (g)	2
Total carbohydrates (g)	24
Dietary fibre (g)	6
Iron (mg)	3
Calcium (mg)	89

I.) Nutritive Value (Kodo Millet Curd Rice)

Nutrients	Per Serve
Energy (Kcal)	181
Protein (g)	9.52
Fat (g)	6.29
Total carbohydrates (g)	21.12
Dietary fibre (g)	6.82
Iron (mg)	6.21
Calcium (mg)	166.29

J.) Nutritive Value (Foxtail Beetroot *Dosa*)

Nutrients	Per Serve
Energy (Kcal)	203
Protein (g)	10
Fat (g)	6.68
Total carbohydrates (g)	34.09
Dietary fibre (g)	8.1
Iron (mg)	2.61
Calcium (mg)	47.04

K.) Nutritive Value (Sorghum *Kadi*)

Nutrients	Per Serve
Energy (Kcal)	104
Protein (g)	3.41
Fat (g)	4.81
Total carbohydrates (g)	11.26
Dietary fibre (g)	2.61
Iron (mg)	2.56
Calcium (mg)	115.06

L.) Nutritive Value per serve (Sorghum *Thalipeeth*)

Nutrients	Per Serve
Energy (Kcal)	109
Protein (g)	2.63
Fat (g)	2.82
Total carbohydrates (g)	18.56
Dietary fibre (g)	3.91
Iron (mg)	1.52
Calcium (mg)	23.12

M.) Nutritive Value (Sorghum *Gattae* Curry)

Nutrients	Per Serve
Energy (Kcal)	238
Protein (g)	5.05
Fat (g)	11.60
Total carbohydrates (g)	27.39
Dietary fibre (g)	5.46
Iron (mg)	2.35
Calcium (mg)	19.32

N.) Nutritive Value (Little Millet Vegetable Pulao)

Nutrients	Per Serve
Energy (Kcal)	232
Protein (g)	6.44
Fat (g)	4.77
Total carbohydrates (g)	36.89
Dietary fibre (g)	7.32
Iron (mg)	5.91
Calcium (mg)	31.06

O.) Nutritive Value (Pearl millet Veggie *Khichdi*)

Nutritive Value	Per Serve
Energy (Kcal)	294
Protein (g)	7.50
Fat (g)	12.94
Total carbohydrates (g)	37.44
Dietary fibre (g)	8.26
Iron (mg)	7.43
Calcium (mg)	38.58

P.) Nutritive Value (Sorghum Tacos)

Nutrients	Per Serve
Energy (Kcal)	145
Protein (g)	4.85
Fat (g)	4.80
Total carbohydrates (g)	20.50
Dietary fibre (g)	3.42
Iron (mg)	1.15
Calcium (mg)	76.48

Q.) Nutritive Value (Finger millet Spiced *Lassi*)

Nutrients	Per Serve
Energy (Kcal)	133
Protein (g)	5.65
Fat (g)	6.05
Total carbohydrates (g)	13.69
Dietary fibre (g)	3.05
Iron (mg)	5.18
Calcium (mg)	278.55

R.) Nutritive Value (Sorghum Choco Pancake)

Nutrients	Per Serve
Energy (Kcal)	194
Protein (g)	4.24
Fat (g)	4.70
Total carbohydrates (g)	33.52
Dietary fibre (g)	4.83
Iron (mg)	2.30
Calcium (mg)	31.41

13.3 CONCLUSION

Reintroduction of millets in our food system represents more than a food re-discovery; it is a sustainable practice rooted in tradition, with the validation of modern science. The collections of recipes presented in this chapter demonstrate how these nutri-cereals can break through diet prototypes and assume the role of nutritional revolution. Through the mindful recipe formulation, in addition to nutrient profiling, this chapter offers a realistic guidance in terms of gut-supportive, diabetes-friendly, bone-nourishing, cardio-protective and culturally applicable meal options. Whether it is the barnyard millet–based heart-friendly dishes, finger millet–based bone-strength foods, every bite of each preparation bring together a positive blend of tradition, flavour, taste and health. As global food system confronts the dual challenges of climate change and nutrition, millet-based diets are emerging as flexible, adaptable, potently nutritious and sustainable options. This portfolio of recipes show meticulous decisions made about routine food can lead to healthier lives.

REFERENCES

Balkrishna, A., Verma, S., Singh, S. K., Dobhal, V., & Arya, V. 2024. Exploring the antioxidant mechanisms of millet polyphenols: regulation of Nrf2 and NF-κB and their impact on gut microbiota. *Discover Food*, *4*(1). https://doi.org/10.1007/s44187-024-00199-0

Bisht, A. 2022. Small-millet-based traditional and unconventional food products. *In Small millet grains: the superfood in human diet*, edited by S. Srivastava. Springer, Singapore, pp. 95–111. https://doi.org/10.1007/978-981-16-9306-9_5

Chandrasekara, A., & Shahidi, F. 2011. Antioxidant phenolics of millet control lipid peroxidation in human LDL cholesterol and food systems. *Journal of the American Oil Chemists Society, 89*(2), 275–285. https://doi.org/10.1007/s11746-011-1918-5

Chaudhuri, S. 2025, July 17. *Grainstorm: Why millets are reshaping resilience strategies.* Agro Spectrum India. https://agrospectrumindia.com/2025/07/17/grainstorm-why-millets-are-reshaping-resilience-strategies.html

ICMR – National Institute of Nutrition, India. n.d. https://nin.res.in/RDA_short_Report_2024.html

Jacob, J., Krishnan, V., Antony, C., Bhavyasri, M., Aruna, C., Mishra, K., Nepolean, T., Satyavathi, C. T., & Visarada, K. B. R. S. 2024. The nutrition and therapeutic potential of millets: an updated narrative review. *Frontiers in Nutrition, 11.* https://doi.org/10.3389/fnut.2024.1346869

Jha, A. 2024, March 26. Millets World: Rediscovering ancient grains for sustainable future. *Times of India Voices.* https://timesofindia.indiatimes.com/blogs/mithila-note/millets-world-rediscovering-ancient-grains-for-sustainable-future/

Kumar, T. S., Nageswari, R., Somasundaram, S., Anantharaju, P., Baskar, M., Ramesh, T., Rathika, S., Vanniarajan, C., & Subrahmaniyan, K. 2024. Significance of millets for food and nutritional security—an overview. *Discover Food, 4*(1). https://doi.org/10.1007/s44187-024-00149-w

Muskan, F., Redhu, M., Redhu, S., & Rahimi, M. 2025. Millets in the global market: a critical review of challenges and opportunities. *Food Production Processing and Nutrition, 7*(1). https://doi.org/10.1186/s43014-025-00316-1

Saleh, A. S., Zhang, Q., Chen, J., & Shen, Q. 2013. Millet grains: nutritional quality, processing, and potential health benefits. *Comprehensive Reviews in Food Science and Food Safety, 12*(3), 281–295. https://doi.org/10.1111/1541-4337.12012

Sharma, S., Anurag, & Garg, A. P. 2023. Effect of germination on the physicochemical and anti-nutritional properties of finger millet (*Eleusine coracana*), pearl millet (*Pennisetum glaucum*), and sorghum (*Sorghum bicolor*). *The Pharma Innovation Journal, 12*(3), 4763–4772. https://www.thepharmajournal.com/archives/2023/vol12issue3/PartAZ/12-3-611-828.pdf

Sowunmi, L. I., Babalola, Y. O., & Ogunbamowo, P. O. 2024. The cultivation, nutritional polyphenolic contents, bioavailability, and health benefits of finger millet (*Eleusine coracana (L.) Gaertn.*). In *Food security and nutrition.* CRC Press eBooks, pp. 97–116. https://doi.org/10.1201/9781003469766-8

Thakur, N., Dishri, M., Nath, A. K., Chahota, R. K., & Ceasar, S. A. 2025. Millets as climate-resilient crops: mitigating food and nutrient insecurity. *Cereal Research Communications.* https://doi.org/10.1007/s42976-025-00680-1

Tripathi, T., & Vyas, S. 2023. From ancient grains to modern solutions: a history of millets and their significance in agriculture and food security. *International Journal of Home Science, 9*(2), 72–78. https://doi.org/10.22271/23957476.2023.v9.i2b.1466

Wale, N. 2024, December 9. *Millets: the super grains that benefit both health and the environment.* Nature Wale. https://www.naturewale.org/blog/millets-the-super-grains-that-benefit-both-health-and-the-environment/

Index

Abrasive mills, 35
Abrasive dehullers, 35
ACE inhibitory activity, 170–171
Acetate, *see* Short-chain fatty acids (SCFAs)
Adaptive immune response, 186–187
Adiponectin, plasma levels, 170
Advanced glycation end products (AGEs), 149
Agricultural challenges, 91
Alkaline-forming foods, 90
Allergic reactions, wheat proteins and, 193
Alpha-amylase, 24, 26
Alternative therapeutic approaches, 189
Amaranth, 9, 66–67
Amino acids
  insulin secretion and, 142
  metabolism of, 86, 91
Amylase inhibition, 15–16, 26, 144–145, 148, 154, 156–157
Ancestral wisdom, 229
Ancient grains, 33
Anemia, 7, 83, 85, 90–91
Angiogenesis, inhibition of, 160, 168, 172–174
Animal studies
  on millets, 139, 150, 154
Antibodies, 95, 97
Anticancer activity
  apoptosis induction, 160, 172–174
Anti-diabetic effects, 144–151
Anti-hypertensive effects, *see* Blood pressure
Anti-inflammatory effects, 114–115, 129–130, 172–173
  cell proliferation inhibition, 160, 172–174
Antioxidant enzymes
  catalase, 171–172
  superoxide dismutase, 171–172
Antioxidants, 1, 8, 11, 39–40, 66, 69, 84, 88, 94, 97–100, 102, 104, 106, 108–109, 119–121, 228–229, 250
  activity, 41, 44, 85
  properties, 140–141, 143, 146–149, 152–157
Anti-nutritional factors, 14, 24, 26, 34–35, 37–38, 39, 42, 91, 238, 240
  alpha-amylase inhibitors, 91
  enzyme inhibitors, 26
  oxalates, 26
  phytates, phytic acid, 8, 14, 26, 37–40, 91, 100, 106–107, 124–126, 143
  protease inhibitors, 26, 91, 196
  saponins, 26–27, 99–101, 108
  tannins, 8, 24, 26, 34, 38, 41, 68, 143, 171
  trypsin inhibitors, 91, 124
APEDA, 75
Apoptosis, 96, 99, 103, 109
Appe pan, 231
Appetite regulation/control, 113–114, 116–118, 147
  dietary fiber and, 112–113, 117–118
Area under the curve (AUC), 150
Arginine, 97, 108–109
Artificial intelligence, 42
Asafoetida, 239, 242, 244–246, 249
Atharva Veda, *see* Veda
Atherosclerosis, 166–170
Awareness campaigns, 70, 76

Baked millet products, 212
Bajra, *see* Pearl millet
Barnyard millet, 3–4, 6, 33, 65–67, 69–70, 74, 88–89, 102, 106, 108
  antioxidant activity, 88
  food preparations, 90
  iron content, 89
Basal Metabolic Rate (BMR), 118
B-group vitamins, 3, 84, 86, 88, 90; *see also* Vitamins
Bio-accessibility, 40, 143, 155–156
Bio-active compounds, 33, 40, 82, 84–85, 89, 125–126, 133, 140–144, 146–147, 150–151, 153–154, 156–157
  catechins, 24, 85, 172–173
  ferulic acid, 85, 172–173
  flavonoids, 24, 33, 40, 44, 81, 85, 88, 119–121, 170–173, 228
  gut microbiota modulation and, 147
  hydroxybenzoic acid, 40
  hydroxycinnamic acids, 40
  kaempferol, 24, 85
  lignans, 159–160
  myricetin, 85
  phenolic compounds, 23–24, 33, 35, 39–41, 119–121, 133
  phytosterols, 99–100, 108, 170–171, 194
  polyphenols, 34–35, 40, 43, 85, 99, 101, 103, 105, 108, 119–121, 133, 141, 143, 159–160, 172–173, 228–229
  quercetin, 24, 85, 172–173
  resistant starch, 40, 113, 116–118, 122, 124, 128–129, 141, 171, 228–229
  studies on, 150
Bioactive peptides (BAPs), 24–25, 140–142, 146, 152, 154, 156–157
  anti-hypertensive activity, 25
  anti-inflammatory, 25
  antioxidant, 23, 25
  DPP-IV inhibition, 25
Bioavailability, 35–36, 38, 40, 65, 68, 90–91, 230, 250
  carbohydrates, 38, 43
  minerals, 33–34, 36, 40
  nutrients, 33–36, 39, 44
Biofortified, 29, 65, 67, 75
Biomarkers
  HDL-C, 170
  LDL cholesterol, 169–171
  total cholesterol, 170
Blood glucose/sugar regulation, 117–118, 121 –123, 146
Blood pressure, 1, 7, 112, 129–130
Blood sugar spikes, 228
Body composition, 127
  body fat percentage, 127–128

body mass index (BMI), 128–129
clinical trials, 127
Body weight reduction, *see* Weight management
Bone mineralization, 86
Bran, 35–36, 40
Breakfast; *see also* Millet-based products
cereals, 210, 211
high-protein, 123–124
millet pancakes, 122
millet porridge, 118, 122
millet smoothie bowls, 122
Breast cancer, 8, 160, 174
Breast milk, 83, 87
Buckwheat, 9, 66–67
Butyrate, *see* Short-chain fatty acids (SCFAs)
Buying behavior, 212
B-vitamins, *see* Vitamins

Calcium, *see* Minerals
finger millet and, 87
recommended intake, 86
Cancer
carcinogenesis, 172–173
colon cancer, 160, 166, 174
liver cancer, 160
prevention mechanisms, 168–174
Carbohydrates, 21–22, 27, 84, 90, 112–113
amylopectin, 21
amylose, 21, 112–113
in diabetes, 141
digestibility, 21, 27
non-glycemic, 141
Cardioprotective, 228, 254
Cardiovascular disease (CVD), 1, 110, 119–121, 159–171
inflammation, 160
management, 170–171
Celiac disease (CD), 7–8, 11, 33–34, 42, 185–190
complications, 189–190
diagnosis, 189
dietary management, 188–189
genetic predisposition, 186
immune response activation, 186–187
mechanism of action, 186–187
signs and symptoms, 187–188
tissue transglutaminase role, 187
Cell-cycle arrest, 172–173
Child malnutrition, 75
Cholesterol metabolism, 169–170
Climate change, 228–229, 254
Climate resilient crops, 55
Cognitive development, infant, 86
Commercial crops, 49
Complement proteins, 95
Complementary feeding, 66–67, 75–76
Complementary foods, 124
high-fiber combinations, 124
high-protein combinations, 124
legumes and, 114, 122, 124, 131–132
Congenital deformities, 86
Constipation, 89–90
Consumers, 210, 211, 219
acceptability, 35–36, 41
acceptance, 219
consumption trends, 111
demand, 210
perception, 226
preference, 210, 211
Copper, *see* Minerals
Crude fiber, 84
Cuisines, 229
Cultural significance, 64
Curd rice *(Kodo Millet)*, 229–230, 239, 252
Cytokines, 96–105, 108, 114, 129–130, 160, 187, 192

Decortication, 35–36, 39–41
bioavailability, 35–36, 38, 40
nutrient losses, 35
Dehulling, 27, 35–36, 39–42
bio-active compounds, 33, 40
dietary fibre, 33–36, 39–40
nutrient loss, 35
traditional methods, 42
Demand for millet products, 211
Dermatitis herpetiformis (DH), 185, 190–191
diagnosis, 190
management, 190–191
signs and symptoms, 190
Desi ghee, 233, 235
Desi khand, 229, 233–237, 250
Diabetes, 1, 7–8, 33, 36, 39–40, 119–120, 139, 228, 254
complications of, 139–142, 144, 146–148, 150–151, 153, 157
Diabetic friendly millet product, 219, 221, 254
Dietary diversity, 46, 75
Dietary fibre, 4–7, 11, 21–22, 24, 28, 33–36, 39–40, 65–66, 69, 87–89, 91, 101, 107, 113, 116–117, 124, 129, 140, 143–144, 146–147, 149–153, 156, 158, 229, 251–254
bile acid reduction, 171
bioactive effect of, 146
constipation management and, 89
fermentation and, 151
gut health and, 112, 116–117, 129–130, 147
health benefits of, 22–23
insoluble fiber, 22, 28–29, 116, 129–131
in vivo studies on, 154
satiety promotion, 169
soluble fiber, 22, 28–29, 116, 129–131
Dietary guidelines, 110
daily millet intake, 131
healthy plate concept, 110, 131–132
ICMR-NIN, 110, 132
Dietary management strategies, 193
Digestibility, 35, 37–39, 41
carbohydrate, 38–39, 43
protein, 33–39, 44
Digital retail, 211
Digital technologies, 41
Dipeptidyl peptidase IV inhibition, 142
Distribution channels, 211
DNA damage, oxidative, 172–173
Dosa, millet-based, 90
Drought-prone regions (conditions), 42, 91
Drought resistant crops, 46, 55
Dyslipidemia, 170

Eco-friendly packaging, 211
E-commerce platforms, 211

Electrolyte balance, 87
Endosperm, 20, 36, 40
Endothelial function, 159–160
Energy (Kcal), 69, 251–254
Entrepreneurs, 210, 211
Enzyme inhibitors, *see* Anti-nutritional factors
Essential fatty acids, 21, 84
Estrogen exposure, 166
Extrusion, 37, 39–42
  bio-active compounds, 33, 40
  HTST, 39
  nutritional quality, 37, 39, 44

FAO, 75
Fats, 21–22
Fermentation, 14, 27–28, 34–35, 37, 39–41, 43, 89, 143, 147, 150–152, 155, 157, 230
  anti-nutritional factors and, 27–28, 34–35, 37–39, 42
  digestibility and, 35, 37–39, 41
  mineral bioavailability and, 38, 40
  nutritional quality and, 37, 39, 44
  processing techniques and, 151
Ferulic acid, *see* Bio-active compounds
Fetal
  development, 84
  growth, 83–86, 88
Finger millet, 2–4, 6–9, 17, 33–34, 38, 41, 43–44, 46, 55–56, 61–69, 70, 72–76, 84, 87, 89–90, 102, 111, 122, 131, 228–230, 233–239, 248–252, 254
  bone health and, 87
  calcium content, 87
  food preparations, 90
  nutrient value, 17, 111
  nutritional benefits, 87
  preeclampsia management and, 89
Flaking, 37
Flavonoids, *see* Bio-active compounds
Foam-cell formation, 171
Folate, *see* B-group vitamins
Food companies, 210, 211
Food security, 33, 41–43, 46
Fortification, 41
Foxtail millet, 2–3, 6–9, 18, v25, 30, 33–34, 44, 63–67, 69, 70, 73–74, 83–84, 87, 90, 102–103, 105–109, 111, 127–128, 229–230, 234–235, 240–241, 251–252
  BMI reduction, 127–128
  calcium content, *see* Minerals
  dietary fiber content, 87
  gestational diabetes management, 87
  iron content, *see* Minerals
Functional foods, 25, 30, 110, 133, 153–155, 157–158, 169–171, 226

Gallic acid, 172–173
Gamma aminobutyric acid (GABA), 4
Garh bhoj, 8
Gastrointestinal disorders, 8
Genetic predisposition, 186
Germination, 14, 26–28, 34, 37, 39–41, 68, 230, 250
  anti-nutrient reduction, 27–28
  mineral bioavailability, 38, 40
  nutrient enhancement, 27–28
  protein digestibility and, 39
Gestational diabetes mellitus (GDM), 84, 88–89
  hypertension, gestational, 86, 88, 90–91
Ghee, 233–237, 241–242, 244–247, 250
Gliadin, 185–186, 193
Global Alliance for Improved Nutrition (GAIN), 75
Global market, 210, 219
Global scenario, 45
GLOBOCAN statistics, 159
GLP-1, 147, 169
Glucose metabolism, 84, 88, 146–147
  magnesium and, 141–142
  postprandial regulation of, 140–141, 144, 146–148, 150, 158
Glutamine, 97, 106
Gluten, 1, 8, 11
  immune responses to, 185–187
  intestinal damage and, 186–187
  intolerance, 42
  neurological effects, 191–192
  wheat allergy and, 193
Gluten ataxia (GA), 185, 191–192
  autoimmune mechanisms, 191
  diagnosis and management, 192
  neurological deficits, 191
  symptoms, 191
Gluten-free diet (GFD), 185, 188–193
  adherence challenges, 188–189
  dietary deficiencies, 188–189
  management of dermatitis herpetiformis, 190–191
  management of gluten ataxia, 192
  management of non-celiac gluten sensitivity, 192–193
  management of wheat allergy, 193
Gluten-free foods, 15, 20, 30, 81, 87, 90, 228–229
Gluten-related disorders (GRDs), 185
Glycemic control, 113, 116–118, 126, 140–141
  insulin sensitivity and, 114–118, 121, 130–131, 141–142, 146–148, 150–151, 154
  millets and, 143
Glycemic index (GI), 4, 8, 33, 117–118, 122, 128–129, 143–144, 151, 229
  low, 143–144, 151
  observational studies on, 150
Glycemic load, 143–144
Government of India, 1, 8, 9
  initiatives and, 42
Green Revolution, 83
Gut
  health, 112, 116–117, 129–130, 147
  hormones, 147
  microbiome, 89, 100, 104–106, 109, 116–117, 129–131, 228
  microbiota, 143, 147–150, 160
  supportive, 254

Halwa (Finger Millet, Foxtail Turmeric), 229, 230, 233–235, 251
Harappan Civilization, 83
HbA1c, 149–150, 158
HDL cholesterol, *see* Lipids
Health, 228–229, 250, 254
Health benefits, 28–29, 33, 41–44
  antioxidant properties, 34, 44
  metabolic disorders, 36, 39
  weight management, 33

Heart disease, *see* Cardiovascular disease
Hemoglobin, 65, 67–68, 75
Hemoglobin production, 83, 87
Hidden hunger, 68
High-pressure processing, 68
HLA-DQ2, 186–187, 190
HLA-DQ8, 186–187, 190
Human leukocyte antigen (HLA), *see* HLA-DQ2; HLA-DQ8
Human trials, 91
Hydrocolloids, 197–201, 203
Hydroxypropyl methyl cellulose (HPMC), 197–198
Hyperglycemia, 8
Hypertension, 170–171
Hypoglycemic properties, 194

ICDS, 70, 75–76
IDA (Iron deficiency anemia), 86–89, 188
IgA deposits, 190–191
IgE sensitization, 193–194
Immune system, 88–89
  activation, 187, 192
  regulation, 160
  response, 185–187, 189, 191–192
Immunity, 94–102, 105–109
  acquired immunity, 95, 96
  antibody mediated immunity, 95, 96
  cell-mediated immunity, 95, 96
  innate immunity, 94, 96, 108
Immunogenic peptides, 185–187
Immunomodulation, 102
Indus Valley Civilization, 82
Industrial feasibility, 41
Infant
  growth, 65–66, 69
  weaning, 63–64
Inflammation, 1, 85, 88, 94–102, 104, 106–109, 114–117, 119–121, 129–130
  chronic, 114, 166–173
  interleukin-6 (IL-6), 114
  systemic, 160
  tumor necrosis factor-alpha (TNF-α), 114
Inflammatory bowel disorders, 7
Instant noodles, 212, 217
Insulin resistance, 171
Insulin response, 117–118
Insulin secretion, 115–116, 141, 142, 147
  amino acids and, 142
Insulin sensitivity, 114–118, 121, 130–131, 142, 146–148
  bioactive compounds and, 146
  gut microbiota modulation and, 146
  observational studies on, 150
Insulin signaling pathways, 112, 115–116, 146, 150
International Year of Millets, 14, 64, 83, 56, 228
Intestinal
barrier, 147
  barrier dysfunction, 186, 189, 192–193
  health, 228
  lymphoma, 186, 190
  permeability, 185, 189, 192
  villi, 188
Intrauterine growth restriction (IUGR), 83
Iron, *see also* Minerals
  barnyard millet and, 89
  deficiency of, 83, 85–86, 88–89, 116
  finger millet and, 87
  foxtail millet and, 87
  recommended intake, 86
Irritable bowel syndrome, 228

JAK/STAT signaling pathway, 187
Jhangora, *see* Barnyard millet
Jowar, *see* Sorghum

Kaempferol, *see* Bio-active compounds
Kakum, 4
Kangni, *see* Foxtail millet
Khichdi (Pearl Millet Vegetable), 18, 19
Kilning, 37
Kodo millet, 3–6, 18, 33–34, 43, 63, 65–66, 69, 72, 84, 90, 105–106, 108, 111, 194, 198, 201–202, 228–230, 232–233, 239–240, 252
Koko, 67
Kutki, *see* Little millet
Kynurenine pathway, 97

Lactation, 82–91
Lactobacillus plantarum, 202–203
Lactogenesis, delayed, 83
LDL cholesterol, *see* Lipids
Leucine, 113–114
  mTORC1 pathway, 113–114
  muscle protein synthesis, 113–114
Lifestyle-related diseases, 194, 228
Linoleic acid, *see* Essential fatty acids
Linolenic acid, *see* Essential fatty acids
Lipids
  cholesterol, 8, 114–115, 121, 129–130, 169–171
  metabolism, 159–170
  nonpolar lipids, 22
  oxidation, 42
  polar lipids, 22
  profile improvement, 169–170
  triglycerides, 114–115, 121
Little millet, 3–6, 18, 33–34, 63–66, 69, 73, 83, 90, 102, 111, 194, 198, 201, 229–230, 245–246, 253
  vegetable *pulao*, 230, 245, 253
Local brands, 210
Low birth weight, 83, 91
Low-glycemic
  foods, 194, 199–200
  index, 63, 66
Lymphoma, 186, 190

Maillard reaction, 38
Malnutrition, 33, 39, 42, 83
Malting, 26–28, 34–35, 37, 39, 41, 43, 66, 68, 90
  digestibility, 35, 37–39, 41
  germination, 34, 37, 39–41
  traditional methods, 42
Market, 210, 212, 219, 226
  accessibility, 42
  linkage, 91
Maternal diet, 82, 83–90
Maternal health, 82–91
  bioactive compounds and, 84–85
  micronutrient deficiencies and, 85–86
  mortality maternal, 85, 89

Meal planning, 131
 breakfast ideas, 122
 complementary foods, 124
 daily intake recommendations, 131–132
 lunch and dinner ideas, 122
 meal timing, 122–123
 portion control, 123–124
 snack ideas, 122
Mechanisms of action, 144–148
Metabolic balance, 83–84
Metabolic health, 169
Metabolic syndrome (MetS), 119–121, 127, 130
Methionine, 97, 108
Micronutrients, 3, 35, 63, 66, 68–69, 83–86, 88–91, 115–116, 228
 deficiencies, 42
 malnutrition, 69
Millet(s), 1–11, 33–44, 228–230, 232–234, 250, 254
 anticancer properties, 159–184
 anti-diabetic effects of, 145–148
 bioactive profile, 85
 cardioprotective properties, 159–171
 classification, 33–34
 consumption, 45, 46, 48, 49, 54–58, 60–62, 83–91
 cultivation, 41–42, 45, 50, 52, 57, 81, 83, 91, 210
 cultural significance and, 83
 major millets, 3, 16–17
 minor millets, 194, 196, 228
 nutritional benefits, 194–196
 nutritional profile, 33–35, 41–42, 81–91, 140–142
 peptides, 148, 149–150
 policies, 45, 46, 49, 58
 product development, 196–198
 production, 45–47, 49, 50, 52–58
 sustainability and, 42, 81, 83, 91
 yield, 44, 46–47, 49–50, 52, 57
Millet-based products, 35, 40–42, 90, 133, 211–219, 221–229, 230, 254
 bars, 122, 133
 bread, 211–212, 215
 crackers, 122
 dalia, 212, 213
 dosa/idli mixes, 212, 217, 229
 drinks, 219, 213
 exports, 211
 fermented product, 122, 219, 221, 228–229
 flakes, 133
 malt, 219, 221, 222, 225
 muesli, 212, 214
 munch, 219, 225
 namkeen, 212, 219, 222, 224, 225
 packaged food, 210, 211
 pancake, 212, 216
 pasta, 133, 185, 196, 200–201, 203
 porridge, 122, 133
 recipes, 64, 69–73, 76
 snacks, 210, 211, 212, 224, 225
Millet composition, 20
 bran, 20
 endosperm, 20
 germ, 20
Millet gluten-free products, 194–198, 212, 215, 216, 218, 222, 224, 225, 226
Millet-processing techniques, 35, 41, 151
 challenges and gaps, 41
 industrial feasibility, 42
 primary processing techniques, 34, 39
 secondary processing techniques, 36
Milling, 27–28
Mindful eating, 132
 behavioral strategies, 132
 meal satisfaction, 132
 portion control, 123
Minerals, 33–34, 36, 40, 64–67, 69, 76, 82–91, 228–229, 251–254
 bioavailability, 35–36, 38, 40
 calcium, 17, 22, 34, 40, 64–67, 69, 76, 87, 111
 copper, 88
 iron, 22, 34, 40, 64–67, 69–70, 76, 83–89, 91, 99–102, 111, 106, 108, 116, 125, 140–142, 188, 202
 magnesium, 7, 22, 34, 40, 65–66, 76, 83, 86–88, 90–91, 115–116, 125, 171
 zinc, 22, 65–66, 69, 70, 75, 84, 86, 99–100, 106, 115–116, 125, 166, 171
Molecular mechanisms
 apoptosis, 172–174
 oxidative stress reduction, 172–173
 vascular protection, 159–160
Morning sickness, 90
 dietary management of, 89

Natural antioxidants, 172–173
Neural tube defects, 84, 86, 88
NF-κB pathway, 146–147
Niacin, 4, 34, 40, 84, 86, 88
Non-alcoholic fatty liver disease (NAFLD), 149
Non-celiac gluten sensitivity (NCGS), 185, 192–193
 diagnosis and treatment, 192–193
 gastrointestinal symptoms, 192
 immune activation, 192
 mechanisms of action, 192
Non-nutrients, 22–27, 97, 108
Noodles, 196, 200–201, 203
Nutri-cereals, 9, 11, 33, 45–46, 49, 56–57, 228–229, 250, 254
Nutrients, 1, 4, 5, 7–8, 11, 250–254
 deficiencies, 81, 83, 85–86, 91, 188–189, 193
 recommendations, 85–86
 retention, 35
Nutrition, 1, 9, 10
Nutritional, 228–230, 236, 250, 254
 insecurity, 1, 11
 profile, 33–35, 41–42, 140–142, 228, 254; *see also* Millets
 requirements, maternal, 83–86
 security, 77, 194
Nutraceutical properties, 159–160
Nutritive value, 236, 250–254

Obesity, 89, 110, 114, 116, 119–121, 127–128, 133, 166, 169, 228
Obesity management, 194
Occasion of consumption, 213–224
Ohmic heating, 68
Oleic acid, 84
Omega-5 gliadin, 193
Osteomalacia, 86
Oxalates, *see* Anti-nutritional factors

Oxidative stress, 70, 85, 88, 112, 115, 119–121, 141, 146–147, 149, 154, 158–160, 172–173, 194
DNA damage and, 172–173
free radicals and, 110, 114, 119–121
protection from, 112, 115–116, 119–121

Packaged food, 210, 211
Palatability, 195–196
Pancake (Sorghum Choco), 229–230, 249–250
Parboiling, 36, 39
starch digestibility, 39
Pasta, *see* Millet-based products
Pathophysiology, 185, 192–193
Pearl millet, 2, 4, 6–7, 9, 33–34, 36, 38, 41, 43–44, 46, 49–50, 52–53, 56, 60–61, 63–71, 73, 75–76, 84, 88, 90, 102–103, 105–107, 111, 124, 131, 150, 194, 197–203, 228–230, 246–247, 250, 253
folate content and, 88
food preparations and, 90
gestational diabetes management and, 88
iron, *see*, Minerals
magnesium, *see* Minerals
Peptide YY (PYY), *see* Satiety hormones
Plasma cells, 95
Phagocytes, 95, 103
Phenolic, 8, 33, 35–36, 40–41, 88, 146–148, 172–173, 199, 202–203
Phytate, *see* Anti-nutritional factors
Phytic acid, *see* Anti-nutritional factors
Phytochemicals, 1, 5, 11, 23–24, 66, 69, 99, 101, 171
Phytonutrients, 194
Phytosterols, *see* Bio-active compounds
Pizza bases, 185, 196
Policy initiatives, 49, 57
Polyphenols, *see also* Bio-active compounds
gut microbiota modulation and, 146–147
in vitro studies on, 148
Popping, 37–40
Porridge, 2, 11, 63, 76
POSHAN Abhiyaan, 64, 75
Postnatal nutrition, 83, 86
Postprandial glucose, 146, 169; *see also* Glucose metabolism
in vitro studies on, 148
observational studies on, 150, 151
Prebiotic
fibre, 229
properties, 194, 202
Preeclampsia, 85–86, 89, 91
Pregnancy complications, 82, 85, 87–91
Preterm birth, 86, 89, 91
Price support, 46, 60
Proanthocyanidins, 23–24
Probiotics, millet beverages and, 202–203
Processed food market, 197
Processing
methods, 68
millet, 196
Processing equipment, 42
Processing techniques, 34–36, 39–43, 89, 91, 151, *see also* Millet-processing techniques
consumer acceptability, 35–36, 41
nutritional quality, 37, 39, 44
Product claims, 213–224
Product visibility, 211
Propionate, *see* Short-chain fatty acids (SCFAs)
Proso millet, 2, 4, 6, 8, 9, 33, 65–66, 69, 71, 83, 90, 103, 107, 194, 197, 199–201, 228–229
Protease, 197
Protease inhibitors, *see* Anti-nutritional factors
Protein, 21, 38–39, 45, 96–104, 106–108, 142
amino acids, 21
digestibility of, 21, 27, 39, 69, 198–199, 202
Pseudocereals, 194, 199–200
Public health, 41–42
Puffing, 38, 40–41
mineral bioavailability, 38, 40
Pyridoxine, *see* B-group vitamins

Quercetin, *see* Bio-active compounds
Quinoa, 67

Ragi, *see* Finger millet
Rancidity, 195
Reactive oxygen species (ROS), 172–173
Ready to cook, 212, 217
Ready-to-drink products, 195, 202
Ready-to-eat, 90, 210, 214, 223, 224
Research and development, 42
Resistant starch, *see* Bio-active compounds
Resource-constrained regions, 42
Response surface methodology (RSM), 201–202
Retinol metabolism, 148–150
Rheological properties, 185, 197–201
Riboflavin, *see* B-group vitamins
Riboflavin metabolism, 148–150
Rice flour, 197–199, 201
Rig Veda, *see* Veda
Risk factors
obesity, 166
smoking, 166
Roasting, 36, 40–41, 67–68, 230
antioxidant activity and, 41, 44
phenolic compounds and, 33, 35–36, 40–41
RUTF, 69

Sales channels, 112–114, 116–118, 124, 212
Saponins, *see* Anti-nutritonal factors
Satiety, 112–114, 116–118, 124, 140
Satiety hormones, 113–114, 116–117, 124
cholecystokinin (CCK), 113–115, 117, 126, 130, 132
glucagon-like peptide-1 (GLP-1), 113, 116–118, 124
peptide YY (PYY), 114, 118, 132, 147, 169
Scottish oat porridge (SOP), 150–151
Sensory acceptability, 197–203
Setaria italica, *see* Foxtail millet
Shayamaka, 83
Shelf life, 27, 68, 70, 195, 200, 202–203
management, 91
Short-chain fatty acids (SCFAs), 116–117, 129–130, 147–150, 160
Shree Anna (Sri ana), 1, 56–57, 228
Signaling pathways, inflammatory, 172–173
Skin prick tests (SPT), 194
Slowly digestible complex carbohydrates, 228
Small-scale farmers, 210
Small millets, 46, 50, 66, 69–70
Small-seeded grains, 82

Smart grains, 33
Smart processing techniques, 42
Smoking, 166
Snacks, *see* Millet-based products
Soaking, 26–28, 34, 37, 39–41, 89, 91
Sorghum, 2–3, 9, 11, 16–17, 33–34, 38, 41, 43–44, 46, 49, 50, 52–53, 56, 62–67, 69, 72–73, 75, 84, 102, 105, 111–112, 148–151, 194, 198, 200–202, 228–231, 241–245, 247–251, 253–254
  antioxidant profile, 88
  food preparations, 90
  nutritional benefits, 88
Sorghum Gattae Curry, 229, 230, 244, 253
Sourdough technology, 198
Sprouting, 37, 39, 68, 125–126, 238–239
  sprouted millets, 219, 223
Starch, 195, 197, 200
  digestibility, 39, 112–113, 141
  enzyme inhibition and, 144–146
  in vitro studies on, 148
  rapidly digestible starch (RDS), 113, 118
  slowly digestible starch (SDS), 113, 118
State millet missions, 57, 61–62
State-wise millets scenario, 50
Stomach emptying, 147, 148
Storage stability, 42
Superfoods, 45, 210, 212, 218
Superoxide dismutase, *see* Antioxidant enzymes
Supply chain, 210
Supply side factors, 46, 55, 57
Sustainability, 42, 63, 82–83, 91, 110
Sustainable, 9–11
  agriculture, 83, 194, 203, 210, 229
  food, 210, 228

Tannins, *see* Anti-nutritional factors
Techno-functional properties, 195, 197
Texture, 66–67, 69, 76
Thalipeeth (Sorghum), 229, 230, 243, 253
Therapeutic, 1, 169, 228–229
Thermic effect of food (TEF), 113, 118–119
Thiamine, *see* B-group vitamins
Tissue transglutaminase (tTG), 186–187, 190–191
Tocopherols, *see* Vitamins
Total carbohydrates, 251–254
Traditional
  diets, 229
  knowledge, 229–230
  processing techniques, 42
  recipes, 68–70, 90
  wisdom, 228
Transglutaminase inhibitors, 189
Triglycerides, 169–170
Triticum aestivum, *see* Wheat
Trypsin inhibitors, *see* Anti-nutritional factors
Tryptophan, 97, 100, 108
Tumor growth inhibition, 160, 172–174
Turmeric, 229–232, 234, 242–245, 247–248, 251
Type 2 Diabetes Mellitus (T2DM), 139
  mechanisms of action in, 144–148
  oxidative stress in, 146–147
  studies on, 148–151
  therapeutic approaches for, 151

Ulcerative jejunitis, 190
Undernutrition, 64, 66, 75
Underutilized, 1, 11
UNICEF, 75
Unsaturated fats, 17, 29, 171
Uronic acid, 146
Urticaria, 193

Validated gluten-testing methods, 203
Value addition, 54, 55, 61, 64, 69, 75
Value chains, 55, 57, 58, 62, 210, 226
Vascular health, 159–171
Vasodilation, 171
Vegetables, 239, 241, 243, 246–248
  pulao (Little Millet), 229–230, 245, 253
Villous atrophy, 190–191
Viscoelastic properties, 185, 197–201
Vitamins, 20, 21, 26–27, 28–30, 33–34, 36, 40, 63, 65–67, 69, 76, 81, 83–86, 88, 90
  A, 86, 97, 106
  B-vitamins, 20, 24, 68, 115; *see also* B-group vitamins
  C, 86, 98–99, 106, 109
  D, 85–86, 98, 106
  E, 20, 22, 24, 98, 107, 115, 171
  K, 98, 107
Veda, 83

Water-holding capacity (WHC), 146
Weaning foods, 63–64, 66–67, 69, 76
Weight management, 16, 20, 29, 33, 110, 112, 122–124, 127–129, 132–133, 169, 147–148
  clinical trials, 127
  millet-based diets, 118, 131–132
  practical inclusion of millets and, 131 –132
Wheat, 185, 192–194, 197, 200–201
Wheat allergy, 185, 193–194
  diagnostic approaches, 194
  dietary management, 193
  IgE sensitization, 193
  symptoms, 193
Wheat proteins, 185, 193
Whole grains, 171
Whole millets, 40

Xanthan gum, 197, 199, 201
Xenobiotic detoxification, 172–173
Xylanase, 197

YY peptide, *see* Peptide YY (PYY)

Zinc, *see* Minerals
Zonulin, 189, 192